"From the very first page Zuna Vesan takes the reader directly into the very essence of this beautiful book. In a humble, yet very clear and at the same time soft and poetic way, one is taken on a journey through the wisdom of the ancient Chinese art of healing and maintaining health. This book is a treasure written by someone with profound knowledge and deep experiential understanding of the topic. I highly recommend this masterpiece to anyone interested in healthy motion from an eastern point of view."

Monika Steinkasserer, physiotherapist, healer, and dancer

"Dance is one of the purest human expressions of Tao. Dancers must know their own bodies and they must be able to heal when needed. Zuna Vesan has given us an erudite book that is profoundly steeped in dance, medicine, healing, culture and nature. She testifies to a life of peak movement and reveals the spirit within dance. An essential book for dancers, martial artists, qigong practitioners, healers and all who follow Tao."

Deng Ming-Dao, author of *365 Tao, The Lunar Tao, Scholar Warrior* and *Chronicles of Tao*

"*The Tao of Movement* is a book rich with information about movement and health specifically aimed at movers. Written from Zuna's seasoned, experienced eyes, we follow her trail of research as she unravels the mysteries of the body and its vulnerabilities. Her writing contains concrete and clear explanations of how our lifestyle can protect our resilience against illnesses with tips, instructions and information. This is a book to be read by everyone, but particularly those in the dance profession who yearn for a healthy, creative and meaningful life."

Susan Quinn, director of Salzburg Experimental Academy of Dance

"This is a groundbreaking guide of Chinese medicine for movers and performers of all backgrounds. Zuna Vesan expertly connects the ancient wisdom of Chinese Medicine and Qigong with dance, movement and the realities of the demanding life of a performer. Highly recommended for all performance professionals to help create an empowering existence of physical and mental health, by honoring the systems of the body and finding harmony with external factors. Finally, an approach for those seeking longevity and sustainability in their performance and physical practices."

Julianna Bloodgood, physical theatre performer, actress, and teacher

The Tao of Movement

THE TAO OF MOVEMENT

CHINESE MEDICINE PRINCIPLES FOR MOVERS

Zuna Vesan Kozánková

Foreword by Charlie Brittain

Translation by Žubra K. Žubretovská

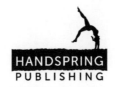

HANDSPRING
PUBLISHING

First published in Great Britain in 2025 by Handspring
Publishing, an imprint of Jessica Kingsley Publishers
Part of John Murray Press

1

Copyright © Zuna Vesan Kozánková 2025

Illustrations: Peter Žuffa
Caligraphies: Seiko Ginsho

Front cover image source: Noro Knap.

The information contained in this book is not intended to replace the services
of trained medical professionals or to be a substitute for medical advice. The
complementary therapy described in this book may not be suitable for everyone to
follow. You are advised to consult a doctor before embarking on any complementary
therapy programme and on any matters relating to your health, and in particular
on any matters that may require diagnosis or medical attention.

A CIP catalogue record for this title is available from the
British Library and the Library of Congress

IBSN: 978 1 80501 269 6
eISBN: 978 1 80501 270 2

Printed and bound in Great Britain by CPI Group

Handspring Publishing
Carmelite House
50 Victoria Embankment
London EC4Y 0DZ

www.handspringpublishing.com

John Murray Press
Part of Hodder & Stoughton Limited
An Hachette UK Company

I dedicate this book to anyone who is interested in deepening the knowledge of the connection between the human body and Taoist wisdom.

Contents

Acknowledgments 11

Foreword by Charlie Brittain 13

About the author 15

1. **The beginning.** 17
   The human body   18
   Energy   19

2. **Taoism: Practical philosophy** 21
   How can Taoist philosophy enrich the
   life of a modern mover?   22
   Taoism and health   25

3. **Qi energy: The basis of the health of
   the mover** 31
   The human body and its energy sources   32
   Three Burners   34
   Three Dantians   35
   The functions of Qi in the body   38
   Blood and Qi   38
   How can we support Qi in our body?   39
   Channels of Qi—meridians   41
   Entrances into the energy system   44
   The power of Qigong in the profession of
   mover   44

4. **Qi obtained from food: Balance
   between expenditure and revenue** 47
   To have or not to have lunch   47
   It is not possible to live without Qi   48
   The importance of warmth   50
   Food quality   51
   Rice as a base   51

Eat too little or overeat   52
Effect of food   52
Methods of preparation   53
In conclusion   54

5. **Organs: Materialized Qi in the body** . . 57
   The organ system as a well-functioning state   57
   Organs—materialized Qi in the body   59
   Functional organ circuits   60
   Surface and interior of the body   61
   Zang-Fu/Yin and Yang in the organ world   62
   Zang-Fu/Five Phases in the organ world   63
   Organ clock   64
   Psychospiritual aspects of organs   67

6. **Yin and Yang: How can these two
   terms help the mover?** 69
   An ancient concept   70
   "Either/or" versus "one and the other"   71
   What is Yin and what is Yang?   73
   There are no absolutes   74
   Sinusoid rate and the golden mean   75
   Culture of Yang and culture of Yin   76
   Yin and Yang and the human body   77
   What is this division for?   80
   The necessity of the crisis   81
   Yin and Yang transformations of the
   needs of body and mind   82

7. **Five Phases of Transformation:
   Five Phases of development and
   cyclicality.** 83
   Yin and Yang in a broader context   83
   A cycle applicable in any process   85
   Relationships between phases   86

8. The WATER phase: The human body in winter time 91

What should a mover do during this period? 91

What is the typical Qi of the WATER phase? 92

Kidneys as a precious royal treasury 93

What exhausts the Qi of the kidneys? 93

Cold 94

The depth of WATER 96

Fear is an emotion associated with the WATER phase 96

What are the kidneys in charge of in the body of the mover? 97

Our hardware in the bones 98

Tune in to how it should be 99

Spine—the "flowing" vertical column 100

Knees of a mover 103

Other connections with the functional circuit of the kidneys 106

Pregnancy, childbirth and subsequent convalescence 107

Moxibustion (moxa) in the mover's first-aid kit 109

Relationship of the WATER phase to other phases 110

Conclusion to the WATER phase 111

Meridians 112

Bladder channel (BL)/Yang 112

Bladder channel in movement 113

Kidney channel (KI)/Yin 113

Kidney channel in movement 114

Diet in winter and for the WATER phase organs 115

A few tips and recipes 119

9. The WOOD phase: The ability to pass through and the elasticity of the human body and mind. 123

The WOOD phase and spring with everything that needs to manifest 124

An emotion that breaks through 124

Liver, the ability to pass through, movement and the realization of our creativity 125

The Hun—the Ethereal Soul and the mental world 127

The gallbladder makes decisions 128

Movement of the wind 128

Movement, tendons, blood quality and physical performance 130

Tendon injuries and their treatment 132

Achilles tendon connects us with the Earth and builds our verticality 133

Tendons and grace of movement 135

Other connections with the liver and its functional circuit 135

Relationship of the WOOD phase to other phases 137

Conclusion to the WOOD phase 137

Meridians 138

Gallbladder channel (GB)/Yang 138

Gallbladder channel in movement 139

Liver channel (LR)/Yin 140

Liver channel in movement 141

Diet in spring and for the WOOD phase organs 141

A few tips and recipes 143

10. The FIRE phase: When the soul has joy in the body. 145

The FIRE phase as an energy peak 145

Openness 146

The FIRE phase in humans 146

Brightness and clarity 147

Heart—our inner emperor 148

The Shen Spirit 148

Let us not deceive our souls 149

Enter-Exit 150

Conscious exit 150

Proportion in everything we do 151

Fire needs to be tamed by its opposite—water 152

Joy belongs to FIRE phase and the heart 152

Here and now 153

Sleep 154

Other connections with the heart and its functional circuit 155

The relationship between the heart and other organs of the FIRE phase 158

Relationship of the FIRE phase to other phases 158

Conclusion to the FIRE phase 159

Meridians 160

Heart channel (HT)/Yin 160

Heart channel in movement 160

Small Intestine channel (SI)/Yang 161

Small Intestine channel in movement 162
Pericardium channel (PC)/Yin 162
Pericardium channel in movement 163
Triple Burner channel (TB)/Yang 164
Triple Burner channel in movement 165
Diet in summer and for the FIRE phase organs 165
A few tips and recipes 168

11. **The EARTH phase: Returning to the center** 171
Earth center 172
Necessity of returning to the center 172
Qi of the EARTH phase builds up stability 172
Transitions between periods and seasons 173
Source of Qi from food 175
Spleen—transport and transformation 176
Muscles—their capacity, but also their shape 176
Support in regularity 181
The spleen and our mental potential 182
Stomach and its master point *Zusanli* 183
A mover on a journey 184
Other connections with the functional circuit of the spleen 188
Relationship of the EARTH phase to other phases 189
Conclusion to the EARTH phase 190
Meridians 190
Stomach channel (ST)/Yang 190
Stomach channel in movement 191
Spleen channel (SP)/Yin 192
Spleen channel in movement 193
Diet in late summer and for the EARTH phase organs 194

Some tips and recipes for breakfast 201
A few more tips and recipes 202

12. **The METAL phase: Moving inwards and acknowledging values.** 205
Autumn is about the journey inwards 205
Metal like a machete 206
Filling and emptying 207
The lungs are the master of Qi 207
Breathing 208
Smoking 209
Supervision of two gates—nose and throat 209
Large intestine 210
"Passability" and healthy intestinal microflora 211
Ability to let go 212
Skin 212
The Po—the Corporeal Soul 216
Sadness 218
Other connections with the functional circuit of the lungs 219
Relationship of the METAL phase to other phases 220
Conclusion to the METAL phase 220
Meridians 221
Lung channel (LU)/Yin 221
Lung channel in movement 221
Large Intestine channel (LI)/Yang 222
Large Intestine channel in movement 223
Diet in autumn and for the METAL phase organs 224
A few tips and recipes 226

13. **The realm of the Five Phases of Transformation** 229

Acknowledgments

I would like to thank my Milan, with whom, for many years, I have been discovering the fantastic world of the human body through dance, anatomy, Qigong and Neigong. I also thank him for our deep philosophical discussions on Chinese philosophy and for the many inspirations for all my books.

While writing this book, I collaborated through questionnaires with colleagues and students of dance and Qigong who participated in my two multi-year research projects—*Dance and Medicine* and *Dancing Qigong*—based on linking the principles of Chinese medicine and Qigong with dance. I am grateful that they were willing to share their experiences, which I was able to include in the text of this book. I thank Peter Žuffa, who has painted the illustrations for all my books, of which you can see only a fraction in this one, and Seiko Ginsho for the calligraphy that also accompanies my books.

I am also grateful to the sacred space of our Pangea Center in the nature of the Eagle Mountains in the Czech Republic, where I wrote most of the text of this book and where I gained most of the vision and inspiration for it. I owe a debt of gratitude to this intensive process over many years, through which I had the opportunity to delve even deeper into the depths of Taoist philosophy and to discover there what I would not have discovered in ordinary life.

Zuna Vesan
Eagle Mountains, September 2023

Foreword

I first met Zuna in Belgium, at an international dance festival where we were both teaching at the invitation of our friend and colleague, Milan Tomášik. Zuna led her workshops on "Dancing Qigong," and I taught workshops on dance improvisation, technique and "Integrated Well-Being for Dancers." I had heard much about Zuna's unique work from Milan over the years and greatly enjoyed our exchanges between workshops. Clearly, our common ground was a passion for sharing our knowledge and experience with dancers and movement practitioners in order to enhance performance and improve health and well-being holistically. While united in these aims, our journeys through dance and healing are different. Alongside my professional career in dance, my healthcare practice is predominantly modern and evidence-based, which spans bodywork, myofascial release, medical acupuncture, human biomechanics, sports rehabilitation, emergency care and acute medicine. As I have journeyed deeper and more broadly into different healing sciences and traditions, I have become increasingly fascinated by the ancient healing arts that predominated for centuries. I was excited to hear of Zuna's new book and touched at the invitation to introduce it. Traditional Chinese medicine, and Taoism, is one of the ancient life sciences that I have long wished to explore and now, through Zuna's vision, I have been able to find a guide that seamlessly traverses my interests as both mover and healer.

The Tao of Movement is a stimulating companion for curious minds and creative bodies. Zuna illuminates the ancient wisdoms of the Tao, while offering the opportunity for modern-day movers to consider such knowledge through the reality of their own practice. Zuna expertly applies her lived experience of a life in movement through the lens of Chinese medicine, and offers a perspective on how we can enrich and support our lives both in and through movement. This book offers both valuable insights for movers who want to become holistically sustainable and departure points for exploring our own work, whether creative, performative or health-focused. Drawing on the rich breadth of the Tao, and its countless connections, it provides foundational knowledge and extrapolates ancient Chinese wisdom into the daily life of movers seeking enriched sensory experiences, digestible practical knowledge and concrete steps towards enhanced health and performance.

Movement is synonymous with life, from the microscopic division of single cells, all the way to our ability as organisms to travel in space, perceive time and express and embody consciousness. We could perceive ourselves in a continuum of movement, an analogy of flow, encompassing the entirety of nature itself: the rushing of water, the flowing of air and the steady growth, and decay, of plants. *The Tao of Movement* relates foundational Taoist principles directly to movement, offering a range of imagery and trailheads which are applicable across the breadth of movement styles and disciplines. It looks at the Tao through the perspective of movement, and movement through the perspective of the Tao, offering guidance for movers to cultivate deeper somatic sensing and awareness of the micro and macro happenings within and around them. Through this lens, we are able to consider the aspirations and potential of our creativity and wellness. The possibilities for application of such knowledge for those working in movement disciplines are vast and equip the reader with original ways to interact with their physicality through the long-respected principles of Traditional Chinese medicine.

The Tao of Movement takes us to the wisdom at the heart of an ancient model of living and makes available teachings which have served people for millennia. Zuna offers a beautiful, nuanced insight, founded on knowledge, philosophy and deep respect for the work, which speaks for itself. Akin to the vast fascial system of the body, human life is a dynamic web of interacting experiences, factors and relationships. The book explores all aspects of life, including the all-too-familiar story of injury and cyclical damage to the body, offering practical guidance underpinned by the theoretical and traditional principles of the discipline.

The more knowledge and experience one accrues in the study of movement, health and physiology, the clearer the link becomes between our holistic wellness and physical articulacy. The many aspects of one's health and well-being are uniquely inter-dependant, and in my experience of both dance and healthcare, the relationship between one's performance and health is intimate and direct. When movers enter the studio, they enter with the whole of themselves.

Zuna expertly guides us through the layers of the body and the factors that affect it, always from the perspective of the whole, whether traversing the challenges of an ageing body or navigating injury, overwhelm and crisis. This book is contextualized in an era of global unrest, undeniable planetary crisis and growing public health concerns. Society urgently needs to consider its approach to the core questions of life to stand any chance of finding balance, health and harmony, for ourselves, our communities and Earth herself. It is an opportune moment to open up to a traditional wisdom that can serve us now and for the future—one where connectedness, calm and creativity can predominate. It is rare to find an author who so expertly weaves the detail of such a rich ancient knowledge while continually honoring its place in the whole; this is part of the magic of this book, and, perhaps, of the Tao itself.

Charlie Brittain

About the author

Zuna Vesan Kozánková has been dancing all her life. She considers dance as one of the ways she expresses her Taoist soul. She graduated from the Dance Conservatory and the University of Performing Arts in Bratislava, Slovakia, and had several internships in Europe and Asia. In addition to dancing, she studied Shiatsu, Classical Chinese medicine, Qigong and Neigong.

Apart from her choreographic work, Zuna is a sought-after teacher working all around the world. She has taught for more than 30 years, during which she developed a unique style of working with the human body, based on experience with the anatomy of the human body and the energy flowing within. Together with her husband, Milan, she connects dance knowledge with the universal principles of Taoism, bringing to her students new information about movement intelligence.

In her multi-year projects *Dancing Qigong* and *Dance and Medicine*, she links dance and artistic creation with the principles of Chinese medicine, Qigong and Neigong. Her work, *Spaces*, which was created using the Dancing Qigong method, was awarded with the 2019 Dosky Slovak Theatre Award. For the last few years, she has been mainly engaged in the teaching of Qigong and Neigong and their use in dance practice. She is a practitioner of Japanese Shiatsu therapy and acupuncture.

Zuna is the author of the books *Tao: The Way to Health*, *Meridians: Pathways of Life*, *Qigong as a Medicine* and *The Wisdom of a Tree*. *The Tao of Movement* is her first book published in English. She lives partly in Bratislava (Slovakia) and partly in Eagle Mountains (Czech Republic).

www.artyci.com
www.shiatsu-terapie.sk

CHAPTER 1

The beginning

In my life, I have had the opportunity to work with hundreds of people whose work depends on the movement of the human body—dancers, physical theater actors, puppeteers, singers, circus performers, aerial dancers, yogis, athletes—and also with various body therapists. I call us *movers*. They were and are my colleagues on stage, students in the studio and also colleagues or clients in therapeutic practice. I always like to talk to them about art and its ability to transform human thinking, and about the human body and its abilities. In debates, we almost always reach the boundaries of the body. These are mainly health problems and the limitations of the body, by which we literally physically touch the great paradox—the strength of the human body in its immense fragility. Although these health limitations are our own, I often see a huge gap between recognizing our limitations and realizing that we are largely responsible for them.

The first impulse to this realization came to me when I was 15. Due to an ugly fracture of my leg, I was faced with a heartbreaking decision whether or not to continue my dance studies at the conservatory with some physical limitations. I continued but did not learn the lesson, so the second impulse came when I was 19. Crazy and uncontrollable, I strained my knee tendons during a rehearsal for a performance, which again separated me from dancing, and the healing of this injury took an unpleasantly long time. It was a clear exclamation point, and I really started to

be more attentive then. I realized that although I had studied dance at the conservatory for eight years, I did not learn anything about the health of my body. I found that it was a kind of ignorance and therefore violence against the human body. Ignorance on the part of this educational institution, but also my own.

Movement and health are phenomena that stand so close to each other and are so strongly influenced by each other that this correlation simply cannot be overlooked. They are eternal companions that influence each other mostly in the mover's profession. When there is no health in the body, there is no movement and joy. And consequently there is no joy in our profession. Later, at the academy, I learned about approaches to the body such as Body-Mind Centering, the Feldenkrais Method and Ideokinesis, which convinced me that with the correct movement and the right amount, it is possible not only to keep my body healthy but even to heal it with movement. This way, my body began to heal old wounds and change to a harmonious integrity. This process started to fascinate me. At first, I understood how important it is for the mover to know and respect the anatomy of the human body; later, I began to realize how important proper regeneration and diet are; and, finally, the appreciation came that the body is not only mass but also energy. So the time came to study Chinese medicine and Shiatsu, during which I began to realize the extraordinary connection between medicine and movement and saw the enormous healing potential in using the principles of Chinese medicine to influence the health of the movers and also to improve the quality of their performance. I have been researching this potential for many years. I lead seminars for different types of movers aimed at realizing the connection between health and their movement, I give lectures, write articles and blogs on this topic, and I discuss with movers all over the world everything about their health. And I am constantly studying.

The profession of mover is unique in the way that it requires unusual extremes from the human body. Professional performers must be athletes and artists at the same time: they basically perform a top sport, but simultaneously they are expected to perform a "striptease of their soul" on stage. It is a real extreme, but it makes us content. "The life of a mover does not offer gratitude. You reach 40 and you seem to have nothing, as if you did not build anything, you just grow old...but still...my work is my happiness and for this I am grateful," writes one of my colleagues. Therefore, we devote ourselves to this profession with full commitment; we train our body so that it can move as we dancers, teachers, coaches, choreographers and directors need. In doing so, we often exceed the limits of our own possibilities and require a very large output of energy from the body. That would be all right if we did it consciously and if we knew how to reconcile these costs with intakes.

The mover's profession directly depends on health. On the one hand, we have a flexible, slim, muscular and nicely moving body that may be envied by those who sit in offices behind computers all day. On the other hand, the intensity of movement harms our health—it depletes and destroys the physical structures of the body. It is a fact that cannot be changed, but it can be slowed down. Physical exertion is always reaching into deep reserves of energy, and if we do not know how to replenish these reserves, how to use our body without excessive physical wear, sooner or later it will affect our vitality, physical performance or mental state. Therefore, if we do not respect certain laws of nature and rob our health by too much movement, we can completely deplete our energy reserves, destroy our body and, as a result, end our career. Do we want this?

THE HUMAN BODY

What if the body is destroyed but the soul still needs to cooperate with it? We have a body in order to use it. But we also have to understand it. Living with it in symbiosis should be in the interest of every person, and this applies to movers even more. The human body is the primary tool for each of us, so it is extremely important that every mover is initiated into the study of the body. Just as a car mechanic should know all the parts of a car so that he can repair it, so the mover should know the parts of his or her body, their functions and connections. Why? It is a question of "equipping" one's own inner wisdom and harmony, which brings several advantages on a practical level. Anatomical knowledge, focused primarily on the locomotor system (skeletal, joint and muscular), helps us to better understand our body, movement mechanisms in it and movement with it. We can locate individual parts of the body, and thus use them more fully and consciously when moving—that is, in a correct and healthier way. We know how to relax our body, remove excess muscle tension, thus saving energy and using it for more substantial movement. When we know what is related to what in the body and how one part affects another, we are able to avoid many unnecessary injuries and at the same time save energy. Anatomical knowledge is also related to the discovery of new body movement possibilities. Thanks to their knowledge of anatomy, many movers have actually discovered a new body and a new vocabulary of movement. Those who have been initiated into the anatomy of movement are able to understand more quickly and clearly what a teacher or choreographer wants from them, and thus they reach a more precise achievement of the movement. They can figure out for themselves why there is tension and pain in any part of the body. They easily realize their badly acquired movement habits and are able to "reprogram" them with time and effort.

ENERGY

In this book, I deal with energetic health connections, which are, of course, also connected with the physical component of the body and the physical side of movement. The basis of my reflections is the knowledge of Chinese medicine, which is part of the overall concept of maintaining health according to Taoist philosophy. Gradually, I will introduce you to the world of universal laws, to the logic of natural transformations of energy in the body related to the development of energy during the seasons, and to the energy system connecting the activities of organs with individual body structures. Only a few movers know that by supporting the kidneys, they will achieve better physical performance or ensure good joint and bone condition; that when they harmonize the liver, they will be more emotionally balanced and their tendons will be elastic and supple; that excessive physical exhaustion can lead to depletion of the quality component of the blood, which can result in depression, for example. I will try to show you that when we learn to accept and use this knowledge in our lives, it can become an endless source of information on how to maintain health for as long as possible, thus making life more pleasant with good health. Last but not least, this will help us extend our career.

Because of my fascination with the principles of Chinese medicine and the whole Taoist philosophy, I decided to run two multi-year research projects—*Dance and Medicine* and *Dancing Qigong*, based on linking the principles of Chinese medicine and Qigong with dance. The research takes place in my pedagogical and choreographic work. So far, almost 500 students from all over the world have participated in practical dance seminars and movement research, lectures and discussions. I was fascinated by how dancers who had not had experience with anything like it before were able to completely change their view of their body through working with these principles and with meridians. They began to physically understand what the body was offering them and to feel Qi energy in their meridians during movement. This concept, which may seem too abstract and philosophical in books, was easily understood and felt through physical experience. The research also included my online communication with many artists and movers around the world, students and colleagues, with whom I was able to verify many things related to health in our profession. I have included this knowledge in this book.

I have written this book over several years, mostly in the lap of mountain nature. Here I had the opportunity to watch and experience the changes in the energy of the seasons in the marrow of my bones and observe what the human body really needs in each season. I was writing the individual chapters focused on the phases— WATER, WOOD, FIRE, EARTH and METAL—which are directly connected to the energy of the seasons, in the given season, and I tried to capture in the lines the message of experiences, perceptions and lessons. I was learning from trees and animals, and I was observing my own feelings, the amount of energy I had or my emotions in each season. At the same time, I traveled to the city, where I taught my students about these energy changes, their power and the possibilities to use them. I taught them to perceive and observe what was happening around us, whether in nature or in the city, and to connect to this cosmic order.

A number of wise books have been written on the Chinese medicine art of healing, which is based on the wisdom of Taoist philosophy. Some of them go back to ancient history. In this book, I include a few quotations from one of the oldest known books, *The Yellow Emperor Classic of Medicine* (*Huandi Neijing*). Many books have been and are being written nowadays, and since, according to Chinese medicine, the world of health is vast and can be viewed from different angles and indefinitely, each opens a different door to understanding. This book has no ambition to compete with them. However, many books are too professional and difficult for an uninitiated mover. I have tried to bring practical and easy-to-read information to this book and to transform my knowledge as experienced by the practice of a performer but also of a pedagogue. The book does not aim to give a recipe for guaranteed health. Its goal is to encourage the reader to think about the fundamental natural things around us and within us, and thus to understand ourselves a little more. So let's embark on a journey of understanding Qi energy, Yin and Yang and the Five Phases, the world of organ logic and the energy network in the body and everything related to it.

CHAPTER 2

Taoism

Practical philosophy

About: the Way we walk / the ancient Taoists / connection with nature's cycles / application of Taoism in the profession of a mover / respect for the body / health from a Tao perspective / Wuwei—action in non-action / prevention / immunity

Before we get into the practical information about how Tao can help us in our profession, let's explain a little bit about what Tao and Taoism actually are.

Taoism is an original Chinese spiritual tradition that has significantly influenced the culture and thinking of the Chinese nation. Along with Buddhism and Confucianism, it is one of the three great philosophical movements that have interwoven traditional Chinese culture. Of these, Taoism is the oldest and the only original Chinese spiritual tradition. Originally, it was not a religion but a philosophy that permeated all areas of Chinese life. The term Tao, and thus the name of this philosophy as Taoism, came into use in connection with the life of the master Laozi and his work *Dao De Jing*, which was written in the sixth century BC. But the origins of this philosophy go back to an ancient period of shamanic alchemical tradition dating back as far as 5000 years.

The word *Tao* (Dao) is not easy to translate in one word. The character for Tao, which you see in the image on the right, consists of two parts. In the upper part of the character we see a head, the hair disheveled. The lower character translates as *walk*. Tao, therefore, tends to be translated as *the*

path or *the path we walk*, or more precisely *the path we walk freely as with loose hair*. A deeper insight into the essence of the character encourages the use of the words *way* or *principle*. It is the path we walk, but also the way we do it, the way we live. However, the Tao also offers ways to learn the lightness of our steps along the way, making it extremely practical and useful for us.

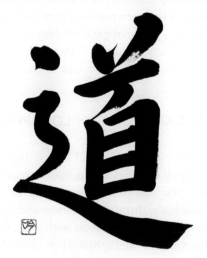

Chinese character for Tao

In a philosophical context, the term Tao is untranslatable. It cannot be expressed; it can only be understood internally and lived practically. It is the original source, the origin of all existence. We come from the Tao and return to it after death. It is a state that precedes the origin of anything, something eternal, unchanging, everywhere present, and at the same time imperceptible. For me personally, the Tao is a path that, in addition to its profound spiritual message, offers a guide to the practical use of life with all that it brings us. I think this is what sets it apart from many religious movements. It is a way of seeking the meaning of life on Earth, but also a way of being able to find possibilities that can be used in this time-space for life on Earth in a harmonious way.

The ancient Taoist masters were doctors, sages, philosophers and artists. Their thinking was strongly connected with nature. They observed it patiently and thoroughly, and although they had no special equipment to make these observations, they found out that there are certain mechanisms, patterns, cycles and rhythms that are constantly repeating in all forms of life. They also found that what happens in nature, outside of human beings, also happens *in* them. Some lived as hermits in the countryside, in the mountains; others lived and carried out their mission in the overcrowded cities. During their search, they gathered great wisdom and came to a deep understanding of human nature. They observed the stars, the cycles of the universe, the energy around us and also within humans; they compiled exercises and meditations to strengthen life energy, and developed methods of healing following these patterns. They were willing to spread their wisdom further to those who were able to perceive it. In times of despotic regimes in China, they were declared rebels and excluded from society. Conversely, in times of more enlightened regimes, they held prominent positions in government; they were teachers, doctors and counselors. They developed their enormous potential for wisdom in several branches, which together form a kind of "philosophical family" of Chinese thinking. The oldest member of this "family" is *The Book of Changes* (in Chinese, *Yi Jing*); other members are Chinese astrology, Feng-shui, Chinese medicine, Qigong exercises, Taijiquan and martial arts. All of these members contain the same philosophical foundation, and each one focuses and develops in a different way. For example, Feng-shui focuses on the arrangement of the space in which we live, Chinese medicine focuses on healing practices, Qigong focuses on physical and meditation exercises.

In the context of this book, I call these sages *Taoists*. For me, this term is a personification of everything that Taoist philosophy brings. Under the term *Taoist*, we will encounter the philosophy and wisdom of Taoism throughout the book.

HOW CAN TAOIST PHILOSOPHY ENRICH THE LIFE OF A MODERN MOVER?

From my own experience, I believe that Taoist philosophy enriches life in many areas—from purely practical health issues related to the physical body, through the power and depth of creativity that lies dormant within us, to deep philosophically metaphysical or cosmological insights into our existence. Taoism is a philosophy that is extremely practical and applicable in everyday life. It is based on the reality of what is happening around us and within us, and it offers its use. Last but not least, it brings us a lot of inspiration.

The path to a healthy and valuable life
Taoism offers the view that being healthy and living a long and fulfilling life are vital factors in building a meaningful, creative and spiritual life. According to the Taoists, the soul and the body are not two separate entities; on the contrary, they are a common continuum. For them,

the human body is not merely here to survive in some way, but it is here to enable us to realize our mission during our lifetime in health. Then we can flow smoothly with our given potential.

Therefore, for Taoists it is important to keep the body in good health, for only then can we carry out what we are meant to carry out, and thus move our soul forward. Such a healthy body and soul are essential for anyone who works with the human body. Taoists focus on how to lead a long, happy, meaningful and productive life. A life in harmony with nature that benefits not only themselves, but also all of humanity and ultimately the entire planet.

Connecting with the rhythms of nature

Taoism follows the patterns of nature. It respects the cycle of day and night, the seasons, planetary cycles and so on. It observes and makes practical use of the logical connections and sequences of these laws. As long as we respect and follow them, we benefit. I experience this with my students, with whom we have a series of seminars each year in which we focus on the qualities of the year, seasons and the needs of the body according to the season. Together, we return to the naturalness that both heals and encourages us to respect these patterns of nature. At the same time, this connection to nature helps us to see nature as the great mother of which we are a part, nourishing, teaching, physically and spiritually shaping us. It teaches us to have a spiritually based reverence for nature, to feel the presence of the Tao in things and creatures and to be in harmony with the great rhythms of the universe. However, even while pursuing its position in the context of the laws of nature, it offers each individual the opportunity to find his or her own personal path. Connecting with the rhythms of nature in cities is more difficult, but still possible. It can even bring us many interesting inspirations to our work.

Respect for the body and partnership with it

Taoism does not suppress the human body. Some religious ideas declare the body to be impure and unworthy of our attention in comparison to the spirit. On the contrary, for Taoists, the human body is a tool for understanding and applying the principles of the Tao. It is a privileged place to experience the Tao, a kind of materialization of Taoist philosophy. But Taoists do not cling to it; rather, they see the endless transformations of the body, ending in death, as a natural fact. Furthermore, Taoism deeply respects the body's existence, perceiving it as an "empire," a space for the cultivation of the spirit and inner alchemy. For Taoists, the body is a microcosm within the macrocosm. It is the embodiment of the forces of energy around us. The principles that take place in the macrocosm are also reflected in the microcosm of the human body. The whole philosophy is thus reflected in it and has the opportunity to be realized and to evolve. For us movers, the human body is a tool for work and at the same time a means of expression. For me personally, the reverence for the body that is felt in many Taoist practices helps me to love my own body and to care for it adequately.

The latent energy of the human body is understood by Taoists as a raw gem that we receive at the beginning of life as a gift. If it is not grounded in a meaningful way, we will fail to fully realize our purpose. In the human body and its processes, we find the principles of Yin and Yang and their interaction. The concept of the Five Phases (Five Elements) is embodied in it in the form of organs and their functions that affect the physical structures of the body (bones, joints, tendons, etc.) that we use directly in our profession. We also find in it a space for various alchemical processes of energy cultivation. Therefore, daily work with body energy—the Qi—is part of Chinese culture, and through Qigong, Taijiquan and various martial arts, we can encounter its essence in countries outside of

China. And, naturally, it is an inspiration to many artists. Taoism thus leads us to respect the body that has been entrusted to us and encourages us to take responsibility to care for it appropriately. That is what this book tries to do.

Simplicity and openness

Taoism is not a theoretical, complicated and over-intellectualized concept. It gets straight to the point, offering realistic advice, the meaningfulness and effectiveness of which have been proven for millennia. And, as is typical of Chinese culture, it often uses poetics, stories and anecdotes, rather than factual theses, to convey this information, advice and practice. In this way, it places its wisdom in a reality close to the human person, but also in a softer world outside the rationale we so prefer in the West.

Taoists avoid extremes or fanaticism; they have no need to stand against people who think differently. They do not impose their teachings on anyone. Thanks to their respect for nature and the universe, they practice a philosophy in life that has a deeply spiritual essence. The Tao offers ways that both an atheist and a religious person can understand. It calls for originality, an individual's experience of it; its interest is an ordinary person—thus also an ordinary mover.

Relativity of everything in constant transformation

One of the oldest and most inspiring books of ancient Chinese thought is the aforementioned *Book of Changes* (*Yi Jing*). It is used for interpretations of oracles or as a guide for the study of knowledge of summarized experiences, making its philosophical basis universal for everyone. Its main theme is the principle of change. The essence of the world is not in something unchanging, but, on the contrary, in constant change and transformation. Change and transformation are present in everything—in natural rhythms and cycles, in the energy around us, but also within us, in our lives and relationships, in

our work and productivity, in opinions or in the evolution of social systems. The book teaches us that trying to preserve anything is always futile. Natural transformations are beyond our power to influence because they happen according to certain laws that are beyond us. And although it is sometimes difficult to accept, in this dynamic of change, it is only a matter of when and how quickly something will change. Personally, the principle of relativity and transiency that Taoism shows helps me to cope more easily with difficult times when I am not so productive compared to other days; it helps me to feel that the crisis is also part of the overall process. So thanks to Tao, I do not fall into negativity and depression, because every cell of me knows that it is only temporary.

Everything is transient and, in its transiency, it is free and paradoxically solid. Thus, the Taoist philosophy interwoven with the ideas of the ancient *Yi Jing* helps us in our ability to detach ourselves from everything: from what is unpleasant to us, but also from what is pleasant to us; from what does not work and worries us, but also from what works and makes us happy. It detaches us from our own failure, because that is only temporary, and on the other hand, it detaches us from our own success—even that is only temporary, and no matter how hard we try to keep it, natural evolution will still bring change. It detaches us from clinging to other beings or things. This will help us from suffering when we lose them. When we learn not to reject what is coming, but also not to hold on to what is leaving, our inner joy will become the same in happiness and unhappiness, and we will be more internally balanced. We will learn to distance ourselves from transient things, to see them as neither more nor less than what they really are, and to behave accordingly.

Wuwei—action in non-action

Related to this is the ability to allow life to flow naturally. This is a Wuwei principle that could be translated as action in non-action. It is one of the most fascinating ideas of Taoist philosophy, and its achievement is not easy, although in essence there is nothing simpler. We humans always need to organize, manage, control; our ego motivates us to do things that are against the laws of nature. In doing so, we often enter the flow of life with unnatural ideas, in a violent way, contrived, hastily, and often as if we are actually fighting with life. Conversely, in our laxity we sometimes let slip through our fingers what needs to be done at that very moment for evolution to occur.

Let's imagine that we are on board a boat that lets us be carried away by the current of the river. We are doing nothing, just enjoying the rocking of the water, the breeze, the flow. We do not switch on the engine, we do not change direction, we do not pull open more sails than necessary. However, if something changes about the condition of the river and it becomes dangerous, we will react immediately to avoid danger. Or imagine that we are gliding on a hang glider drifting on a current of air. Of course, we had to make an effort to get the hang glider into the current, and we will have to use our wits and skill to land it on the ground. But when we glide, we should do nothing. Just watch, enjoy, let it flow, slightly navigate, because if we interfere too much, it will not end well.

Wuwei is not real non-action, absolute do-nothingness or total passivity. Rather, it is a kind of receptivity to what is to come, what is to be done, which is predetermined by the flow of the Tao. The state of Wuwei is about observing natural changes; it teaches us not to interfere with the flow of life with our own ego. It is not a state of nothingness; it is rather a promising space in which there are many possibilities. And all it asks of us is to do what is needed in the very moment. But the main precondition for us to be able to merge with the Tao is our complete openness. Its condition is inner emptiness. Not emptiness in the sense of insensitivity and aridity, but freedom from opinions and ideas on how things should be, and from the various tensions that force us to intervene continuously. Such openness is led by cultivating a *state of silence* within us, which is a prerequisite for accepting simplicity and naturalness. It is not a matter of putting aside all intentions, visions and plans, but of not being overly full of them. To get rid of compulsions and not to let ourselves be controlled by them. It doesn't mean that we should totally give up the achievements of modern times and go to the forest, but that we should not be enslaved by them. *Emptiness* or a *state of silence* within us also means detachment from the pressures of the outside world, from all possible opinions of the environment, so that we can discover our real needs. The way to this emptiness and state of silence is through meditation practice, an ancient way of practicing the Tao. In this way, we learn to be independent of external circumstances, healthily flexible and adaptively resilient, yet continually fulfilled and strengthened from the inner depths of ourselves.

TAOISM AND HEALTH

Everything mentioned in the previous section leads in essence to health. For Taoists, health is a harmonious state of body and spirit. Since ancient times, Chinese people who have cultivated the Tao have also been practicing medicine. Thus, Chinese medicine could be said to be a Taoist philosophy applied in medical practice. It is a teaching about the unity of a human with the laws of nature, about the unification of the energies of body and mind, and about finding the true nature of a human.

According to the Taoists, real health can only be achieved if our inner microcosm is in harmonious balance with the outer macrocosm. In acupuncture, for example, different points on the body are used in therapy in each season, Chinese dietetics—the science of eating—adapts what we have on the plate to the weather conditions of the season and what is available during the season. Treatment as well as prevention are adapted to the individual, his or her specific constitution and condition, but also to what kind of work he or she does during that period and his or her age. And all this in balance with the whole external environment.

For us movers, health is a primordial prerequisite for practicing our profession. So, what are the health issues we are most concerned about and interested in? Since the tool of dancers is the body, most often it is about problems with the body itself. These can be acute injuries or chronic physical problems. However, no accident is a coincidence; it is often caused completely unnecessarily. We weaken the body with poor nutrition, extreme exertion and disrespect for the anatomical possibilities and conditions of a particular body. In addition to these acute accidents, we also suffer from chronic problems with the joints, spine or tendons, which are caused by the same causes, but also by natural overloading.

However, movers also suffer from digestive problems. Many of these problems come from schools where the "you are fat, lose weight" type of bullying has led to pointless fasting and often to bulimia. All of this disturbs the digestive tract and consequently the whole immune system, psychological balance or ability to reproduce. Many female movers suffer from irregular and painful menstruation. This is commonly considered a normal condition, but it is not normal, and it indicates a woman's overall health. Psychological problems are no exception—due to various pressures on achievement, due to huge ambition and the need for realization, we often suffer from anxiety or depression. Related to this is mental and physical exhaustion, which severely weakens the kidneys. Since the kidneys are our "batteries" and, among other things, nourish the bones,

joints and spine, we get back to physical ailments and injuries, so it is a kind of vicious cycle.

The way of prevention

Taoism has a wide and varied list of techniques for maintaining health. Based on the observation of natural principles, it developed an amazing system of healing practices, which include acupuncture, phytotherapy, moxibustion, tuina massages, medical Qigong and the like. However, it places the importance of preventive healthcare first. Prevention includes many effective methods of using Qigong, Taijiquan, breathing, relaxation and meditation techniques, moxibustion and harmonious eating. In the complexity of the whole Taoist philosophy, we could also include Feng-shui in prevention, which helps people to maintain harmony by maintaining the correct flow of Qi in the environment in which they live and work.

Taoism is interwoven with the pursuit of a healthy life. The primary essence of Chinese medicine is not to cure the disease, but to prevent the disease. Chinese physicians were mainly concerned with this art. If someone fell ill, it was a sign that the doctor in charge had failed. He lost his right to reward and had to treat the patient without claiming it until the patient was cured. If he was a physician of an influential person, or even an emperor, news of his failure spread very quickly across the country, and then he had to work for a long time to renew the trust. I remember the image from *The Last Emperor* movie, where a doctor smells a potty with the morning stool of a little emperor and states from the smell what the emperor lacks in his body and what he has in excess, and then dictates to the chefs how to adjust the emperor's diet. "Start digging a well before you're thirsty," says an old Chinese proverb. And Chinese medicine warns us in this way to be careful about what is not yet. Therefore, when diagnosing, the doctor must be interested not only in what is apparent in the patient but also in what is not yet visible, what has not manifested, but what can be expected in the patient. He must listen attentively, observe and even read from the date of birth what medical ailments the patient will be susceptible to. In this way, the Taoist view of health significantly differs from the Western one. In our countries, we usually deal with the disease when it has already occurred, and it is often too late. Therefore, in recent years, many movers have turned to Chinese medicine or Shiatsu therapists with their problems.

Circulation of Qi

An important prerequisite for health is the smooth and even circulation of energy in the body, which the Taoists call Qi. When it does not circulate evenly and regularly, stagnation from excess or deficiency of Qi occurs in the body. If such stagnations are not removed in time, or deficiencies treated, they generate disease. In this way, all the methods offered by Chinese medicine are used to circulate Qi in the body and get it wherever it should go to nourish the body, in order for the body to have an energy balance, which is the basis of the success of Chinese medicine. It also includes various meditations and Qigong exercises that the Chinese always practice to improve health and avoid disease. In China, one can experience this first-hand and with one's own eyes. Every morning, before the start of the daily rush, the parks in any large modern city are filled with training people. They are full of actively moving people, enjoying the new day with the movement of their body. They practice Qigong, Taijiquan or martial arts, recharge themselves with the energy of trees, dance, sing or play ping-pong. Here you can see old ladies who have no problem kicking their leg to the level of their breasts or leaning it against a tree and stretching the hamstrings and the tendons below the knees, or competing to see who can do more "sit-ups." By no means does any of this seem like some obligatory Spartakiad; on the contrary, you can sense that everyone enjoys this morning

ritual. In a quieter mode, this is repeated in the evening. In such activities, they can also enjoy the folly of the big cities with the joy of their bodies. The movement that ensures the circulation of Qi throughout the body, and thus strengthens health, is an enduring part of Chinese culture.

Supporting the Upright Qi

The body has the ability to heal itself. By nature, we possess within us mechanisms that can fight various influences and pollutants that would like to disturb our health balance. However, a prerequisite for this strength is a sufficiently strong immunity. However, we do not find the word *immunity* in the terminology of Chinese medicine. The basis of our strong immunity is called, in Chinese medicine, *Upright Qi* (in Chinese, *Zhengqi*). It is Qi that is created, cultivated and maintained throughout our lives from several sources. The first is the energy input of our parents—the constitution with which we were born, the proverbial "root" that is either strong or weak. People with strong roots have stronger health and nothing breaks them easily. They can afford to gamble with their health a little more, but if they overdo it, their strong roots can weaken or can even be destroyed. People with weaker roots have to take more care of themselves and their health during their lives, because they feel that they are more susceptible to diseases, and their predispositions do not allow them to draw too much from their energy. This is a matter of constitution. Both types of people have to take care of their condition. It is daily self-care, from a proper and regular diet, through the choice of work we do in life, regular exercise and "psycho-hygiene" to sufficient rest and regeneration. The constitution with which we were born and the condition we maintain on a daily basis together form the Upright Qi. This is the basis of the fight against pathogens. Thus, Upright Qi is something that we are partly predestined to have but which we are also able to cultivate and strengthen throughout our lives. Regardless of heredity and the quality of the surrounding environment, we always have the choice to spend our natural life force faster or slower, and thus influence the course and length of our life.

Basis in energy balance

At its core, Chinese medicine aims to activate the body's self-healing mechanisms without excessive outside help. It does it in a very sophisticated way—by establishing energy balance in the body. And thousands of years of observation and successful practice only confirm that balance of Qi in the body means health, and imbalance is the way to disease.

So what does Chinese medicine do when, for example, the flu viruses attack us? It does not deploy an army in the form of pills or vaccinations from the outside. Conversely, it supports the army we have—the army of Upright Qi. Ideally, it does this preventively, even before the flu season occurs. However, depending on the situation, it is able to fight back in the same way even when the flu has already struck.

And against whom is the army fighting? Every disease is described as a struggle between two forces—between the body's resistance (i.e. Upright Qi) and various other factors, the pathogens, that cause the disease. This is harmful Qi, called *Pathogenic Qi* (in Chinese, *Xieqi*). Pathogenic Qi can come from outside or inside. External pathogens mainly include weather factors. They are cold, wind, heat, summer heat, drought and humidity. They are typical of different seasons, subject to certain rules and have their limits. When this balance is disturbed—when they are excessively strong or weak—they can become harmful. If we are not sufficiently protected from them, they will invade our body, upset its balance and cause disease. Once they penetrate the body, the fight begins. Pathogens want to get as deep as possible into the body and disrupt it, so there is a struggle between them and our Upright Qi. It depends on its quality whether the pathogen wins or is defeated and eliminated from the body. This

explains, for example, the fact that among people living in the same environment for influenza, some get sick and others do not. Thus, Chinese medicine begins a direct fight against the pathogens that want to attack the body. It works on their elimination, but at the same time it helps the body to fight for itself—by supporting the Upright Qi in it. Therefore, Upright Qi is crucial: it is a defense, a kind of armor and, in Western terms, we call it sufficiently functioning immunity.

These pathogens can also enter us in different ways. Most often it is through diet. Each food has an effect on us. It can cool us, warm us, create dryness or moisture and so on. All of these effects are fine, because when there is excessive heat outside, we need to refresh ourselves internally. On the other hand, when it is cold outside, we need to warm up internally. However, if we favor a food with such a specific effect to the detriment of others, it will obviously turn out to be harmful, because, in principle, anything that can help us can also harm us. It depends on the situation and the level of consumption. For example, yogurt, which contains many of the bacteria needed for the intestines, is essentially a cooling and moisturizing food; if we overdo it with yogurt, we will create cold and dampness in ourselves to such an extent that, after a while, we will be unusually susceptible to colds, our congestion will manifest itself in frequent coughs and bronchitis, and, in women, in gynecological discharge. In general, improper or insufficient nutrition is an internal pathogen.

Emotions are also internal pathogens. Chinese medicine deals thoroughly with our emotional world. It considers emotions to be normal states of mind that depend on mental and emotional activity, but also maintain close relationships with the functions of the internal organs. Taoists have observed and noticed how individual emotions interfere with our organism, what they cause in it, and how they affect organ function and vice versa. Anger, for example, causes the rise of Qi—when we get angry, we feel a surge of energy in our faces. Worries can "knot" the flow of our Qi, causing it to stagnate. Fear, in turn, causes a decline of Qi, which can cause our knees to buckle from fear. Emotions can cross natural boundaries in cases of strong, sudden or prolonged stimuli. This disrupts the flow of Qi in the body and the functions of the internal organs. Therefore, emotions can trigger a variety of diseases. They also have a significant impact on the development of diseases: existing diseases can alleviate or worsen. And Taoism has a lot to teach us about how to handle emotions wisely. We will gradually analyze the basic emotions and the world of our psyche with individual organs.

Overloading is considered as another internal pathogen. This may be exhaustion of any kind—physical, mental or sexual. Of course, an unbalanced diet, but also an excess or lack of it, can also harm us. Rest is an equally important condition of good health. The art of relaxation is part of the art of working. When this wholeness is disturbed, diseases appear.

Table 2.1 Pathogens—causes of diseases

Internal pathogens	External pathogens	Others
Weak constitution Poor living conditions Emotions Overwork, excessive sexual activity Dietetic defects Malnutrition or overeating	Climatic influences: cold, wind, heat, fire, humidity, dryness	Epidemic Injuries Parasites Incorrect treatment

When we are already sick

We can never be 100 percent healthy, and fighting tooth and nail to stay healthy all the time is not a harmonious state of mind. Sometimes we just get sick. However, illness can always give us good feedback so that we realize what we have neglected, or so that we understand that taking care of ourselves is predominant and we learn from our mistakes.

Chinese medicine, of course, intervenes even when the disease has already occurred. It has different mechanisms for this compared to Western medicine. The key is always to establish balance, so it focuses more on how to balance the states of Qi energy in the body. It replenishes where there is a lack of Qi, and it takes away where there is an excess. The basis is the balance between Yin and Yang, the blood and Qi of the individual; these words are too abstract for us to understand right away. In this book, I will attempt to make them understandable, even though they are different from what we commonly encounter in the Western view of health.

In Chinese medicine, there is no such thing as broad-spectrum treatment. Chinese medicine focuses on each individual aspect of the origin and course of each individual patient's disease. This means that it does not treat patients with the same disease in the same way. It takes into account not only what the disease is and how it originated, but also how the organs of a particular patient work, in what condition they are, and what constitutional potential they have. All organs are taken into account, even those that at first glance have nothing to do with the problem. Chinese medicine also takes into account the way in which the individual thinks, his or her emotional world, the state of life, age and so on, because these are also aspects that will accompany the treatment process. In addition, the original medical practices—so-called Classical Chinese Medicine—also relied on cosmology and astrology. Based on the impact of various cosmic constellations on life on Earth, it is possible to predict from the date of birth how they affect an individual's life and health. For example, a person with influenza who was born with weaker energy of the kidneys will be treated differently compared to a person who was born with weaker energy of lungs. At the same time, it can foresee what a person's predisposed health tendencies will be, and so, as a preventive measure, it can assist the person in ensuring that his or her as-yet-secret illness may not manifest itself in his or her life at all. Classical Chinese Medicine works with the belief that everyone brings completely different input data into their lives, and this diversity makes Chinese medicine a true art. In treatment, it is very important to know the tendencies, imbalances and the cause of the occurrence of a disease. And when the disease is cured, it is not enough to name the condition in which the patient is now, but it is necessary to understand how the disease originated and how it can be avoided in the future. The disease is always approached individually, depending on the specific patient. It is not uncommon for the same disease to be treated differently in two or three different patients. Conversely, the different manifestations of two or three patients can be treated in the same way. For example, we will always treat a person who is healing a broken bone or a person suffering from fatigue or a person with lumbar spine pain in a way that supports the energy of the kidneys.

CHAPTER 3

Qi energy

The basis of the health of the mover

About: the Prenatal and Postnatal Qi / Jing essence / Qi function / care for Qi / the Three Burners / the Three Dantians / upper and lower brain / meridians and acupuncture points / Qigong in the profession of mover

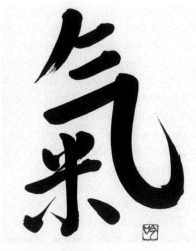

Chinese character for Qi

We use the term *energy* in the world of dancers, performers, or other movers, for example, in connection with urging to better performance using words such as "Put more energy into it." We know about energy when we feel it within us or when we do not have it and we feel tired. We perceive energy among the performers at a rehearsal, during the performance on the stage, but we also feel the energy of the spectators in the auditorium and the energy of music. However, energy is also deeply connected with the health of the movers. According to Taoist philosophy, it is its basis.

However, the term *energy* is not entirely correct when talking about health, as it has some connotations in our Western culture that can be misleading. Therefore, let's rather use the Chinese term *Qi*. It appears, for example, in the word *Qigong* (translated as "cultivation of Qi"), or in the Japanese version *ki*, it can be recognized in the name of the Japanese martial art of *Aikido* (translated as "the way of Qi harmony").

The Chinese character for Qi consists of two parts. We can see them in this calligraphy. The lower part shows a grain of rice in a pot, and the upper part shows the steam above that pot. This is important information because it implies that Qi can be material, tangible, but also very subtle, intangible, but perceptible by thinking and feeling. It is almost impossible to define Qi satisfactorily. It cannot be understood by the analytical mind. It is an immanent cosmic substance, a basic, pervasive principle. It is invisible in itself; it cannot be grasped, disassembled or cut out. But all we can see and name is Qi manifesting in different densities and thus in different forms. It is in the human body, healing herb, air, animal, movement, dance, music, tides, thought, word, inspiration, etc. Qi is also the time we spend somewhere, or what we feel when we are with a loved one, when we are at a pleasant place, or even a place where we do not feel well. The physical process of healing a wound or mending a broken bone is also the result of Qi. Taoists believe that the world is continuously forming itself by constant development, constant emergence and extinction, from a single material—from primordial, Original Qi. They claim that everything is just one of its aspects and states of greater or smaller condensation. The Taoist philosopher Zhuangzi says, "One is grateful for one's life to the condensation of Qi—as long as it is condensed, it is life; as it suddenly disperses, it is death." However, this death cannot be understood as the absolute end; it is only the return of Qi to a state of undetermined potentiality, from which there will be a new condensation into a new form. So Qi is constantly changing and never ceases to be. A drop of dew, which condenses in the cold of the night, then heats and evaporates during the day, rises to become part of a cloud in which it can freeze, and then falls to Earth as hail, where it melts again into a drop of water. It is still the same force, but it acquires different densities and shapes due to different processes.

THE HUMAN BODY AND ITS ENERGY SOURCES

The same thing happens with the human body. During conception, "nothing" becomes something huge. Two people, who may not have known an hour ago that something serious was going to happen, combine two of their tiny, visually invisible cells to create a new human being. They give it the power to concentrate Qi into cells, which gradually form all the material structures of the body. During pregnancy, Qi gradually thickens into strong bones, flexible tendons and muscles, protective waterproof skin, an adaptable nervous system, or a number of different organs until the baby is born. However, in the human body, cells are constantly dying and regenerating, so if we think in terms of the cellular composition of tissues, the adult is not actually the same as the original child. The cells are exchanged, but it is still the same person.

At the beginning of our lives, we are all endowed with a huge amount of Qi, which we spend by living. But where does it come from, where does it go and what is it?

We are born with an abundance of Qi, which the Taoists call the primordial energy—*the Jing essence*. This primary life force of a human arises at conception, by combining the essence of the mother and father, the egg and the sperm. From the moment of conception, Qi starts to accumulate in the kidneys, and although the organ does not yet fully exist, energetically the material is already being worked on. The Jing essence is stored in them throughout life and, with the help of organs and energy pathways—meridians—it is distributed throughout the body. After birth, this Qi is supplemented by the Qi of the air that a person breathes and the Qi of the food one consumes. Together, these two resources create the *Original Qi* (in Chinese, *Yuanqi*)—our life force, vitality, which is the basic premise of life.

In a figurative sense, we can imagine that we live on two "batteries," two sources of Qi—on the prenatal and postnatal "batteries" between which there is a relationship. Together, they create the Yuanqi.

Prenatal Qi
Prenatal Qi, the aforementioned Jing essence, is a non-renewable source of Qi or a very difficult one to recover. We inherited it from our parents. Its quality is given, and it determines our power, talent, intelligence, predisposition to diseases, life expectancy, the overall "drive" of a person; it

is a carrier of DNA. What genetic preconditions a child receives depends on the state of previous generations of its family, and also directly on how its mother and father live, because they give it this Qi. If the parents have enough Qi, they give the child a real spark in life. However, the role of the mother after fertilization does not end. It is important for the new being how the mother eats during the whole pregnancy and breastfeeding, and to what extent she exhausts her body. But the state of her psyche is also vital, because emotions are related to the state of Qi and affect its quantity. Prenatal Qi is like a supply of underground oil. It is sufficient, but we are draining it, and it will eventually run out! And when it happens, it is no longer possible to recover, and death occurs. We can also liken it to a savings bank account in which we have an inheritance; we do not use these funds for routine matters, but rather keep them as a reserve.

While we are young, we live very well on this Qi because we have enough of it, but we seldom realize its shortness, volatility, and fragility in its paradoxically enormous power. It is exhausted mainly by extremes—late nights, extremely demanding work, excessive work, excessive fasting, excessive sex, constant travel, frequent diving, movement at high altitudes, etc. As movers, we exhaust it just when it becomes the rule for us to overcome the limits of our fatigue. It is when we very often do not give our body rest and relaxation that we feel physical and mental exhaustion. Or when we work too often at night, or when our lives do not respect the nature of the changes of the seasons and the different needs of the body associated with those changes.

Postnatal Qi

Postnatal Qi is the second source of human Qi. We could compare it rather non-poetically to car care—from refueling, through the change of quality oil, technical inspections, to cleaning the interior and exterior. It is daily maintenance, preservation of what works, which gives us the possibilities of transport, implementation and communication. We can also liken it to a current bank account, from which we draw for current needs; we must constantly receive a "salary" so that we have something to live on. The "salary" is the intake of the food and fluids we receive, the quality of the inhaled air, but also the quality of the thoughts we deal with. However, the quality of interpersonal relationships and the handling of one's own emotions also affect the state of Qi. A person who lives in harmony with nature, eats properly and regularly, has enough activity, but also rests and is not too exhausted emotionally has enough of this Qi. The stomach and spleen are responsible for its processing.

Both sources of *Yuanqi* are equally important, and as the amount of Qi from one source decreases, the source of the other will naturally be depleted more than normally. Taoist sages viewed Qi circulating in the human body as perfect unity. In one day, a young and healthy person gets 100 percent of the necessary energy from food, air, physical activity and rest. And spends about 60–70 percent on their daily lives—work, digestion, breathing, walking, thinking, etc. We consume Postnatal Qi almost to the bottom every day and recharge it daily. Feeling hungry is one of the signals that this battery is running low and needs to be recharged. We eat and thus replenish it again. If we did not recharge it, we would have to reach for another source, the source of Prenatal Qi. Fatigue is also a signal that Qi is running out and needs to be recharged. If we did not do so and continued, we would already be drawing from Prenatal Qi. And, as I mentioned, it is not easy to recharge.

The good news, however, is that it works the other way around. The higher the quality of Postnatal Qi—the quality of food, water, air, relaxation and other aspects of life—the less we draw from Prenatal Qi. There is harmony in the body, in which all processes can run smoothly; the organs work smoothly and are able to regenerate. If this does not happen, the organism will be exhausted more than necessary at a young age, and health problems and limitations will be reported earlier than we would expect. Ultimately, however, the body may not decline at all. Qigong and Taijiquan masters are vital even at a very old age, precisely because they work economically with their Qi and cultivate it through exercise, breathing and meditation.

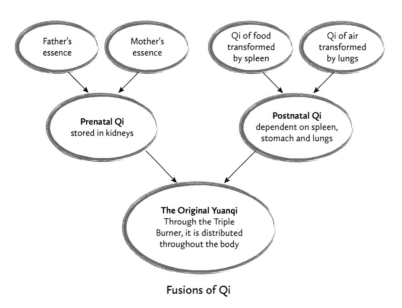

Fusions of Qi

THREE BURNERS

These two sources of Qi work together for us, ensuring the functioning of the body, its metabolic processes and the ability to assimilate and regenerate. What is the mechanism by which these two sources of Qi are interconnected in the body and what ensures their distribution to the body? The activator of this fusion of Qi, as well as its distributor throughout the body, is the *Three Burners* (in Chinese, *Sanjiao*).

The Three Burners, also known as the *Triple Burner*, *Three Heaters*, *Triple Heater* or *Triple Energizer*, are kinds of powerful alchemical chambers in our torso. Together, they form a system of cooperation between the organs in order to interconnect and distribute Qi throughout the body. In Western terminology, we would call their joint activity absorption, metabolism and excretion. The Three Burners do not have a specific shape; they are three areas in the torso separated by the navel and the diaphragm. Each of these areas incorporates certain organs and also participates in their function. In the terminology of Chinese medicine, we say that the Three Burners are the trigger for the merging of the Qi from the Prenatal Qi (the Jing essence) with the Postnatal Qi, which we obtain from food and air. By merging, they create the *Yuanqi*, the Original Qi. At the same time, they transport it to the whole body and distribute it to all organs, tissues and parts of the body. The quality and flow of Qi in our body is therefore determined by the quality of cooperation between the Three Burners. In the figure below, I show the relevant organs and a simplified description of principle of what happens between the Three Burners.

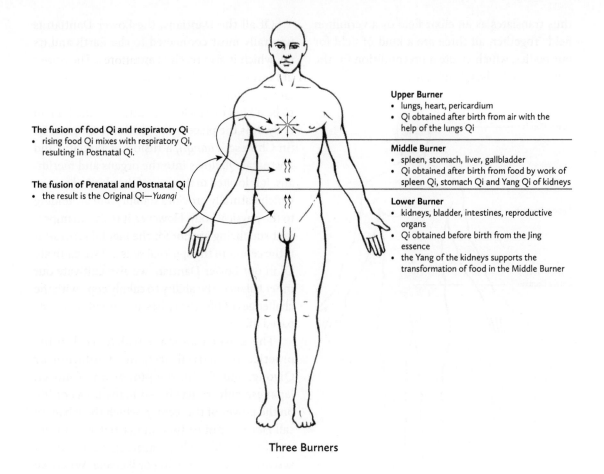

The fusion of food Qi and respiratory Qi
- rising food Qi mixes with respiratory Qi, resulting in Postnatal Qi.

The fusion of Prenatal and Postnatal Qi
- the result is the Original Qi—*Yuanqi*

Upper Burner
- lungs, heart, pericardium
- Qi obtained after birth from air with the help of the lungs Qi

Middle Burner
- spleen, stomach, liver, gallbladder
- Qi obtained after birth from food by work of spleen Qi, stomach Qi and Yang Qi of kidneys

Lower Burner
- kidneys, bladder, intestines, reproductive organs
- Qi obtained before birth from the Jing essence
- the Yang of the kidneys supports the transformation of food in the Middle Burner

Three Burners

THREE DANTIANS

An important part of the energy anatomy is the three energy centers in the torso, the *Three Dantians*. They function as storehouses of Qi, but also as distribution centers, from where Qi is transmitted to the entire system. Let us not confuse them with the Three Burners just described. The Three Dantians have different locations as well as different abilities and roles. They are positioned along the central axis of the body, which is the *Taiji Pole*. The Taiji Pole acts as a communication channel between the Earth and Heaven in the human body. It has a connection with the spine, spinal cord and brain, and thus the nervous system and the whole network of energy channels—the meridians.

Understanding the concept of the Three Dantians is not easy due to its immense complexity. The Chinese character for *Dan* translates as "red" or "cinnabar." Cinnabar—mercury sulfide, a rare type of mineral in ancient China—was the material used for the production of special vermilion ink reserved exclusively for the emperor's affairs. It was also used as a remedy to calm the spirit and for heart problems, but only in very small amounts, because mercury is poisonous. In alchemical terminology, *Dan* is also called "elixir." For the character of the word *Tian*, the most appropriate translation is "field." In Chinese philosophy, the field is of great importance because it provides us with sustenance. Dantian thus translates as an elixir field or a vermilion field. Together, all three are a kind of field for our bodies, which create a precondition for the nutrition of body, Qi and spirit.

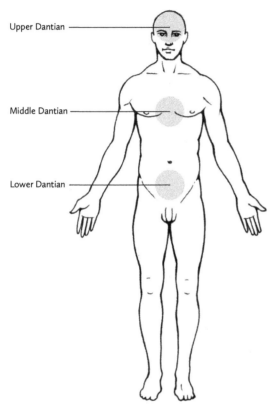

Upper Dantian

Middle Dantian

Lower Dantian

Three Dantians

The Lower Dantian

The *Lower Dantian* (in Chinese, *Xiadantian*) is located in the area around the navel, and the navel itself is part of it. It is the energy space in the physical "container" of the body, which includes the intestines, kidneys, bladder and genitals. In the back area, it is connected to the kidneys and to the strong energy point between them, the *Mingmen*, which we will mention in the chapter about the WATER phase. Below, it is connected with the perineum, where the acupuncture point is located through which the Yin Earth Qi flows into the body. It is called very appropriately the *Meeting of Yin* (in Chinese, *Huiyin*)—CV1.

Of all the Dantians, the Lower Dantian is naturally most connected to the Earth and its Qi, which it also receives and stores. The power of Lower Dantian lies in storing the Jing essence and Qi, often called the *Sea of Qi*. It is considered to be a kind of bioelectric battery of the human body. It is the place from which the Original Qi (in Chinese, *Yuanqi*), a fusion of Prenatal and Postnatal Qi, flows into the organs and meridians. It is located in the area of the physical center, which naturally provides stability and grounding to the physical body. However, it is also an important stabilizing anchor for the mental process; it is the center in the spiritual sense. If we cultivate Qi in our Lower Dantian, we also cultivate our inner balance, the ability to calmly cope with the challenges of life, the twists and pitfalls of a fast-paced life.

The Lower Dantian is widely used in the practice of martial arts, in meditation or Qigong, and also in the profession of mover. Japanese culture has based many areas of life on the power of this center, which the Japanese call *Hara*. It can be used in martial arts, zazen, archery, calligraphy, painting or common activities such as cooking or ikebana. When we are connected to the Lower Dantian in doing something, everything is easier for us, we save a lot of Qi and, at the same time, we have more power for the activity. Even utterly prosaic activities, such as opening a tightly closed bottle or pushing something heavy, are much easier if we connect to the Lower Dantian and send the force into the hands from there. In a mover's practice, working with this Dantian and drawing strength from it is very important. We use it to gain perfect stability and to use the body effectively—for example, during contact improvisation or partnering. It is also a support for coping with various turbulent life circumstances.

This center of physical strength is considered to be a source of kinetic receptivity. To understand what is meant by kinetic receptivity, imagine the sensitivity of the body, its physical capabilities and abilities, and at the same time a kind of intuition of the physical body. It is the source of our ability to instinctively perceive and respond to the environment in which we find ourselves and to what is happening around us. In many situations, we can rely on this bodily sensibility, which is strongly connected to our subconscious mind, more than on the logical mind. Modern research shows that a person has two brains. One is in the head, the other in the Lower Dantian area. Dr. Michael D. Gershon, in his book *The Second Brain*,[1] presents the results of studies that have shown that the nervous system of the intestines and the digestive system has a vast supply of nerve cells that receive and transmit information and respond to our emotions independently of the brain. He states that the brain in the abdomen is even more accurate in emotional responses than the brain in the head. The upper brain (in the head) is able to think and has memory, so it is able to store data. The lower brain also has memory, but is unable to think. Both brains are connected through the spinal cord. This modern research confirms what the Taoists said long ago.

The Middle Dantian

The Middle Dantian (in Chinese, *Zhongdantian*) is a kind of reservoir for mental and emotional Qi and its vibrations. In its space are the heart, the pericardium, the lungs and the thymus. It is also called the *home of emotional feeling and empathy*. It is the source of our ability to communicate and pay attention. As children, we are born very empathetic, but as the years and our life experiences increase, the ability to communicate empathically becomes weaker. This is done through parental education, education in the school environment and adaptation to the rules of the society in which we live. Emotional communication is connected to the heart. If we cultivate Qi in the Middle Dantian, our heart is open and able to communicate straightforwardly, manifest, feel and register.

Some sources point to two Middle Dantian locations. The second location is positioned at the level of the solar plexus. However, the size of this dantian is such that it extends to the level of the solar plexus, so the solar plexus is part of it.

The Upper Dantian

The Upper Dantian (in Chinese, *Shangdantian*) represents the spiritual aspect of human beings and their connection to Heaven, Tao. The brain and its two important glands—the pineal gland and the pituitary gland—belong to this area:. In the front part, it is connected with the *Yintang* point, translated as *the Hall of Impression*, which is the entrance to the third eye. At the back of the head, it is connected with the cavity under the skull, called the elongated spinal cord (medulla oblongata), and at the top of the head, where the *Bahui* point is located, translated as *One Hundred Meetings*, GV20. It is the highest point of the body connecting us with Heaven, with Yang. Its very center is located in the center of the brain. The Upper Dantian thus has the shape of a pyramid directed to Heaven, ready to receive *Heavenly Qi*. The Upper Dantian is responsible for mental activity and mental clarity. When this dantian is filled with Qi, our spiritual intuition and psychic receptivity increase. It is home to spiritual and intuitive communication and wakefulness.

However, the Three Dantians become real elixirs only through the cultivation of Qi, for example through Qigong, Neigong and meditation.

---

1   Gershon, M.D. (1999) *The Second Brain: A Groundbreaking New Understanding of Nervous Disorders of the Stomach and Intestine.* New York, NY: HarperPerennial.

THE FUNCTIONS OF QI IN THE BODY

We can describe and classify Qi in various ways. However, it can be said that in the human body it carries out the function of the driving force—it is the "engine" of the functioning of vital organs.

Qi warms the body, thanks to which we do not suffer from cold; in addition, the warmth also provides suitable conditions for many vital functions that need a certain temperature for their operation—for example, digestion.

Qi is involved in various types of transformation, such as the conversion of food into energy.

Qi nourishes the body and protects it from external influences. Its one component, the *Defensive Qi* (in Chinese, *Weiqi*), which will be mentioned in the chapter on the METAL phase, flows in the space between the muscles and the skin and forms a kind of armor. Its quality depends on how quickly an external pathogen penetrates us—for example, how quickly we catch a cold, but also how successfully or unsuccessfully we will be able to resist a virus.

Qi is constantly moving in the body, circulating through the body without ceasing. It enters and exits, rises and falls, sometimes moves fast and fluently, at other times slowly. Its quality and quantity vary according to the time of day, the age of the person, their state of mind, the season, the weather, social and other factors. If we do not care for it, it may be low or its quality may be insufficient. This can be manifested, for example, by a tendency to catch a cold or succumb to infectious diseases. In this case, not enough Qi gets into the layer of defensive "armor" under the skin. Another example of its deficiency may be digestive problems, when the Qi of the digestive organs is weakened and does not allow them to perform their functions properly.

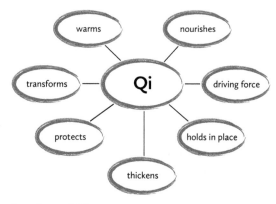

Functions of Qi

BLOOD AND QI

Circulation of blood is evident for Westerners, but we do not realize that it is connected with the circulation of Qi. However, blood flow is one of the most important physiological manifestations of the body's energetic functioning. The relationship between blood and Qi is key to health. Together and continuously, they circulate through the body to nourish, warm, maintain its functions and moisturize tissues. Thanks to Qi, the blood moves, so the movement of blood depends on the movement of Qi. Qi, on the other hand, needs blood as a kind of material substrate through which nutrition can circulate through the body. Qi carries the Yang aspect of their cooperation; it is the driving force. Blood, on the other hand, is a material substance, Yin—a liquid form of Qi that carries nutrients and information. They cannot exist without each other, and together they form an inseparable pair.

You may say that blood flows in the veins due to the heartbeat. Yes, that is exactly it! The heartbeat is a clear manifestation of the movement of Qi. It is one of the forms of Qi, manifested in the contractions and relaxation of the heart muscles, thanks to which the blood is distributed throughout the body.

In Chinese medicine terms, blood and Qi are used in the sense of overall health. A decrease in the quality and quantity of blood and Qi is a decrease in overall vitality. If the quality of Qi and blood remains sufficient even in a serious illness, the prognosis for recovery is favorable. Conversely, if a disease or lifestyle significantly weakens Qi and blood, recovery is difficult, sometimes impossible. The human being is regulated by blood and Qi and all changes in the balance between them.

However, what we call blood and Qi in the Taoist context is much more than just a red fluid and the dynamics of its circulation. The presence of blood also means a platform for the presence of spiritual energies, consciousness, perception and knowledge. According to Taoist philosophy, blood is the residence of the spirit. Blood is like a material substrate in which the soul can have its "roots" so that we feel sufficiently grounded in life on Earth. Therefore, excessive blood loss—for example, during childbirth or injury—can cause loss of consciousness and delirium. The "roots" of our soul lose the solid ground beneath their feet and seek it in delusion. However, the quality of

blood can also be lost by neglecting a harmonious and nutritionally balanced diet, excessive physical or mental overload of the body, lack of sleep and rest, and excessive experience of emotions.

Sufficiency of blood is reflected in everything—in our efficiency but also our ability to switch off; in a calm but also creative mind; in good-quality sleep or the speed of regeneration. It is clearly reflected in the appearance of the skin, which should be its natural color and smooth; in the quality of the muscles, which should be firm and full; in the condition of the tendons, which should be flexible; in the strength of the bones and the good condition of the joints—so in all the body structures that our profession needs. In addition to nutrition, the blood also provides moisturization. For example, it moisturizes the skin, thus ensuring its suppleness and defense.

Replenishing and nourishing blood is extremely important. And this is not just about blood donors who voluntarily lose a certain amount of blood. This applies to anyone who has physically or mentally demanding work.

HOW CAN WE SUPPORT QI IN OUR BODY?

We need to care for both "batteries"—both prenatal and postnatal sources of Qi. Postnatal Qi is nourished with a high-quality and regular diet, proper breathing, being in fresh air, detoxification of the organism, and psycho-hygiene. We can take care of Prenatal Qi with enough rest, by practicing Qigong and Taijiquan and by avoiding any extremes. At the same time, it would be appropriate to be aware of a kind of energy economy. The more demanding the performance, the greater the consumption of Qi in the body. In the profession of mover, it is not only our limbs that move, but all the organs of the body work while moving. For example, the liver is the organ responsible for storing blood, among

other things. This means that when the body is at rest, most of the blood is in this organ. Once the body starts to move, the liver is responsible for distributing blood to the parts of the body and the structures involved. The harder and faster the movement, the more work the liver has to do. The lungs pump enough air for the body to move, and the heart pumps blood to ensure the circulation of oxygen and nutrition to the body, and so on. We will describe these connections in more detail in the chapters on the individual phases and related organs.

On the one hand, the movement charges us mentally and physically, and thanks to it, Qi circulates in the body, which also activates endorphins that have a positive effect on the psyche. On the other hand, the intensive movement of the mover requires large contributions of Qi. For this reason, it is necessary to give the body, but also the mind, enough rest after exercise, to be able to draw on new doses of Qi and thus regenerate. It is important to plan performances, pedagogical or other work activities so that Qi has enough time and space to regenerate. The body to which we pay such care will repay us by the fact that it will function for a long time and will also guarantee the quick repair of damaged tissues after an injury. Ankle sprains, fractures, tendon strains, ruptured menisci, as well as common diseases such as colds, are easier and faster to treat with enough Qi. The more exhausted the Qi in the body, the longer a person takes to resolves health problems or the faster they succumb to them.

Emotions

Economically, it is advisable to work on our emotions, because from the point of view of Chinese medicine, emotions are a strong consumer of Qi. Outbursts of anger, resentment, a feeling of strong malignancy against someone or something, gossip, or constant judgment of others, negativity, or even excessive joy are factors that affect the quantity and quality of Qi in the body. Qi is confused and aroused in anger, disappears in grief, decreases in fear, and stagnates and becomes knotted by excessive thinking so that it cannot flow continuously. Qi participates in all the physical and mental functions that naturally consume it.

Travel

Movers travel a lot, often across time zones. These travels demand large Qi contributions, which we often do not even know about. The Taoists have observed that excessive travel depletes the prenatal "battery" and weakens the kidneys. Therefore, it is extremely important to provide the body with sufficient rest after such trips. When planning a journey, it is necessary to include time for sufficient acclimatization and rest after the traveling before we start performing in a new place. We will deal with the topic of travel in detail in the chapter on the EARTH phase.

Regularity

The postnatal "battery" needs regularity for its harmonic state. Therefore, it is appropriate to think about a regular supply of food, regular sleep, regularity in training, etc. Just the fact of regularity will lessen the depletion of this battery. However, adhering to regularity excessively strictly and in all circumstances is an extreme that can be counterproductive.

Connecting to the Qi of nature

Last but not least, the Taoists' advice on how to save Qi is to connect to the flow of Qi in nature, because what happens in nature during the seasons naturally affects us. One feels different in the winter, when everything around is resting, and differently in the spring, when the rested Qi wants to grow and act again. We feel differently in the summer, when Qi culminates in its greatest activity, and differently in the autumn, when Qi calms down and begins to prepare for winter relaxation. Taoist philosophy advises us to begin to register these changes and follow them in our lives. Thus, Qi will not be unnecessarily depleted and can be renewed like the nature around us. This means, for example, realizing that winter is a period when it is not appropriate to be physically exhausted. Or to accept that at present we can no longer deal with the same load as we did 20 or even ten years ago, and that we need to transform this new state into something else and not harm ourselves. How wonderfully nourishing it would be for the bodies and minds of students if the school curriculum also provided a connection to the cycles of nature!

Qi and mind

So far, there has been talk of Qi in relation to the body. However, Qi is also part of the mind. The body and the mind cannot be separated; the state and attunement of the mind clearly affect the state of the body, and vice versa. Qi can be mind-guided and is able to respond to our imagination. And this is a thing that can also be used in dance, performance, yoga or any other physical activity. An excellent result in an exam or in rehearsal, a good delivery of a performance, success in a competition or anything else can be achieved by visualizing the situation before the achievement. "When the intention (Yi) arrives, the Qi arrives," says a Chinese idiom. Visualization is also a suitable treatment. Thanks to suggestion, endorphin secretion occurs in the brain, which can reduce physical pain or change perceptions of the world and circumstances. Endorphin secretion, on the other hand, is also stimulated by dynamic physical exercise—that is, intense movement can awaken Qi in us and can also heal. Our vitality is nourished by receiving Qi from a universal source. But even so, we all influence it and make a difference in it by thinking about how we perceive the world around us and ourselves in it.

Basic principles for Qi support

- regular and quality diet
- balance between work and rest
- sufficient and good-quality sleep
- being in fresh air
- regular detoxification
- a calmer emotional life
- avoiding extremes
- rest after travel
- regularity
- being in nature for regeneration
- sufficient movement
- time for yourself

CHANNELS OF QI—MERIDIANS

Our Qi system consists of an active network of pathways—meridians, or channels—which extend throughout the body. They pass through the limbs and head and inside the body, where they connect with internal organs and energy centers. They create a network of pathways, thanks to which energetic communication takes place throughout the body.

In the West, the idea of meridians is not considered relevant because they cannot be seen, measured or dissected. Energetic communication takes place in them, and Chinese medicine, Qigong and Taijiquan is based on this principle. The flow of Qi in the meridians will be felt by anyone who is treated with acupuncture or Shiatsu. A needle or finger acts on a point, but Qi spreads from it along the entire meridian or a shorter section of it. One can feel this stream of Qi as a light electric shock, vibration, filling or expanding. The flow of Qi in the meridians can also be felt during the practice of Qigong and yoga, but it is also perceptible during dance, if we work on the flow of Qi consciously.

The ancient Taoists looked at the meridians in a very poetic yet practical way. The pathways are called *Jing Luo*, where *Jing* could be translated as "moving through something" or "stream of water underground" and *Luo* is translated as "network." Meridians are thus like a network of deep water passages, pathways, underground rivers, streams that energetically intertwine the internal structures of the human body, including the organs, and put them into interaction with the external structures.

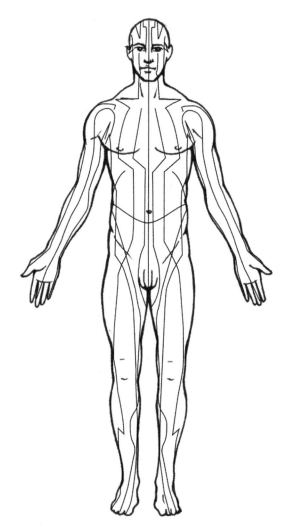

Meridians—Pathways of Qi

According to Chinese medicine, the system of meridians integrates all parts of the body and its functions into a single organism. The meridians are of great importance for the energetic as well as the physical system of the body. They are the main trunk of the tree of Qi circulation and are considered to be the basic energy support of the internal organs. They act as means of communication between the external and internal environment of the body, ensuring communication between internal organs and sensory organs and other components of the body surface, such as the skin or body orifices. They distribute the Qi of the organs throughout the body—they are like extended arms of the organs. They also ensure communication and harmonious cooperation between the upper and lower parts of the body and harmonize the Yin and Yang polarity of the body, which will be discussed later. In addition, they provide the connection and integration of Earth Qi with Heavenly Qi within the human body. And last but not least, they protect the body from external pathogens with a Qi shield under the skin.

Qi flows in a continuous circuit in these channels. Its flow has its source, but its circulation has neither a beginning nor an end. We divide this continuous flow into sections, because each of these specific sections affects other parts of the body, other organs, their functional relationships, which will be discussed in the chapter on organs and their functions. This division also provides us with an easier overview. We know 12 main channels. They are paired, symmetrically, on both sides of the body. They are so-called organ meridians, because each one of them corresponds to one of the 12 basic organs of the body and its functions, and also bears the name after this organ. They are *Kidney channel*, *Heart channel*, *Spleen channel*, *Liver channel*, *Lung channel*, *Pericardium channel*, *Bladder channel*, *Small Intestine channel*, *Stomach channel*, *Gallbladder channel*, *Large Intestine channel* and *Triple Burner channel*. In addition, Qi flows in eight extraordinary meridians – the *Governing Vessel (Dumai)*, the *Conception Vessel (Renmai)*, the *Penetrating Vessel (Chong Mai)*, the *Girdle Vessel (Daimai)*, the *Yin Linking Vessel*, the *Yang Linking Vessel*, the *Yin Motility Vessel* and the *Yang Motility Vessel*. All meridians run vertically, with the exception of one—the Girdle Vessel, which is horizontal. They are also divided according to the principles of Yin and Yang, according to the Five Phases (Five Elements) and according to their function.

Table 3.1 Yin and Yang organ meridians

Yin meridians	Yang meridians
Lung channel (arm)	Large Intestine channel (arm)
Spleen channel (leg)	Stomach channel (leg)
Heart channel (arm)	Small Intestine channel (arm)
Kidney channel (leg)	Bladder channel (leg)
Pericardium channel (arm)	Triple Burner channel (arm)
Liver channel (leg)	Gallbladder channel (leg)

We will get acquainted with the 12 organ meridians in this book step by step. We will also get to know the possibilities of how to work with them while moving. The meridians naturally participate in every movement that a person does. Therefore, of course, they move and are activated during dance, yoga, sports and any kind of movement. After all, the Qigong and Taijiquan movement exercises are based on the sense of Qi flow. I work with them through Qigong and dance. But not any kind of dance! We work with meridians in dance improvisation, in which the mind is also involved, consciousness is sent into the body, and we can perceive what is happening there from an energetic point of view. Based on my experience and the experience of my students, I can say that working with meridians through movement is an excellent way to feel the flow of Qi in one's body and at the same time a good way to remember these pathways of Qi—and not just mentally, but remember them in the physical memory. One can look at them in the image above, but there is nothing better than experiencing them in your own body, when each cell remembers them through movement. Such movement improvisation is thus a suitable way of enabling the flow Qi in the meridians. In this book, I offer some ideas on how to work with the meridians in movement improvisation. You can find these after the description of each meridian.

If we work consciously with meridians during movement improvisation, this has a huge impact on the quality of movement, and also on health. During my years of researching the connection between the principles of Chinese medicine and dance, I naturally began to work with meridians in dance improvisations. In this work, it is possible to include several aspects in the movement: the section of the particular channel and the anatomical areas of the body where the Qi of this channel passes; the direction and intensity of the Qi flow in it; areas of higher concentration of acupuncture points on a particular channel; its Yin or Yang qualities; and also the qualities of some of the Five Phases (WOOD, FIRE, EARTH, METAL, WATER), to which the channel is related. Students also work with their own ideas that the meridian associates in them. The results are interesting in the field of movement expression. This work brings students new movement possibilities, and their movement becomes more interesting and conscious. From a health point of view, we can also experience interesting changes. After a week of experimenting, one student began menstruating again after more than six months of absence of her period. She chose the Liver and Kidney channels, which are, among other things, closely related to the menstruation cycle. Improvisation with the Bladder and Kidney channels can lead to the release of stagnation in the spine. When working with the Stomach and Spleen channels, we can correct digestion, and so on. Thus it could be said that conscious dance improvisation can be a form of Qigong capable of harmonizing the organism and even healing it. I consider the basic knowledge of meridians to be a part of the basic "equipment" of every person who works with the human body.

ENTRANCES INTO THE ENERGY SYSTEM

The meridians are connected to the body surface via acupuncture points (in Chinese, *Xue*), which are used in therapeutic practice (application of a needle, pressure of a finger, palm, foot or elbow, or by applying a seed, a magnet or electric discharge). They act as a kind of gateway through which the energetic system can be entered and influenced. The word *point* is a very limited translation of Xue because it encourages us to imagine it as a surface. However, it is rather a multidimensional place where, in addition to space, time and dynamics take place between them.

Xue are found on various body structures—in the crevices of bones and cartilage, under the bones, or in places where the bones connect to each other. We can also find them on the muscles, in places where two or more muscles, tendons, ligaments or fascia meet, but also in areas where nerves protrude closer to the surface. They even occur on the bones. In certain areas of the body, such as the joints, more of them are located. The joints thus function as "meeting and communication stations." The spine and the area next to the spine are literally full of them.

Xue can be deep or shallow, wide or narrow. These possibilities are mostly conditioned by the anatomical structures through which the meridian passes and the places where they are located. One located on the thigh muscle, for example, has a different depth and spaciousness than one located on the bone, or in the gaps between the bones or between the tendons. The quantity and quality of Qi in an individual Xue also depends on the spaciousness and depth, but it can also reflect the quantity and quality of the Qi of a particular organ to which the Xue is related. The therapist using acupuncture, acupressure, medical Qigong or Shiatsu is able to connect with the Xue mentally, feel it through touch or meditation and find out what the space and quality of Qi is in it, and adjust it if necessary to restore health. In our experiments with working with meridians in movement, we were able to feel the culmination of Qi in an individual Xue very significantly.

THE POWER OF QIGONG IN THE PROFESSION OF MOVER

For several years now, Qigong has been a part of my lifestyle. Naturally, I also involve it in my pedagogical and interpretive work. I am more and more amazed by its effects. It has changed my approach to the body, but it has also changed my own body. I would even say it cured my body. I perceive how it helps me maintain the right body tone and relationship between individual body structures and organs, but also how it keeps me in a harmonious emotional state. Last but not least, it has increased my amount of Qi and keeps me healthy. However, it also changed my approach to choreography—through Qigong, I discovered such movement principles and possibilities that I would not have discovered otherwise.

Cultivation and mastering vital life force
Qigong is one of the ancient Chinese practices aimed at balancing body and mind. It is grounded in the theory of Chinese medicine. One of its main principles is the fact that a person is healthy

if his or her Qi circulates through the body uninhibited, evenly and regularly. Qigong literally means *work with Qi*. We already know what *Qi* means. *Gong* means activity, work, ability and also the time and attention we spend on using something. Thus, Qigong means the art of cultivation and mastering vital life force Qi. It is a way to secure its circulation throughout the body.

Qigong exercises are usually simple and done at a slow pace. They improve our sense of Qi and its circulation throughout the body. They are the basis for martial arts and, at the same time, for the ability to heal. Qigong comprises sets of exercises, inspired by ancient Taoists, which have been gradually adjusted to a form accessible to the broad public. Practicing these exercises leads to balancing Qi in the body, which is expressed by increased immunity, better hormonal stability, stability of the lymphatic system, and overall balance and cooperation between inner organs. Qigong also helps to get rid of problems such as back pain, tiredness, stress and concentration and sleeping disorders. Qigong cultivates well-being, emotional stability and peace of mind. The main benefit for healthy people is that Qigong harmonizes the human organism before an illness appears on a physical level.

Matter of consciousness

The key in Qigong is our conscious work because the amount of Qi depends on our conscious focus and ability to connect and concentrate inwards. The amount of generated Qi depends on our consciousness. I do not compel students to memorize any complicated forms of Qigong (series of exercises). On the contrary, I use elementary and essential exercises focused on carrying out and sensing Qi in one's own body rather than on the exact sequence. The exercises are very simple but extremely effective. They always focus on a specific body part, body center or body structure, which is, afterwards, important in movement training. I usually open my lessons with Qigong to wake up energy in movers'

meridians, to activate their bodies and prepare them for further work during the dance training or dance improvisation. However, Qigong, in its essence, can be parallel to dance as a subconscious part of dance and movement expression, both during dance training or improvisation and even during performance on stage. The physical effort during dancing usually leads to exhaustion. However, if the principles of Qigong are applied to dance, it results in charging the body and soul.

Originally, the aim of Qigong was not just for health and stamina cultivation; above all, it was for self-knowledge, getting to know one's own body and mind and achieving its natural condition, a state of harmonious body–mind connection. Such Qigong, which leads to the cultivation of mental power, is known as *Inner Qigong* (*Neigong*) and it is a very important part of my work. We also use Qigong in my dance practice because it cultivates patience and persistence. It is not possible to expect immediate effects and especially not those that are visible at first sight. Therefore, students learn both to be humble and to trust their bodies and their processes, as well as their own focus and ability to concentrate.

Wuwei

Another fascinating aspect of Qigong, which I use and offer to my students, is the principle of Wuwei—action in non-action. To put it simply, it means "letting nature take its course." We aim to achieve a peaceful state of mind when we do not strive for success and perfection or when we do not make efforts to be better than others. Such states of mind often prevent dancers from moving naturally and can even lead to injuries. Wuwei also teaches us not to get confused by various physical or mental states that may occur during exercises. Although we can feel discomfort, pain or, on the contrary, extreme pleasure, we learn not to cling to any sensations or feelings at all. We try to let the present moment flow freely, accepting anything it can bring along. Many of our feelings are illusions anyway. Qigong can teach us to let go of these illusions. It is a long-term process, cultivating our persistence and modesty.

Strengthening the body

Last but not least, Qigong can be an amazing way to help strengthen the body for dance or any kind of movement. Practicing Qigong can strengthen bones, joints, tendons, muscles and inner organs, and, according to Chinese medicine, nourish those structures with beneficial Qi. For this purpose, we use various exercises—for example, *breathing to the bones*, *breathing to the kidneys*, *rubbing tendons*, etc. In fact, those exercises wake up new life in body structures which are nourished thanks to Qi circulation. Moreover, absorbing and recycling Qi strengthens the immune system, and Qigong is a perfect means to expedite healing injuries as well. I have a personal and intense experience with it. I used internal Qigong to regenerate the injured structures caused by the dislocation of the collarbone and two ribs, and the rupture of small tendons next to the sternum. With this injury, regular doctors sent me to the operating table. But following three precise treatments received from an osteopath, and thanks to my intensive Qigong practice focused on healing those structures, I performed on stage again a month after the injury.

Connecting to inner spirit

Qigong also develops our ability to connect to our inner spirit. Conscious work with Qi is the basis of Qigong. We can use this skill to calm ourselves, tune us to the current situation or our state, but also as a way of concentration before a performance or before a difficult test. The power of a calm mind together with focus on physical structures can sometimes prepare the body for performance more thoroughly than physical exercises themselves. I, myself, practice this art before performing. I no longer do such an intense warm-up focused on muscles and tendons, but I do warm up mentally through Qigong.

Inspiration

It is possible to consciously work with the meridians and Qi flowing in them through various exercises and also through Taijiquan, or other Eastern martial arts, working with the guidance of Qi. In martial arts, the focus is primarily on defense against the attacker. Their defense does not rely on muscle strength but on the strength of directing Qi. This guidance of Qi creates physical fluency—an interesting form of the body, often similar to the cultivated movement of animals, but also to the cultivated human movement expression. Not surprisingly, these techniques, whether martial arts or cultivation of Qi by the aforementioned exercises, are a frequent inspiration for dancers and movers, and many of them practice them. Aikido, for example, is a good way to grasp the basic principles of contact improvisation.

Thermal adjustment of the body

A completely prosaic and practical advantage of Qigong is that it is an excellent way to warm up the body in the cold season. Activated Qi generates warmth. From my own practice, I have attested with the students that a good Qigong before training can generate an ideal thermal adjustment of the body even in a very cold room, and is therefore a suitable preparation for performance.

CHAPTER 4

Qi obtained from food

Balance between expenditure and revenue

About: breatharianism / the art and specifics of Chinese dietetics / the importance of heat for digestion / food quality / effect of food / the importance of chewing / overeating / the harmfulness of the microwave

Many of us in this hectic world are not sufficiently aware that food is not about filling our bellies and getting rid of hunger; rather it is, above all, about getting the most nutrients and Qi needed for life. The lives of movers are mostly hurried and full of tension. They rush from rehearsal to rehearsal or the lessons they teach. They either eat food in a hurry during breaks or at the end of the day, when they remember that they have not actually eaten all day. So they eat something before they go to bed, and thus actually prevent their body from finally relaxing at night after their busy day. The digestive tract is fully awake and it works all night, instead of resting. In addition, we often travel and do not always have suitable eating conditions.

Our way of life requires a great deal of energy. We work extremely hard physically and, many of us, mentally, too. Both ways consume a lot of Qi. Therefore, it is up to us to learn to manage it wisely, because only we decide whether we spend our Qi in the immediate years ahead or save it for all our life. In the previous chapter on Postnatal Qi, I emphasized that food is an important source of human Qi, and due to its quality and quantity, Prenatal Qi does not have to be consumed faster than necessary.

Qi, which is converted from food by metabolic processes, is the basic material substance of the blood. It is a nutrient that is distributed by the blood to all structures of the body. We need it for muscles, tendons, bones, joints—all the parts of the body that we use in motion. However, we also need blood of sufficient quality for the well-being of our psyche. The blood, which contains all the necessary nutrients and Qi, is like a substrate in which the psyche finds its support. And you will certainly agree with me that a relaxed psyche is also extremely important in our profession. So it is important for us to start valuing our own Qi more and learning to treat it wisely. In my research, I have noticed that many colleagues have realized that we can pursue our profession better if it is supported by a healthy diet.

TO HAVE OR NOT TO HAVE LUNCH

In my therapeutic practice, I had a young woman who had not eaten for several weeks. She came to me because she felt exhausted, and even though she was young, she developed significant health problems. When asked if she was experimenting with becoming a breatharian, the answer was that she was not. It was just that she did not have time to eat because of so much work. In the world of movers, we commonly encounter skinny, even malnourished dancers or yoga instructors, whose physical condition borders on or suffers from an eating disorder. How alarming! We expend so much energy in our profession, and at the same time we do not feel the need to supplement it sufficiently. When the car runs out of petrol, we refuel so we can continue on our journey. However, we often neglect the need for our own good-quality "refueling."

I think it starts in schools. I had the opportunity to work at several dance schools and monitor the students' relationship to food, but also the relationship of schools to their students' diet. The range of approaches is really wide—from enviable to alarming. There are schools in which the importance of a balanced diet is part of their holistic concept, and they provide their students with quality lunches—some even a macrobiotic diet, or a diet according to Chinese dietetics. There are schools that do not provide meals for students but give them enough time to have lunch and to digest it. Unfortunately, there are also schools whose schedules provide students with a lunch break of less than an hour. And if the canteen is not in the school building, the students not only do not have time to get there but also cannot eat in peace and digest their lunch. After lunch, they tend to have physically demanding lessons in the schedule, so the students think twice about whether to have lunch and feel sick or not eat at all.

Paradoxically, this actually suits many students. For them, food intake equals calorie intake, and calories equal extra kilograms. I know this from my own experience. The fear of excess weight has been rooted in us since the beginning of our studies. I started studying at a dance conservatory at the age of ten. One of the first things we had to do after starting school was stand on a scale and the teacher recorded our weight. This was repeated every month, and woe betide us if it did not fit the standards in the tables. The natural development of the body and associated hormonal changes during puberty were also not taken into account.

The young people thus learn to deny their bodies and their needs, and even to deny their physical and hormonal development. They learn to suppress many feelings, including the feeling of hunger. And in the pursuit of perfection, in the effort to avoid criticism or even open remorse about their body shape, students decide not to eat. This can naturally develop into an eating disorder such as bulimia or anorexia nervosa, but at the very least it can cause malnutrition, the consequences of which can be manifested in osteoporosis, joint pain, tendon stiffening and so on—basically, weakening those parts of the body that we need for movement. Another consequence may be a delayed onset of the menstrual cycle, or its irregularity or even its loss. Gradually, this can lead to infertility at a later age. Of course, the weakening of the function of all the organs is also a consequence.

IT IS NOT POSSIBLE TO LIVE WITHOUT QI

Unless we are breatharians—that is, people who obtain Qi directly from the source—we must receive food in order to get Qi. You can live without food, but not without Qi. Who is able to receive Qi directly from the source does not have to eat. But who can do it so easily?

Taoism has something to do with the modern term *breatharianism*. The oldest cases of the art of living without food come from the Taoist tradition. More than 2000 years ago, people who practiced the art of *Bigu* lived in the Chinese mountains. *Gu* is simply translated as "food," and *Bi* means "to avoid." They claimed that one does not have to consume food at all, and yet one can be healthy and vital. However, these people achieved the state of Bigu by practicing Qigong and Neigong (Inner Qigong)—that is, by receiving Qi in a direct way. They were able to survive years without food. However, they claimed that for the practice of Bigu, it was necessary to achieve a level of some kind of *full unity*. If a person is in good condition and healthy, Bigu comes naturally. However, if we try to achieve Bigu by force just because we want to master it, we can harm our body. Bigu is therefore possible, but it does not mean that everyone can practice it at will. It is necessary to learn this technique in the right way. At the same time, the environment is very important for practicing Bigu. Our cities are full of chaos and various types of energy that are harmful to humans—electromagnetic smog, stress, pathogenic energy fields, various pollutants in the air and in relationships, etc. Obtaining Qi directly from the source is all the more challenging for us.

Since the art of Bigu cannot be practiced by anyone, the Taoists have also developed the art of understanding the Qi of food—that is, how diet affects our health. And this means not only the state of the physical body, but also emotions, mental processes and overall energy balance. Each food has its own Qi, which resonates in the body in a specific way. In principle, food can energize us, but it can also make us dull and tired; it can relax or awaken us to an activity, cool or heat us, and so on. Food can help us concentrate better, it can cause us to lose our concentration, or it can even darken our mind. It can draw us into ourselves and encourage contemplation or release us to be more sociable. For example, certain foods can help get rid of excessive internal moisture or cold, but others can accumulate moisture and cold in the body when consumed excessively. With long-term intake, foods are able to influence emotions and mental processes. In addition, food contains information codes of the sources from which it comes, and these also affect us when consumed. Different energy will be radiated by a person who has a piece of meat on the table every day compared to a person who eats mainly vegetables, cereals and fruits. A person will have different energy if they eat the meat of a fast and agile animal, and different energy if they eat the meat of a slow, robust animal. We are talking about the so-called Chinese dietetics, which developed this topic into complex dimensions of a very detailed nature. The framework of this book naturally provides space for basic information only.

The Chinese concept of healthy eating has little to do with the eating style prevalent in Europe. Therefore, I emphasize that modern Chinese fast food cannot be included in this art. Most has adapted to Western customs and thus does not offer the interplay of flavors and effects that characterize Chinese cuisine. The art of Chinese dietetics is how to respect and strengthen various aspects of health through food, and thus meet different needs. Several factors play a role.

Our *constitution*—that is, our hereditary predispositions—but also our *condition*—that is, the state in which we are now. For example, *age* is decisive, because in each period of life and development, the body has different requirements for choosing the right diet. Of course, children need a different diet compared to adults, but, in general, not much is known about the fact that with increasing age, the human digestive tract naturally weakens, so older people should consume lighter food, which is therefore easier to digest. The *time of day* also has certain specific rules, which can be followed by the selection of suitable foods, their quantity and their preparation. As our Qi develops during the day—that is, in the morning it is strongest and it gradually weakens from lunch to dinner—breakfast should be hearty, lunch normal and dinner light. Likewise, *gender* is decisive, because a woman who has more Yin essence needs something different compared to a man who has more Yang essence. The *season* that we are currently in naturally offers options for choosing food according to what is in season, but it also encourages us to choose foods that will harmonize the temperature changes that each season brings. In the winter, it would be illogical to consume large quantities of cooling foods, such as tropical fruits and raw vegetables; conversely, in the summer, overwarming from the inside with warming food or food prepared in a very warming way, such as baking or grilling, would be detrimental. And, of course, it is also dependent upon how much Qi we spend in our profession. If we have periods of extremely strenuous physical expenditure, it is wise to consume more food, and it is recommended to include meat or broth from meat or animal bones and more fat in the diet. If we have a period of less physical or mental expenditure, the diet should be lighter.

> In this book, I offer an overview of what is appropriate to consume according to the Qi of the seasons and, for inspiration, several recipes for these seasons. You will find them in the chapters focused on the Five Phases.

THE IMPORTANCE OF WARMTH

One of the most important views held by Chinese medicine in connection with digestion is that the digestive organs need warmth to be able to actually process food and get as many nutrients from it as possible and turn it into Qi. Therefore, it prefers warm preparation (cooking), which provides a kind of external pre-digestion. Because of this, food becomes more digestible for the body. The master of our organ digestion is the stomach. It can perfectly digest food only when the food is about 38°C (100°F). In a warm environment, the stomach can function as a heated cauldron in which food can be processed immediately, so it consumes Qi only for this processing. However, if we put something cold in the stomach, the stomach must first warm the food and only then can it start digestion. It naturally consumes more Qi because it has extra work to do.

Taoists have observed that in the digestive process, warming by food causes Qi to be activated and, conversely, cooling by food causes the opposite. In China, it is customary to always have hot, boiled water on hand. In restaurants and hotels, but also in various public spaces, such as theaters, cinemas, museums, transport stations, or even on some means of transport, there are large thermoses with hot water. Drinking something cold, and thus cooling their stomach, is unthinkable in Chinese traditional subconsciousness, because Taoists know that the stomach needs to be always warm. When we imagine Western eating habits, in which the consumption of food is associated with drinking a cold or often even an iced drink, it is not surprising that we suffer from digestive problems to such an extent. Unfortunately, this trend can already be seen in China.

Cooking also releases the taste and smell of food. When a wonderful smell spreads through the kitchen, our appetite is stimulated, which is an important mechanism that supports digestion itself. Another process that helps the stomach in processing is the pre-digestion of food in the oral cavity. So chewing is very important. Before food enters the stomach, it needs to be ground and mixed with saliva. Mixing with saliva during chewing adds an important alkalinizing component to the digestive process. Since the stomach does not have saliva and teeth, we have to do it in our mouths. When we swallow ingested food directly into the stomach, we deprive it of its Qi. Why? Because the stomach has to deal with this condition by creating more juices to digest large pieces of food, for example. Consequently, it will have less Qi left for digestion itself, which will reduce the nutrients we could absorb. To exaggerate slightly, we flush the money put into food down the toilet.

FOOD QUALITY

There is no food that can be considered healthy or unhealthy. A Chinese proverb says, "Anything that can help us can also hurt us." It depends on the amount, but also on a particular person's digestive tract or the conditions in which he or she consumes a meal. What helps one can harm another. Even what one considers healthy may not suit another person or the season of the year. For example, fruit is commonly considered healthy because it contains many vitamins. That is true, but it is only a narrow understanding of the benefits of fruit. Fruit cools us, and if a person with a weak spleen Qi consumes an excess of raw fruit, it weakens the spleen Qi and stomach Qi even more, and thus weakens the digestive tract. Therefore, Chinese dietetics does not apply any strict general principles; instead, it encourages us to think about food, about combining it, and encourages us to observe what is happening in us and to respect the natural predetermination of the seasons. However, certain principles do apply because they have been proven over years of experience.

In any case, the food we consume must be of good quality. The production and sale of food in ordinary food chains is often alarming. The shelves are filled with lots of unripe fruits and vegetables; eggs from hens kept in cages naturally carry information of stressed hens, and meat also contains information of the environment in which the animal lived. If the animal suffered and felt fear and stress at the time of its death, this information is stored in the cells of its flesh, and we then consume it. If crops come from an environment where pesticides are used, we take in all these substances, too. Foods are full of stabilizers, preservatives and dyes. All these affect our health, and modern research confirms this. There are many adverse health effects, such as disruption of the endocrine system and disruption of the organs themselves, and including the cause of cancer. Therefore, it is important to choose foods that are as little contaminated as possible with these chemicals. It is natural that many people today are focused on obtaining organically grown food and free-range animals. Various small supply chains for such foods are emerging, which really needs to be supported. Today you can find a local producer whom you may know personally. Home-grown fruits and vegetables taste and smell quite different and are several times higher in Qi compared to those conventionally produced.

RICE AS A BASE

We are used to associating Chinese food with rice. It is no coincidence, because cereals should really make up the majority of our diet. And it is not just the Chinese domain; grain has always been an important part of the diet of all ancient cultures. Archaeological finds of cereal grains in some tombs also prove this. During my travels around the world, when I had the opportunity to get close to the elderly, I was often offered various kinds of cereal porridge for breakfast. In the European environment where I come from, this has also been the case in the past. Grains are not limited only to rice. There are many other types of grains: millet, barley, rye, oats, wheat, buckwheat, corn, kamut, sorghum, quinoa, amaranth and the like.

Cereal grain contains the information and potential of the whole plant. It is a huge source of carbohydrates— substances that transform into Qi, harmonize and strengthen the Yin and Yang balance in the body, create Qi and body fluids, help to eliminate toxic substances from the body and calm the emotional world with their harmonizing effect. However, not every cereal grain is easily digestible for us. Therefore, it is recommended to pre-soak some harder grains such as wheat, rye or barley. For the same reason, there are also versions such as groats, flakes, grits and the like.

> Information on carbohydrates, sugar, grains, breakfast porridge and some recipes can be found in Chapter 11 on the EARTH phase.

In addition to grains, of course, other ingredients are needed, such as protein in the form of legumes and meat, and vegetables in large quantities, but also fruit for its vitamins, minerals and trace elements.

EAT TOO LITTLE OR OVEREAT

When it comes to quantity, the appropriate amount is decisive. The amount of food can show signs of sufficiency, scarcity or excess. Dietary doses that are lower but well adapted to our needs will strengthen the functioning of the digestive tract. Chinese medicine teaches that we should not fill our stomachs completely with food. We can fill two-thirds of its volume, but one-third should remain empty. The empty third is there to leave room in the stomach and Qi for digestive processes. Eating until full is therefore extremely burdensome for stomach Qi. It is also not appropriate to starve all day and then eat excessively only once a day, and God forbid in the evening. In general, however, we feel that we need to eat a lot to have energy. Therefore, we get used to overeating to some extent and thus burden the digestive tract. Nutrients cannot be fully extracted and benefit the body. Excess food weakens the digestive organs because they have to work harder than they should. At the same time, waste accumulates in the body, which also causes the consumption of Qi, because the body must process it and then eliminate it.

EFFECT OF FOOD

One of the specifics of Chinese dietetics is the division of foods according to their *taste* and *character*. Each of the tastes has some quality and ability to influence a person's Qi. Every taste belongs to a different organ, which we can either support and nourish with it or harm with it. It depends on whether we consume a certain taste in normal, limited or excessive amounts. All tastes should be present in the diet. If we eliminate or prefer one, we upset the balance, which can later result in disease.

Table 4.1 Effect of tastes

Taste	Functioning	Influences organ	Effect	Excessive influence	Contraindicated
Sweet	Harmonizes	Spleen	Nourishes, moisturizes.	It harms the spleen in sudden excess and harms the kidneys in chronic excess.	In the case of excessive moisture in the body.
Bitter	Dries	Heart	Laxative, dries moisture in the body, releases stagnation of food.	It harms the heart in sudden excess and harms the lungs in chronic excess.	In the case of dryness and bone disorders
Sour	Draws inwards	Liver	It accelerates the penetration of flavors and effects of food into the body.	It harms the liver in sudden excess and harms the spleen in chronic excess.	In the case of dry mucous membranes and skin.
Salty	Softens	Kidneys	Laxative, moisturizes, softens.	It harms the kidneys in sudden excess and harms the heart in chronic excess.	In the case of diarrhea and weakened blood.
Piquant	Dispels	Lungs	It supports the circulation of vital Qi, brings pathogens to the surface from the inside, and initiates sweating.	It harms the lungs in sudden excess and it harms the liver in chronic excess, causing premature wilting of the body.	In the case of weak lungs, because it irritates the cough.

The character of food means what thermal effect the food will have on the body. Here it is necessary to realize the difference between the temperature of the food itself and its thermal effect on the body after digestion. Tofu, for example, can be consumed raw, warm, cooked, stewed or even grilled, but it will always have a cooling effect on the body. On the other hand, drinking warm mint tea in the summer is ideal, because mint itself has a cooling effect, and even if we drink the tea warm, it cools us. In this manner, we divide food into *cold*, *refreshing*, *neutral*, *warm* and *hot*.

METHODS OF PREPARATION

The method of preparation also affects digestion and Qi. There are a number of preparation methods that can be used to adapt to the needs of an individual or the season. In winter, we should prefer the preparation that will help the body to warm up, and in the summer the preparation that will refresh us. Here is a list of preparation methods from the coldest to the hottest.

The way of creating a fire under the pot is also important because it determines the Yang Qi that we get into our digestion. Fire produced from wood is the best option for cooking. However, not everyone can afford that, especially in cities.

Therefore, the closest variant to it is cooking on a fire achieved by using gas (i.e. gas stoves). Creating Yang with electricity is no longer a real fire, so there is no real Yang that would provide quality Qi for prepared meals.

In general, it is not recommended to prepare food or heat it in a microwave oven, because this process kills almost all life in food. Microwaves vibrate atoms, causing them to warm up. Therefore, the food can be cold on the surface and boiling in the middle. This vibration also vibrates the organs and their Qi, and this is unsuitable for our body.

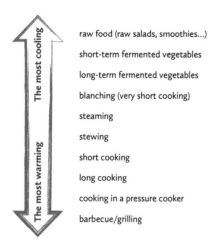

Preparation methods

Frozen foods contain less Qi than fresh, fermented or dried. Frozen semi-finished products are sometimes a quick solution to quenching hunger, but from an energy point of view they do not give us much Qi because they contain little of it. The freezing process takes place at a temperature of –40°C and the frozen pieces of food are shaken on vibrating tables during this process, so that the individual pieces do not stick to each other. Thus, not only extreme cold but also wind gets into them. As we will read later in the chapters on the WOOD and WATER phases, both of these influences, cold and wind, are challenging for us.

During the freezing and subsequent thawing of meat, the cellular structure of the meat changes, which can have an impact on health with increased consumption. So consume frozen food sparingly. Today, freezing is also a common part of bakery products, which are baked from pre-frozen semi-finished products. Likewise, butter in normal distribution is no longer a fresh food, because until it became butter, it went through a freezing process at the cream stage.

IN CONCLUSION

You might say that I promote Chinese cuisine and that it does not suit you. And why should it when you come from a different environment? If you are healthy, I can only agree with you. However, certain principles offered by Chinese dietetics should be of benefit to any diet. Whether we eat according to Chinese dietetics, macrobiotics, Ayurveda, vegetarianism, veganism, modern raw food or we leave it to "classics," for the greatest benefit from eating, we can follow a few universal tips:

Take time to eat
When we eat, we should not rush anywhere but devote that time to ourselves. It is said that it is healthier to eat something unhealthy in peace than something extremely healthy but stressed. Even after eating, let's not rush to work again. Taoists recommend having a real rest after eating.

Sit down
Eating while standing, or, worse still, while walking, is very inappropriate. Only when our body is in a relaxed state (i.e. sitting quietly) is our digestive system able to receive nutrition. A sitting position helps the blood flow more smoothly into the digestive tract and makes it easier to transport nutrients to the cells.

Eliminate distractions while eating
Let's pay full attention to food intake. It will help good digestion if we really enjoy the food that we have prepared or has been prepared for us. If we focus on it, we perceive its taste, texture, etc. When we overwhelm the digestive organs with our problems during the processing of food, we prevent them from digesting properly. If we solve work

problems at a business lunch, we will also burden our stomachs with these problems. It is also not advisable to eat while working on a computer, watching TV or even driving a car. If we do this regularly, the digestive tract will eventually resign. Only in a calm state is the body able to perceive the amount of food ingested and naturally regulate it. When it feels it has had enough, it instructs us to stop.

Don't eat when emotionally excited

Emotions significantly disrupt the flow of Qi in the body, and therefore the flow of Qi in the digestive tract. In a strong emotional state, digestion cannot take place in full. In such situations, food commonly stagnates in the stomach, leading to stomach pain. Sometimes the digestive tract vomits ingested food if it is consumed during emotional disturbance. It is better to eat only when we have calmed down enough.

Don't solve problems when preparing food

Food is also affected by the Qi that was used for its preparation. If we cook food with love and joy, this Qi will also be reflected in the Qi of the prepared food. If we argue with family members during cooking, attempt to solve a problem or work on something else, we will serve this Qi on a plate.

Avoid preferring certain foods

Our diet should be colorful. Every food has an effect on the body and mind. If we prefer something, we supply our body with an excess Qi of this food and, for the most part, there is no room left for other options that could balance it. At the same time, if we prefer something because of a taste that we like, it may indicate a weakness of an organ, because tastes are directly connected to the Qi of individual organs. So it can be information for us about what we should pay attention to.

Be grateful for the food

Any food is a gift from the Earth. Saying "thank you" before consumption expresses gratitude for this gift. Such gratitude is also a factor that influences the processing of food into Qi.

Eat daily at regular times

Regularity causes the regulation and synchronization of all bodily functions. This will improve all our cycles: blood sugar intake, hormone balance, menstrual cycle in women, sleeping patterns, overall vitality, but also mood. Of course, sometimes regularity cannot be adhered to and trying to cling to it like a limpet can also be counterproductive.

Chew each bite 30–50 times

This may sound like a joke or science fiction, but let's at least try to chew food sufficiently in our mouths. Only in the mouth does food have the opportunity to mix with saliva, which helps to break down food completely and thus improve digestion and nutrient intake. One proverb says, "Liquid food should be chewed, solid food must be drunk." This means that the solid food must be chewed so that it almost pours into our stomachs, and the liquids and soups are to be mixed in the mouth with saliva as if we were chewing them. Whatever valuable food we eat, if we do not chew it sufficiently and mix it with saliva, it is actually a burden to us.

Don't overeat

As already mentioned, filling the stomach to complete fullness is very burdensome. If we pay attention to food, we are able to learn to recognize when we have had enough.

Give the stomach time to rest

The stomach needs time and peace after eating. It is damaging when we put something in it all day long. We may not eat much but continuous snacking during a whole day is very burdensome for the stomach. The stomach needs at least a two-hour break devoted to digestion itself, but also rest. It is therefore advisable to eat only two to three times a day with breaks between meals. After lunch, a small walk is recommended to help the digestion and strengthen the transformational and transport function of the digestive organs.

Don't eat later than three hours before bedtime

Sleep is a time of rest and recovery. If the body has to work at night by digesting food, we rob it of the possibility of regeneration. In addition, food that remains in the intestines overnight rots and prevents the body's natural detoxification. Daytime hours are a good time to digest food. It is a time when our body, including the digestive tract, is in the activity phase. Even digestion needs rest at night. From the point of view of Chinese medicine, late dinners are therefore not suitable. We force digestion to work at night instead of relaxing with us. It is ideal to eat the last meal three to four hours before we fall asleep, but no later than 8 p.m. Of course, this is not always possible. Occasional late dinners with friends or during the holidays or after a performance will not completely derail us, but Chinese medicine does not recommend it as a habit, especially for those who have impaired digestion or suffer from being overweight, for example.

Give food a purpose

We can also enrich food intake with information. We can determine what effect we want to receive from a particular food. It can be the treatment of a specific organ, improving our condition, receiving joy, energy or vitality, or relaxation. Let's prepare and consume our food with this purpose. It can turn everything we eat into a healing experience.

Relax after a meal

Some sources claim that up to 40 percent of the Qi we consume through food is used to digest it—to break it down into individual components, to absorb them into the blood. We need another amount of Qi to select unnecessary components and eliminate them. Digestion is a complicated process; the first bite will start a complex factory in us. Therefore, peace is important during meals as well as rest and relaxation after meals, in order to provide the body with the conditions for it to be able to process food in peace.

CHAPTER 5

Organs

Materialized Qi in the body

About: organ "hierarchy" / cooperation and functional relationships between the internal organs / connecting the organs with emotions and body tissues / connecting the surface with the inside of the body / 12 ordinary and six extraordinary organs / the organ clock / psychospiritual aspects of organs

When a fellow dancer had an accident at a rehearsal some time ago and ended up at orthopedics with partially torn tendons, I commented that she would have to get her liver treated. She looked at me blankly and said, "Liver? But I don't drink." I smiled, but at the same time I realized that it was a pity that people who work with the body on a daily basis know so little about it or have such narrow awareness about it. "The liver will help the tendons regenerate faster," I added. She was still puzzled, so I continued, "The kidneys nourish the bones. They are also in charge of the condition of cartilage, joints, joint fluid, intervertebral discs, bone marrow and spinal cord. The spleen is in charge of the muscle mass and thus the overall shape of the body. The liver nourishes the tendons and ligaments with its Qi and is responsible for their elasticity. As the muscles are attached to the bones by tendons, the quality of the tendons also affects the movement of the muscles. Thus, the liver is also in charge of muscle performance and endurance. The heart is responsible for the condition of the blood vessels through which blood flows and through which nutrition is distributed throughout the body. It also participates in sweating—the cooling of the body's surface during exercise and the removal of pathogens through sweat from the body. Lung Qi nourishes the skin. It contributes to the excretion of harmful substances from the body, but also to the protection of the muscles beneath it. At the same time, the lungs constantly take in Qi from the air, thanks to which they supply the body with the necessary oxygen, which we need more of during physical activities. Simultaneously, they carry away carbon dioxide to prevent internal poisoning. Thus, all these organs cooperate with us in our physical activities. How our body feels, but also the soul within it, depends on their good condition."

THE ORGAN SYSTEM AS A WELL-FUNCTIONING STATE

In the Western conception of the organ system, each of the organs is a separate unit. It can be removed, implanted, but we do not deal much with what happens in the body after that. Chinese medicine perceives organs from a different perspective. Based on long-term observations of the body, its processes, cycles and tendencies, the Taoists have come to realize that our organ system is naturally designed to function as a well-organized grouping or "government." A government in which each member is responsible for something—from the emperor, through ministers, to ordinary officials. Symbolically minded Taoists have given various organs certain attributes according to what they are in charge of in our body or, poetically speaking, *in our empire*. There is even a hierarchy among them, but here there is no fight for power. On the contrary, everything is based on cooperation.

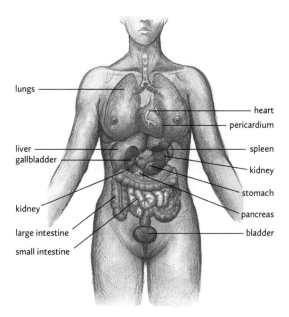

lungs

heart

pericardium

liver
gallbladder

spleen

kidney

kidney

stomach

pancreas

large intestine

bladder

small intestine

Main organs

The heart is the emperor, the ruler of all organs. It is responsible for clear judgment and communication with the world. It is the residence of the psyche and consciousness. *The lungs* are located in close proximity to the heart; thus, they are its chief chancellor, or the supreme dignitary for the rhythmic arrangement of all life processes and the flow of Qi throughout the body. *The spleen* is the source of life for other organs. It must, therefore, be the controller which has oversight of what enters the body through food. The spleen

is also involved in the transformation of food in the body and its transformation into Qi. *The kidneys* are called the *Source of Life*, overseeing the storage of Qi, and are therefore the council responsible for increasing Qi in the body. Their assistant is *the bladder*, which is responsible for the final transformation of fluids. The clean part, in the form of vapor, is left in the body for irrigation, and the unnecessary, turbid part is returned to the Earth. *The liver* is the general of other organs. It is responsible for the overall strategy and planning; it is the origin of the considerations and tactical plans of the entire organ system. *The stomach* is the official responsible for the public food store. *The large intestine* is the chief movement officer in collaboration with the lungs. It is the keeper of the sewers; the things that have been transformed exit through it. *The small intestine* is the court supplier of nutrients to the body. It has the ability to recognize what is essential and what the body must absorb. It takes in, distinguishes and transforms so that it is possible to build blood from the components. *The gallbladder* is a reliable and faithful assistant to the emperor, a kind of clerk for justice and good decision making. It directs and controls our judgment, estimations, discernment and opinions, but also how we pursue them. It controls what decisions we make, gives those decisions vigor and gives energy to our actions. It provides the ability to orientate oneself in situations and to make decisions accordingly.

I am convinced that if we learned to look at the body in this way, our relationship with it would change. Let us look at the uterus, for example. The uterus is considered by Taoists to be the heart of the lower abdomen. The words *heart* and *lower abdomen* immediately bring up associations other than a piece of muscle. Each of us has a beginning in the womb, and at the same time the womb has given us the space to develop. Therefore, the womb holds an important place in our lives. It is like the temple of the entrance of the human soul into the human body, and therefore it is considered to be the heart of the lower abdomen. For Taoists, the lower abdomen is a powerful Qi center, the above-mentioned Lower Dantian. The womb and Lower Dantian are the main storehouses of Qi, and therefore this area is often called *the Sea of Qi*. Thus, the uterus is not just a muscle that can be cut out of a woman's body after the end of her reproductive life. A literal translation of another Chinese character for uterus—*Nuzhibao*—means "woman-child-palace." They therefore call it *the Womb Palace* or *the Children's Palace*, or even *the Heavenly Palace*. Naturally, with the word *palace*, our respect for the womb multiplies and we begin to perceive it differently and thus treat it as such.

Each of these organs is in charge of certain body structures that movers use in their profession and without which they would not be able to do anything physically. These are the bones, joints, tendons, muscles, skin, but also the blood vessels that distribute nutrients via the blood throughout the body. In this way, it is not only what is obviously visible that is involved in the movement of the human body, but also what is in the internal organs that are hidden. It is therefore important for movers to know at least the basic context, because if, for example, they rupture a tendon, then, on the basis of this information, they know how they can contribute to its faster regeneration. It also means that

if we have weaker kidneys, for example, and this was diagnosed also by Western medicine, we will be able to orient ourselves better in our abilities through our knowledge of Qi. We will know that we cannot afford extreme physical exertion and will respect our abilities, instead of trying to do something that neither our constitution nor our condition will allow. We would be hurting ourselves by doing so. We should use our assumptions and possibilities in an adequate way, and thus we may discover something in our possibilities that we would not have discovered during normal use of the body. Thanks to the knowledge of organ contexts that Chinese medicine has observed and works successfully with, we have the opportunity to learn to respect our body and eliminate its excessive wear and tear.

This knowledge also gives us the space to respect the possibilities of others. In schools, for example, we cannot demand the same performance from every student or, worse, humiliate someone for being weaker.

Table 5.1 Organs and body tissues

Kidneys	bones, cartilage, joints, synovial fluid
Liver	tendons, ligaments, fascia
Spleen	muscles
Lungs	skin
Heart	blood vessels

ORGANS—MATERIALIZED QI IN THE BODY

As we already know, Qi travels through the body via a network of meridians. As it passes through the torso, it materializes in the form of single organs. It is a kind of condensation of Qi, or a denser grouping of atoms that form organs out of Qi. In the context of Chinese medicine, the organ is not just anatomical matter. It is a kind of central point that registers not only the needs of the body, its intakes in the form of food, water and air, and consequently the possible expenditures

of Qi for our daily metabolic activities, but also the activities that we consciously do. Qi provides the central point (organ) with information about the condition of the various body parts, tissues and structures which are related to a given meridian and which belong to a given organ. From the organ, Qi is sent to the body and its individual structures and parts to nourish them. The Qi of an organ is thus embodied in its shape, but it is also related to its function and influence on other parts of the body. Modern research has proven that each organ vibrates at different frequencies. And frequencies are ways for an organ to influence other parts and structures of the body that match with them frequently. When people are healthy, their internal organs vibrate at the necessary frequencies, work well and maintain a harmonious relationship with each other. If the activity of one organ is excessive or diminished, the frequency changes and no longer corresponds to the "original plan," and if this condition is not brought back into balance, the result will be disease.

FUNCTIONAL ORGAN CIRCUITS

When talking about an organ in the context of Chinese medicine—for example, when talking about the kidneys—we do not consider only the kidneys themselves, but the *kidney Qi* with the sum of the corresponding body parts and functional relationships that the kidneys are in charge of. Taoist thinking is complex and in an organ system no organ is a separate unit, but part of a whole functional system, a kind of functional circuit. So when we think in terms of Chinese medicine, by *kidneys* and *kidney Qi* we mean *the whole and its functions for the kidneys, bladder, bones, joints, cartilage, teeth, spine, urine, hair, ears, hearing, prenatal essence, ability to reproduce, fear, will to live, inner wisdom*. This means that when it is said that the kidneys are weakened, it is not just the kidneys themselves that are included, but the whole functional circuit. Therefore, it is necessary to focus on the whole sum of functional relationships in the circuit. The kidneys, among other things, are related to fear and hearing. If the problem is in the kidneys themselves, then by understanding the fear we are experiencing and by working to alleviate it, we will help them. If we expose the ears and hearing to excessive cold or noise, the kidneys suffer and lose Qi for their regeneration. Conversely, if we eliminate these influences, we will help the kidneys. We will comprehensively address the functional circuits in the chapters about the individual phases—WATER, WOOD, FIRE, EARTH and METAL.

Table 5.2 Functional organ circuits

Functional circuit of the heart	heart, small intestine, pericardium, Three Burners, blood vessels, circulatory system, tongue, speech, sweat, the Shen Spirit, sleep, emotion of joy
Functional circuit of the kidneys	kidneys, bladder, bones, joints, cartilage, teeth, hair, ears, hearing, urine, thick saliva, the Will-Power Zhi, vitality, wisdom, emotion of fear
Functional circuit of the liver	liver, gallbladder, tendons, ligaments, nails, eyes, eyesight, tears, bile, the Ethereal Soul Hun, emotion of anger, the need to break stagnation
Functional circuit of the lungs	lungs, large intestine, skin, breathing, body hair, nose, sense of smell, mucus, the Corporeal Soul Po, integrity, emotion of sadness
Functional circuit of the spleen	spleen, stomach, pancreas, muscles, mouth, lips, digestion, taste, saliva, the Intellect Yi, emotion of thoughtfulness

Of course, the psyche also belongs to every functional circuit. Every emotion, psychic impulse, or tendency to think is associated with some and functional relationship to which it relates. Chinese medicine has a detailed understanding of the intersection of the emotional world of a person and the state of his or her organs. Conversely, according to Chinese medicine, the condition of organs significantly influences emotional experience. We will get to know the individual aspects of the psyche at the end of this chapter and in full detail in the chapters about the phases. Likewise, the meridian is not only associated with the organ as such. For example, the large intestine takes care of the excretion of digestive residues. On an emotional level, it is associated with loss, separation, the ability to get rid of problems, and so on. If someone does not know how to let go of something on an emotional-mental level, they may start to suffer from constipation. On the other hand, large financial spending can affect the condition of the large intestine. By harmonizing the meridian of the stomach, we can harmonize the stomach itself, but we can also help an unconcentrated person, who needs to be grounded. Or a person who cannot digest the opinions or behavior of another—someone who "is" in one's stomach.

SURFACE AND INTERIOR OF THE BODY

It would seem that we cannot observe the condition of the organs as they are hidden in the depths of the body. However, the Taoists noticed certain specific connections between the interior of the body and its surface. For example, they observed that each sensory organ is connected to a certain internal organ. Even that every orifice (eyes, ears, mouth, nose, etc.) or various parts of the body on the periphery (nails, hair, body hair, etc.) are under the supervision of a certain organ. This means that the condition of these parts of the body can report a certain imbalance in the organ system, and, conversely, the good condition of the internal organs will affect the good condition of these superficial parts. The condition of the kidneys is recognizable by the hair, the condition of the liver by the nails, the heart is shown by the condition of the complexion of the face, the spleen by the color of the lips, and the lungs by the condition of the skin and body hair. They also observed that the ears and hearing are governed by the kidney Qi, the eyes and sight are in the charge of the liver, the tongue and speech belong to the heart, the mouth and taste are under the supervision of the spleen, and the lungs are responsible for the nose and smell. You can see this again in Table 5.2 (Functional organ circuits) or in Table 7.1 (Basic correlations of the Five Transformations of Qi).

Thorough diagnostic conclusions have been developed, according to which various parts of the body can provide us with information about the condition of organs. It is not the aim of this book to address everything, although we will cover many in the following chapters. The most striking signals can be seen quickly; in a conversation with a person, we can see them on his or her face, or on our own face in the mirror. Circles under the eyes indicate kidney fatigue, wrinkles between the eyebrows indicate tension in the liver, the lower lip reports the condition of the colon, the upper lip the condition of the stomach and so on. Even the tone of speech or the intensity of the voice can reveal a lot. The body is simply a map. Master healers know how to orient themselves in this map thoroughly. They know how to read the information needed to make a diagnosis and treatment plan. This map can tell the average person that something is going on and encourage one's own responsibility for it so that he or she can deal with it promptly with an experienced professional.

ZANG-FU/YIN AND YANG IN THE ORGAN WORLD

We will discuss the Yin and Yang theory and the theory of Five Phases thoroughly later. With regard to the organs, however, I will mention here that the basis of Taoist philosophy is the relationship between Yin and Yang, which also divides the organs of the body according to their Yin or Yang nature. *Yin organs*, in the terminology of Chinese medicine called *Zang* organs, are referred to as dense organs. These are the lungs, kidneys, liver, heart, pericardium and spleen—that is, organs with specific tissue, or organs of dense structures. They store substances and, if necessary, they have them available in the form of nutrition. They are in charge of transforming, creating and storing Qi. They are absolutely fundamental to the body, and their weakness often leads to death. They are most often affected by long-term chronic weaknesses, and usually their problems are caused by a lack of Qi (e.g. lack of nutrition, rest, etc.).

Yang organs in the Chinese medicine terminology are called *Fu*. They are the so-called hollow organs. These include the large intestine, bladder, gallbladder, small intestine, stomach and Triple Burner. They are kinds of tubes or pouches through which Qi and substances (urine, bile, blood, food, etc.) flow. This substance is kept in them for a while, it is processed, and then the organs move it further. The content of these organs thus moves and is not stored there for a long time, so Qi is constantly changing in them—sometimes they are full, sometimes they are empty. They play an important role in digestion and excretion. They can be removed from the body without causing death. They are often involved in the early acute stages of the disease, and usually their problems are caused by an excess of Qi (e.g. excess of food or some of its components, excess of physical work, stress, etc.).

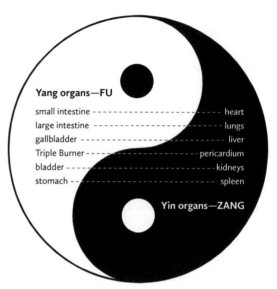

Yin and Yang organs

Two organs, which in the Western context are not considered to be organs, have appeared in the list—the pericardium and the Three Burners. We will deal with them in Chapter 10 on the FIRE phase.

The Yin and Yang organs cooperate with each other within a certain functional relation system. Since Yin and Yang are the basis of balance in everything, the organs also follow the Yin and Yang connection. Each Yin organ forms a pair with a Yang organ. The Yang organ, by its function, helps the Yin organ; thus, it is a kind of assistant to it. The *Yin lungs* cooperate with the *Yang large intestine*; the *Yin spleen* cooperates with the *Yang stomach*; the Yin kidneys cooperate with the *Yang bladder*; the *Yin heart* cooperates with the *Yang small intestine*; and the *Yin liver* cooperates with the *Yang gallbladder*. Some Yin and Yang pairs of organs are also anatomically connected, such as the kidneys (Yin) with the bladder (Yang) or the liver (Yin) with the gallbladder (Yang). Others are connected energetically through internal meridian branches—for example, the heart (Yin) with the small intestine (Yang), the lungs (Yin) with the large intestine (Yang). In the same way, the meridians belonging to the organs are in a close Yin and Yang relationship. We will analyze the relationships between them thoroughly.

ZANG-FU/FIVE PHASES IN THE ORGAN WORLD

In addition to the Yin and Yang connections, the organ pairs mentioned above are also linked to the influence of the seasons and the development of Qi within the seasons. These are the so-called Five Elements—more precisely, the *Five Phases of Qi transformation*, known as WATER, WOOD, FIRE, EARTH, METAL. This division has been developed by long-term observations of the qualities, functions and tendencies of individual organs. The organs are based on the specifics and qualities of the different phases of the year. They have thus become a kind of embodiment of the different seasonal qualities in our body. Each pair of organs is associated with and influenced by one of the phases. The kidneys are associated with the WATER phase (winter), the liver falls under the WOOD phase (spring), the heart belongs to the FIRE phase (summer), the spleen to the EARTH phase (Indian summer), and the lungs are related to the METAL phase (autumn).

Five Phases and organs

However, in the context of the Five Phases, it is not just about the connection to the development of Qi within the seasons. The phases are the embodiment of all the attributes, specific qualities and contexts. Thus, for example, the WOOD phase, which includes the liver and gallbladder, is related to spring. However, it is also the embodiment of the new fresh Qi that represents spring. The new comes from the east, so the east, as the world side, belongs here as well. We use such fresh Qi when we begin any new project or activity. After all, it is also typical for the beginning of a new day, a cycle, a lifetime in which our birth and childhood are involved. It is the spark used by the *Hun* aspect of our psyche to encourage us to constantly learn new things, plan for the future, etc. The liver, which falls under the WOOD phase, is the residence of the Hun aspect and has similar qualities to this sparkly energy. It is also the source of our anger when something stands in our way, which is why the emotion of anger is also associated with the WOOD phase. Spring is also linked to young plants, flexible sprouts, such as tree sprouts, and that flexibility should also be available to our tendons. The tendons fall under the WOOD phase and are controlled and nurtured by the liver.

In this division, however, each phase is cyclically linked to the other phases, and each organ is thus linked to the other organs. The strength of an individual organ lies in the fact that it relates to everything; each organ complements the whole and, in turn, the whole cooperates with each organ. If one organ has a problem, it will affect the others.

In addition to these basic 12 organs, Chinese medicine also works with the concept of *extraordinary organs*. Their peculiarity is that although they are shaped like *Fu* organs—that is, they are hollow and passable—their functions are more in line with the *Zang* organs because they contain some vital substance. Among the extraordinary organs are the brain, the uterus, the marrow, the bones, the blood vessels and the gallbladder. You are not mistaken: we had the gallbladder in the *Fu* group of organs. This is another aspect of Taoist thinking—nothing is absolute; Qi penetrations work everywhere.

ORGAN CLOCK

Most of the metabolic processes in our body take place without our effort. Many of them are tied to the rhythms of nature, and their main trigger is the rotation of the Earth. The rotation of the Earth brings the changes of the seasons, which are the basis for the development of Qi and its subsequent renewal. The basic principle of the Earth's rotation is circulation, rhythm, repetition. Circulation is continuous; it takes place in regular rhythms and it establishes a kind of order. The main means of renewal is alternation—alternation between tension and relaxation, giving and receiving, day and night, activity and rest, Yin and Yang. This organization provides the support that enables all processes to take place harmoniously. Since we are part of life on the Earth, this regularity taking place around us affects the regularity within us. The so-called organ clock also functions on this principle. The organs are regulated by internal mechanisms, but they are also influenced by earthly and cosmic happenings. They are registered and processed by the pituitary gland, the pineal gland and the hypothalamus—a kind of organ chronometer in our brain.

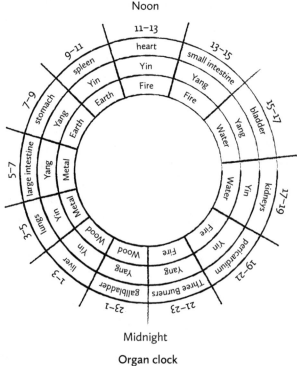

Organ clock

Time: 3 a.m. to 5 a.m.—lungs

Although we are usually fast asleep at this time, there is a deepening of the breath and internal preparation of the body for the day's activity. The lungs are active now so smokers, asthmatics and people with bronchial diseases, colds or respiratory infections usually wake up at this time. The lungs get rid of toxins by coughing.

Time: 5 a.m. to 7 a.m.—large intestine

The start of the day's activity begins with cleansing the body of toxins and metabolic waste in the form of stool. Automatic morning emptying at this time is indicative of good condition of colon and lung Qi and good function of the entire digestive system. People who have problems with excretion should get up no later than 6 a.m. in order to defecate by about 7 a.m. It is advisable to drink a full glass of warm water in the morning; a few drops of lemon juice can be added to eliminate candida from the digestive tract.

Time: 7 a.m. to 9 a.m.—stomach

The stomach is activated and the secretion of digestive juices is increased; now is a good time for a healthy breakfast, because the body is most able to absorb the necessary nutrients. It is ideal to have breakfast by 9 a.m., so that in the next two hours the spleen can process the essences from the food, thus transforming the food into Qi.

Time: 9 a.m. to 11 a.m.—spleen

There is increased production of enzymes intended for digestion, blood purification, red blood cell breakdown and new blood cell formation. Alcohol consumption is not recommended at this time. Excessive physical activity should also be avoided, as this is the time of peak mental capacity. Thus, it is an ideal time for studying or writing a script for a play, etc.

Time: 11 a.m. to 1 p.m.—heart

This is a time of active heart activity when it is not advisable to load the body with large amounts of food. There is a slight energetic slowdown. A walk or short sleep is appropriate. On hot days, we should not expose ourselves to much heat at this time. Drinking coffee at this time is harmful for the heart. Heavy meals should not be consumed either.

Time: 1 p.m. to 3 p.m.—small intestine

This is the time of digestion and absorption of nutrients. After slowing down, physical activity gradually increases. There is a partial reduction in tooth sensitivity, so people who are afraid of dentists should make an appointment for this time.

Time: 3 p.m. to 5 p.m.—bladder

This organ is responsible for the management of water and minerals as well as the elimination of toxins. In the event of bladder problems, it is advisable to drink herbal urological teas at this time. Qi reaches its second peak, activity rises, and it is advisable to engage in sports, yoga, Qigong or dance. The digestive system is able to ingest a hearty meal.

Time: 5 p.m. to 7 p.m.—kidneys

Blood is purified from metabolic products, and liquid wastes are excreted. In the case of kidney problems, it is advisable to drink herbal urological teas at this time. This is also a good time for kidney cleansing treatments. When preparing and consuming dinner, we should avoid what burdens the kidneys, such as white sugar, excessive salt or foods with added chemicals. It is not advisable to drink coffee or alcohol either. If we forgot to drink during the day and only remembered during this two-hour period, it is advised not to overdo it with fluids at this time. It is recommended to reduce stress and slowly start a calm regime in preparation for a good night's sleep.

Time: 7 p.m. to 9 p.m.—pericardium

The body continues to cleanse the blood and lymph; oxygen, minerals and other nutrients are distributed. An energy base is created for the next day. At this time, one is very perceptive, so it is a good time for moderate study, meditation, going to the theater or cinema, etc. It is ideal for the body when we do not consume food after 7 p.m.; our organism would not be able to process it without increased effort before sleep.

Time: 9 p.m. to 11 p.m.—Three Burners

During this period there is a rearrangement of hormonal ratios and information about the thermoregulation of the body. The nervous system needs a calm mode in order to restart its regeneration. The body controls basic life functions in this two-hour period. Either we are already sinking into sleep or we are calmly preparing for it. Therefore, it is not advisable to activate the organism in any way, or to eat or smoke. Watching thrillers before going to bed equally hinders this process.

Time: 11 p.m. to 1 a.m.—gallbladder

In the digestive tract, metabolic and transformation processes take place during sleep at this time. Those with gallbladder problems are usually awake or unable to sleep. It is a time of increased gallbladder attacks. At this time, we should no longer eat anything. Oxygenation of the brain is at its lowest in this two-hour period. Therefore, night driving at this time is dangerous because microsleep can occur. Studying at night has no effect and significantly disrupts the biological clock, which drains a lot of Qi.

Time: 1 a.m. to 3 a.m.—liver

Metabolic, detoxification and transformation processes take place. Attenuation occurs, and the oxygenation of the brain is at its lowest. If we do not sleep at this time, we need to be very careful. If we are at a party that lasts until late at night, it is not advisable to drink alcohol or coffee, smoke or consume fats (e.g. nuts or chips). Normally, we should sleep at this time to give our liver a chance to detoxify. It will not have the opportunity to do so within the following 24 hours.

This inner clock is in line with the outer clock. There is perhaps no need to discuss the main information about this principle—the alternation of activity with relaxation. All common sense suggests that it is natural to be active during the day and to rest at night. Since the invention and introduction of electricity, however, this basic principle has not been easy for people to follow. Cities are lit all night long, and the intensity of electric light allows us to do the same activities at night as we do during the day. We invented night shifts; economically, they seem to us to be advantageous. The existence of TV and computers allows us to stir our mind with various movies and shows at night. Cars are equipped with lights so we can travel and drive at night. It is not easy to resist these possibilities.

The system of an achievement-oriented society forces us to be equally productive whether it is winter or summer. Modern life gives us the opportunity not to respect winter, because some people do not like the cold and darkness that encourage us to slow down and function on a different principle. From the minus temperatures of resting nature, we are able to find ourselves in the tropical temperatures of countries on the other side of the world in just a few hours. When we come back, we may take a long time to recover and struggle with colds or fatigue, but we just wave our hand because we do not see the connection, and the next year we do the same.

Of course, it does not make sense to follow the organ clock strictly. Sometimes even staying up late at a party adds spice to life. Performers commonly perform in theaters late into the night. Nothing terrible happens to us when we have to finish a project and we work on it till late at night because it has to be handed in the next day. However, if the disruption of biorhythms happens frequently and regularly, it will fundamentally affect a person's health. An attuned rhythm is a prerequisite for the harmonious function of the autonomic nervous system. And our physical and mental well-being as well as our professional well-being depend on it.

Related to this topic, people often ask whether they should follow daylight saving time or standard time. The answer is simple. Be more aware of nature and be more in harmony with it. If the change occurs suddenly, it takes about a week to ten days for the body to accept the change and readjust its "program" and its metabolic processes to adapt to the new time. The change from daylight saving time to standard time and vice versa occurs suddenly. We either lose or gain an hour at a time. Since we are not machines, we experience a slight shock, and the body needs time to adjust. It should be noted, however, that a person who lives more connected to the flow of Qi in nature, or who lives in nature and works consciously with its rhythms, a person who perceives how nature naturally changes around us and tunes his or her biorhythm continuously to these natural transformations, adapts beautifully to the change of time several weeks before it "officially" occurs in a given time zone. So when the time change occurs, he or she has actually already realigned. In cities, however, it is harder.

We need about a week or ten days to adapt if we fly to a different time zone. The body has to adapt and start functioning according to the time of a given country. The body has to deal with these adaptations, so if these changes happen too often, it will affect our condition.

> How to help your body with time changes and during jet lag can be found in Chapter 11 dedicated to the EARTH phase.

PSYCHOSPIRITUAL ASPECTS OF ORGANS

We have already mentioned the connection of organs with emotions. However, there is something associated with the psyche other than just emotions. As I see it, the psyche is also linked to inner attunement, to patterns of thinking, to tendencies to adopt certain standpoints, and in our profession, to creativity, perseverance, the ability to finalize projects to their completion, the ability to handle success or failure, and so on. The holistic approach of Chinese medicine says that mental processes, consciousness and thinking mirror the physiological activities of the organs—that the organ is actually a manifestation of the psychospiritual essence, a kind of carrier that stores our psychic predestination. The psyche thus comprises the five aspects which correspond to the five organs, and therefore they govern our mental and spiritual life. Each of these aspects of the soul resides in one of the five vital Yin organs and is responsible for linking its physical component with the psyche. The state of a particular aspect of the soul influences the state of that organ and vice versa.

The heart preserves *the Shen Spirit*—in simple terms, the mind or consciousness, but also our radiance or charisma. It is the consciousness that gives direction to our path, a kind of inner spiritual guide that also helps us to love what we are dedicated to. The lungs preserve *the Corporeal Soul Po*, the so-called *sensitive soul*, or *soul of the body*. It is in charge of the ability to feel through the body, its sensors, and to make use of all that the body has learned so far. It is a kind of preserving and disposing of all the automatisms that the body has acquired and the kinetic experiences that the body has gone through in life. The Corporeal Soul Po plays a huge role in the physicality and movement memory of the mover. But it is also instincts taking care of our survival, a kind of genetic memory of a human being, but also the memory of a particular body in this particular life. The liver preserves the *Ethereal Soul Hun*, the basis of our progress and creativity. The Ethereal Soul Hun is the source of ideas, visions, dreams, inspiration. It is responsible for imagination and creativity, as well as the ability to foresee or see into the future. The spleen preserves the Intellect Yi—the principle of mental processes, a kind of flexible framework that gives structure to our thoughts. The kidneys house *the Will-Power Zhi*—the will, the desire to realize one's goals in life and also to accomplish them.

In the context of a mover's life and work, the quality of each aspect of the soul is of great importance. We can clarify the interaction between them in the following example. Everything we do in life receives its initial impulse. This is given by the Hun, residing in the liver. It is the primal spark, the idea, the inspiration. The Hun presents it to the Shen in the heart to judge whether the idea agrees with our philosophy of life and our mission in life. If it does not, the healthy Shen will reject the idea. If the Shen approves it, it will move it on to an aspect of our intellect—the Yi, residing in the spleen. The Yi will begin to gather all the necessary information to put the idea into action. This is followed by cooperation with the Po, residing in the lungs. The latter will engage all its previous experiences and use them to bring the idea to fruition, helping it to materialize into reality. The Zhi, residing in the kidneys, will give the whole process profound wisdom and strength to face any obstacles, and faith and will to see the idea through to the end.

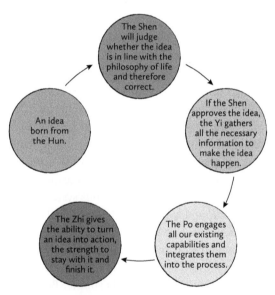

Psychospiritual aspects of the organs

We will deal in detail with the various psychospiritual aspects of the soul in the following chapters. According to the Taoists, the psyche has its basis in the Qi of the five organs and depends on their condition. Each of these aspects of the soul is responsible for linking the physical component with the psyche. Therefore, psychic balance is important for physical health and, conversely, the psyche can greatly affect the health of our organs.

CHAPTER 6

Yin and Yang

How can these two terms help the mover?

陰陽

About: the relativity of opposites / the golden mean / the importance of complementarity / Taijitu symbol / activity vs "involved passivity" / right amount and extremes / the culture of Yang and culture of Yin / Yin and Yang within the human body / the necessity of the crisis

The human being is subject to a flow of constant change and alternation. The in-breath is followed by the out-breath, the systole of the heart is succeeded by the diastole, after the contraction of a muscle, its relaxation occurs, the intake of food and its digestion is followed by its emptying. The cells of the body die and are replaced by new ones, activity during the day is naturally followed by rest at night. Our body is constantly involved in transformations between opposite but interrelated phenomena, which we should not perceive as contradictory, yet as complementary and forming one interrelated whole. Separate inhalation and separate exhalation will not keep us alive, activity without rest would destroy us, and a step with only one foot would get us nowhere if it were not followed by a step with the other foot. One needs the other and vice versa. These transformations of opposite actions and their complementary relationship with each other were defined by the Taoists as Yin and Yang.

This alternation, complementation and influence is also happening outside of humans all around, including the whole universe. On Earth, the cycle of day and night is considered

an example of the interrelationship between Yin and Yang. Day is considered Yang, night Yin. The transition between the two is a process of Qi development in which as one increases, the other decreases. Yin and Yang are not in an unchanging relationship, but they are constantly evolving and alternating dynamically with each other.

On the basis of this principle of constant transformation and their perception as a whole, the human organism also has the capacity for natural regeneration. If the body becomes ill because we have stepped too far out of our balance, it seeks for ways to heal itself. Then it does so naturally, without the help of medications. However, we often make it difficult for it by our actions, because we do not listen to it; we tend to ignore what the body is telling us and expose it to extremes. Serious illness or injury is already the consequence of such a long-term approach. We do not have to get into such a state as long as we learn to listen to and respect our own body, its needs and the environment it is in. If movers feel that they are already going beyond their limits during training or rehearsal, they should also look for space to recover sufficiently and to rest, so as not to hurt themselves. It is necessary to stop and perceive what is happening to the body and what would be appropriate to do for it.

For example, we feel knee pain. We can ignore it or we can be attentive to it. By observing the pain signal in this way, we can understand what is causing it, discover the cause and do something to eliminate or at least alleviate it. In this way, we have the opportunity to learn something new about the knee, to correct its use, to heal it and thus to ensure its longer and healthier use. However, we can choose the other path—the path of ignoring the pain. For a moment, we seem to rise above the problem, numb the pain with medication and continue to use the knee. This can take us all the way to surgery, and from there it is a longer return to our profession.

The Taoist concept of Yin and Yang can be very helpful in such cases. It teaches us a sense of balance and ratio. In this case, physical work is the Yang principle and rest is the Yin principle. After the activity (Yang), the body needs to rest (Yin); it needs the attention and care of its "owner." Observation and attention is the Yin principle in this case; doing—action—is the Yang principle. Only in this way can balance occur. In the case of ignoring pain, however, there is no room for the Yin principle, and after Yang activity comes Yang again—disproportionate activity, which in turn leads to greater activity. There is an obvious overreaching, which can result in weakening and, in the worst case, injury. This extreme Yang is naturally followed by extreme Yin—extended rest periods where recovery takes longer. Ignorance is simply something that has little to do with a sense of balance. The concept of Yin and Yang teaches us to avoid extremes before they occur and cause problems, and thus to enjoy active movement for a long time.

All of us, to some extent, naturally and subconsciously work with the principles of Yin and Yang, even though we have not named it as such and we are not aware of it. If we eat something very salty (Yang), we feel like having a sweet dessert (Yin) afterwards or washing it down with more liquids (Yin). If the room is cold (Yin), we heat it (Yang), or start dancing, jumping or moving around in other ways—we start to create warmth by moving (Yang).

AN ANCIENT CONCEPT

The concept of Yin and Yang is the foundation of Taoist philosophy, and throughout history other philosophies and concepts of ancient China have been influenced by it. It arose from the empirical observation of nature and the changes in it and the perception of the world and phenomena as a whole. An important insight of this observation is the fact that everything in the universe is in a state of constant change. All things in nature, and therefore in our life, are made up of the existence of oppositional forces, where their interconnectedness and complementarity play an important role.

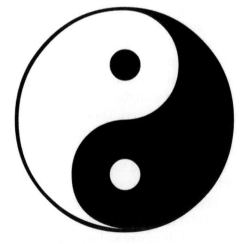

Taijitu symbol

We can perceive Yin and Yang everywhere. Through the interaction between Yin and Yang, we can constantly transform, evolve and live. Understanding Yin and Yang can help us see life as a constantly changing continuum in which everything has its place, its purpose and its time for realization. It can help us to understand the changes within us, which we then do not resist. Changes in our productivity and creativity, changes in the body, changes in society or in the conditions in which we live. It helps us even to understand economic or relationship crises. The concept of Yin and Yang unity has become the basis for the martial arts, Qigong and Taijiquan, and the art of Feng-shui. In Chinese medicine, it is a helping hand in both diagnosis and treatment.

"EITHER/OR" VERSUS "ONE AND THE OTHER"

The symbol associated with Yin and Yang that you see in the image above is the Taijitu symbol. Although there are only black and white, it is not a black-and-white view. Our life and everything that happens in it is not black and white, although it may seem that way. It contains a wide range of colors and possibilities, ranging from one end of the spectrum to the other. Life is about constant transformation and harmonization; life is a continuous evolution where nothing is actually stable.

Unlike European dualistic philosophy, where black is black and white is white, and there is a fixed and unchanging dividing line between them, the contradictory nature of the concepts of Yin and Yang lies in their complementarity and mutual dependence. The Chinese characters for Yin and Yang that you see in the picture contain a mountain within them. The mountain represents existence as such, illustrating a particular symbol, but also the environment with which one is confronted on a daily basis. While one side of the mountain is in light, the other is necessarily in shadow. The Yin is the shadowed, mysterious side of the mountain. The Yang is the dazzling, bright, shining side of the mountain. Yet these states are not final or unchanging. The side of the mountain that was sunlit in the morning will be in shadow in the afternoon, and vice versa. Light and shadow are constantly alternating, and yet they are never separated from each other. Thus, nothing can be definitively Yin or Yang. They contain within themselves the seed of the opposite: Yin changes into Yang, Yang changes into Yin. It is constant transformation and complementation; it is the dynamics of life. Yin and Yang are part of everything, and every movement, every change takes place between them. This is life.

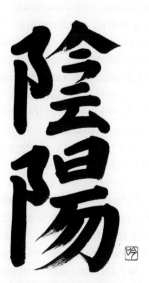

Chinese characters for Yin and Yang

For Yin and Yang, as for many Chinese expressions, there is no adequate expression in Western language to capture the essence. In the white part, we see the seed of the black and vice versa. Yin and Yang are thus not definitions, but rather states and methods of expressing the change, the process, the development between them. When one decreases, the other increases; when one increases, the other decreases. Nothing can last forever—neither joy nor worry, neither success nor failure, neither health nor sickness. Everything that appears to us as "bad" can ultimately bring about a positive, and vice versa—something that we a priori consider "good" may not always be a real win. There are no absolutes, no final state.

Now let us look at the Taijitu symbol in more detail. What does it tell us?

The *circle* symbolizes wholeness and boundlessness. There are no ends or edges, so it can also represent the Qi, which is in everything and has no beginning or end. Although Yin and Yang are two entities, together they are within the circle and so together they form one whole. Together they express the phases of changes of Qi in this whole.

The *dividing line* is not a straight line but is formed by a curve. This evokes constant movement, evolution and dynamism, rather than something static, unchanging. At the same time, that curve indicates the progression of growth and decline, the constant passing of the Yin principle into the Yang principle and vice versa. It is the principle that when something is increasing, the other is inevitably decreasing, that nothing can be permanent.

The *seed of the opposite* can be seen in a small dot located in the field of the opposite color. This indicates that everything contains within itself the seed of the opposite. This small detail foretells that interconnectedness and interweaving that we call complementarity. Even though the parts in the picture appear to us as opposites, together they are the essence of unity. They fit together like a puzzle, where one piece of the puzzle makes no sense without the other. At the same time, the seed of the opposite tells us that everything taken to the extreme turns into the opposite. For example, in the practice of everyday life, it is the fever that is generated from the cold we expose ourselves to. In extreme cold, there was the seed of heat.

The repeating cycle of day and night is considered to be the clearest indicator of the interrelationship between Yin and Yang. However, if the day (Yang) did not contain within itself the seed of night (Yin), the night could not really come. The maximum Yang energy of the day is at noon. By mid-afternoon, the Yin—the darkness that we do not even feel yet—is already pushing in. The Yin darkness, however, is slowly but surely working its way to realization—by evening, we can already feel and see its power, and by the time it gets dark, it is already in full command. Yet in the darkness, in the night, in the Yin, sleeps the little seed of day, light and Yang. It begins to manifest slowly at the time when we are still asleep and it is dark everywhere, but as soon as dawn breaks, the work of Yang coming to the surface finally begins to become fully visible. It is the same with the transformations of Qi qualities in the cycle of the year, with the maximum Yin occurring at the winter solstice (around December 21) and the maximum Yang at the summer solstice (around June 21). Everything in-between is transition; there is the increase of one and the decrease of the other. Without summer, there could be no winter. Without darkness, there could not be day. All that is in-between is a transformation, a process, an infinitely changing Qi.

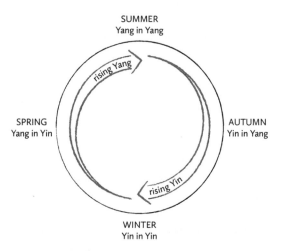

Development of Yin and Yang

WHAT IS YIN AND WHAT IS YANG?

Although Yin and Yang together form a whole, this couple also serves to help us sort and classify all space–time phenomena. Therefore, let us look at the demonstration of a few basic distinctions and put them side by side for greater clarity and understanding of their interconnectedness. Let us now look at this table with the basic examples of Yin and Yang and try not to see these qualities as separate from each other, but combined into a whole.

The list could go on and on. However, it is not necessary; with a little reflection and feeling, we are able to recognize for ourselves what is Yin and what is Yang, how they are related and how they complement each other. And most importantly, we are not concerned with categorizing and separating, but with understanding the inter-relationships between them. It is by no means about sorting into the boxes of "positive or con-structive" and on the one hand and "negative or destructive" on the other. For example, if a sunny day, which we consider to be a wonderful time, were to last uninterruptedly, we would soon die of thirst and hunger. Thus, the concept of Yin and Yang does not show the opposites of things or phenomena, but the interaction between them and the action of these forces.

I will explain the relativity of our Western approach of the opposite with the example of dialogue, a process in which one speaks and the other listens. Yang here represents the active component—the expression of the word, the projection of the thoughts of the one who is speaking. Yin represents passivity—listening. Listening, however, is not an absolute passivity. If it were total passivity, the dialogue would not work. It is a passivity in which the processing of what comes to us takes place. According to our narrowed view, the opposite of activity is pas-sivity. Passivity with everything we can imagine. Yin, however, means something else. We can only understand it when we relate it to Yang.

Table 6.1 Yin and Yang

Yin	Yang
Darkness	Light
Night	Day
Cold	Heat
Winter, autumn	Spring, summer
Water	Fire
Earth	Sky
Moon	Sun
Passivity	Activity
Rest	Action
Stability	Mobility
Slow	Fast
Contraction	Expansion
Inside	Outside
Receive	Give
Female	Male
Female egg	Male sperm
Subconsciousness	Consciousness
Philosophy	Science
Spirituality	Science
Upwards	Downwards
Mass	Energy
Intuitive approach	Rational approach
Plants	Animals
Mental activity	Physical activity
West, north	East, south
Process	Result
Space	Time
Spectator	Performer
Silence, perception of the performance	Spectators' applause
Reprises of the performance	Performance creation and premiere

We could say that listening is passivity because the listener does not put activity into the speech and the expression. However, his or her Yin in listening is another form of activity—the kind of activity that is directed inward. One might call it "involved passivity." And that is important, as long as we do not let what we receive dissolve and we really want to listen, not just hear. Life, then, depends on the interaction of interrelated phenomena, which we have called Yin and Yang. This principle is clearly applied in dance—for example, in contact improvisation and in partnering. In a pair, one dancer leads the movement and the other participatively "listens" and follows. If one did not listen and follow, the connection would be broken, and if both were leading, the dance would turn into a kind of fight.

THERE ARE NO ABSOLUTES

The initial division we see in the table is relatively generalizable. Everything can be further subdivided into the smallest nuances. If we are not referring to some unchangeable shape or object, but to some phenomenon, activity or event, it cannot be exclusively Yin or Yang. Everything, even Yin and Yang itself, always includes both of these principles. The seed of the opposite in the Taijitu symbol indicates it. For example, heat can be mild (more Yin) or hot (more Yang), cold can be mild (more Yang) or icy (more Yin).

Even if Yin is connected with the feminine principle, it does not mean that it will automatically be a quality associated only with women and that men should not use it. Every person, whether female or male, works with both qualities. Just as Yang is connected with masculine qualities, it cannot be associated exclusively with men. Life situations, lifestyles, habits, ways of doing things, or linguistic expression bring one of these two qualities to the fore in every person. A woman is inherently Yin, but she can be more Yang or more Yin. Conversely, a man, who is inherently Yang, may be more Yang or Yin. These shades are influenced by many circumstances of a person's nature, upbringing and body constitution, as well as the condition of each person. But urgent circumstances in life, as well as situations in our profession, sometimes force us to behave differently than we are normally accustomed to—to do something in a more Yin way and sometimes in a more Yang way. For example, if a woman who is of a more Yin, softer, weaker nature happens to think that someone wants to threaten her child, she will engage her Yang, in which she finds tremendous strength and hardness, to protect it. Without this Yang, she might lose the child. Conversely, a man who is of a more active Yang nature, and who achieves whatever he wants, as a result, must sometimes calm his Yang, because he might begin to destroy himself with it. In order to harmonize with the situation, he needs to act with more Yin.

Yang is the engine to make things happen, but some things in life cannot happen and cannot be achieved without the Yin quality. Life is about constant transformation and harmonization; it is a continuous evolution that requires us to be able to adapt.

Therefore, the division of the concepts of Yin and Yang that we see in the table must always be taken in the context of the whole and in the context of some particular situation. We see, for example, that plants are Yin and animals are Yang. This is because animals are more active in using movement in their search for food. At first glance, plants do not seem to use much apparent movement in their search for food. This, however, is only a general division. When we look at it more specifically, we find that certain plants have much more active Yang in them than certain animals. Some plants grow at a tremendous speed or, with the help of the wind, can move very quickly compared to some animals. Conversely, there are some very slow and lazy animals that seem to have not even a pinch of Yang Qi in them. Thus, the terms Yin and Yang in no way serve to describe any patterns of behavior.

SINUSOID RATE AND THE GOLDEN MEAN

The idea of harmony seen in the Taijitu symbol can, through the eyes of a Westerner, be seen as an ideal where black and white and even the shapes are in a 50:50 ratio. However, this does not correspond to the reality. It is not possible to permanently achieve complete balance. Life is dynamic; it brings different situations, surprises, challenges. And even if we strive for perfect harmony, it will rather lead us to blockage, because it is striving for something that is inherently impossible. There is no such thing as complete stability; nothing in our life is inherently stable. What was true yesterday may not be true today, what we were convinced of in our youth may not work for us in our old age; our principles should be updated depending on specific life situations. And that is okay—everything is constantly evolving. Getting out of balance is natural and even sometimes beneficial to the dynamics of life. However, the rate must always be kept in mind. We should know how far we are moving away from the center and whether we are able to bear it—for the further we move away from the center, the more time and energy it takes to come back to the center. I will give a concrete example from the practice of the mover. We all know that the mover's body needs regular training, and any long break is not good for the body. Taking a break is certainly good for the body, but the longer the break is, the harder it is to get back into the previous condition. The length of the break is adequately matched by the length of the return into this condition.

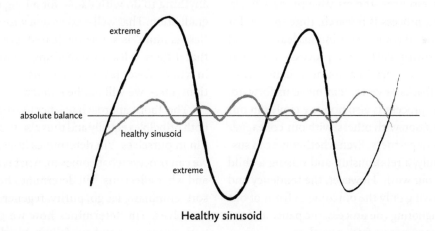

Healthy sinusoid

The term *staying in the center* cannot be understood as immobility. It expresses a degree of oscillation around the center, a measure of our awareness of our distance from it. Thus, the *golden mean* applies here, and the theory of Yin and Yang is actually a teaching about finding paths to the center. So that slight undulating sinusoid on the journey through life is what we are actually looking for. The knee example I gave at the beginning of this chapter is a very prosaic example of moving away from the center. Another example is the Western world, which is far too Yang-oriented. It focuses primarily on outward-looking abilities. What is valued above all is speed, purposefulness, immediate results, and then there is nothing left to do but to put a certain amount of aggression into everything. This approach can also be important in some situations, but it will not be enough for a good and healthy result. Some things naturally evolve slowly; they cannot be sped up. Sometimes it is better to let them develop at their own pace, to let them happen naturally. Accepting things also bears fruit. It is the other side of the coin, the Yin aspect. We consider resting or just being, as wasted time. We consider stopping, contemplating, thinking, meditating as something unproductive. Eastern thought is more process-oriented. A process that results in an outcome. Western cultures often tend to speed up the process, or even skip the process, because we desire the result. We often feel a kind of delay when we have to dedicate our time to something. We want everything right away, quickly, well, efficiently. We lack the cultivation of Yin; we do not even have a developed sense of being able to perceive that we need Yin.

CULTURE OF YANG AND CULTURE OF YIN

Creating performances quickly and presenting them at as many festivals as possible is the measure of a successful creator. Often a piece of art is created just because it has to be done, because there is funding for it, because it is expected and for many other similar reasons. And the time for the creation tends to be desperately short. We forget the essence—the creative process itself. Part of that process is research, time to look for the new and, of course, continuous learning and internal growth. Part of the process—thus part of the Yin—is a certain amount of pause, evaluation, setbacks or crises that move us forward. Part of the process is also how we evolve in our communication with others, with our colleagues and with our partners. Even whether we can sustain a family, a relationship and raising a child alongside our work. However, the tendency and habit of having only the outcome in front of our eyes, and ignoring the process, the pause and the crisis, disconnects us from ourselves.

Unfortunately, we start learning all this in elementary school and then it goes on from there. Studying is often about the quantum of information. Students are in a loop where they just take in more and more information, with no opportunity to process it and therefore reinforce it within themselves. They do not have the opportunity to apply it in practice, or to sort out what they will retain and develop, and what they will let go of. The result of such study, for example, in dance schools, is physical injuries, but also psychological injuries. I often encounter the fact that many students do not want to have anything to do with dance for a long time after graduation. That well-known and wise statement "less is more" is somehow feared. We are afraid that if there is less of something—fewer courses in school, fewer results or awards, fewer productions, etc.—we will not be enough.

The Taoist approach teaches us to strengthen both principles equally and thus also to strengthen Yin in ourselves. Yin determines how effectively we can process what comes in, what is around us and what affects us. Yin determines how we can sort, eliminate, let go, purify, regenerate within ourselves. Yin determines how we can digest both our success and our failure. Yin determines whether we can perceive progress or stagnation in ourselves. Yin determines how we can benefit from all that we do and all that we learn. Yin is the substrate in which the plant of our life takes root and receives nourishment through it. Yang is the watering of the plant. We are taught to just water all the time. We water, we water until we overflow, and we do not care in what condition the soil we grow in is from all that watering. And, as we know, when we overwater a plant, the roots paradoxically dry out and the plant dies.

YIN AND YANG AND THE HUMAN BODY

Taoists regard the human body as a microcosm of the Universe, claiming that human nature is also governed by the ever-changing opposing forces of Yin and Yang. Within the body, there are endless processes of alternation, waves of ebb and flow, use and renewal, or the many manifestations of cyclicity.

Our body has received a basic dose of Yin and Yang from our parents. Our mother gave us some of her Yin energy, and our father gave us some of his Yang energy. But humans are a balanced combination of Yin and Yang also in terms of the action of Earth and Heaven upon them. Heaven's Yang Qi descends to the Earth, and humans receive it continuously through the crown of their heads, a point called *One Hundred Meetings*, (in Chinese, *Bahui*, GV20). The Yin Qi of the Earth ascends from the Earth's core and projects outward to the surface. One receives it through the feet with every step or posture. In the middle of the feet are points called Gushing springs (in Chinese, *Yongquan*, KI1). Through them, we are able to connect to the Earth Qi whenever it is needed—for example, when we need to ground ourselves in various stressful life situations, or when we need to push into something, maintain balance, etc. When we dance, we connect to the floor through these points and their cooperation with the center of gravity in the Lower Dantian area, grounding ourselves to create stability in posture or movement. This keeps our feet stable and makes us feel confident in them: the floor is a strong support, we are able to connect our center of gravity to the ground and we can draw strength into the jumps. This helps us—for example, in contact improvisation or in partnering—to transform the weight of our partner into the Earth, instead of holding it in our body with the muscles. This would unnecessarily exhaust us, so by grounding we save our energy.

The activity of each organ also follows a certain ebb-and-flow principle—each organ has a time when it can work to its full potential, but it also needs time to rest and regenerate. It is simply as the aforementioned Taoist philosopher Zhuang Zhi aptly put it: "Life is a harmonious blend of Yin and Yang."

Let us now look at the Yin and Yang context concerning the human body. The information in Table 6.2 cannot be taken as absolute, however. Everything depends on the circumstances, the context or the overall perspective, so we will discuss some parts of the table in the commentary below.

Table 6.2 Yin and Yang and the human body

Yin	Yang
Lower body (from navel down)	Upper body (from navel up)
Organ	Organ function
Organ	Meridian
Meridians	Collaterals
Meridians through which Qi ascends—meridians of the heart, lungs, spleen, kidneys, liver and pericardium	Meridians through which Qi descends—meridians of the small intestine, large intestine, stomach, bladder, gallbladder and the Three Burners
Zang organs—organs with dense tissue: heart, lungs, spleen, kidneys, liver, pericardium	Fu organs—hollow organs through which matter and Qi move: small intestine, large intestine, stomach, bladder, gallbladder
The material basis of the body, the tissues	The transformative power of the body to reorganize and regenerate

Yin	Yang
Soft body parts	Hard body parts
Front part of the body (soft, internal)	Back part of the body (harder, external)
What needs to be protected (that which is inside and is softer and weaker)	What is capable of protecting (that which is on the surface and is harder and stronger)
Bones, muscles, tendons, fascia (they are inside)	Skin (it is on the surface)
Muscles (they are softer)	Bones (they are harder)
Bones (they are denser)	Muscles (they are less dense compared to bones and more on the surface)
Inside	Surface
Hidden	Visible
Medial (inner) sides and parts of the body	Lateral (external) sides and parts of the body
Torso	Limbs
Lower limbs, legs	Upper limbs, arms
Inner, softer sides of limbs	Outer, rougher sides of limbs
Mass of the body	Qi
Blood	Qi
The food we take in	Metabolic activity to process food
Flexibility	Firmness (to stiffness)
Weakness	Strength
Pregnancy	Birth

For a better understanding, it is also important to understand the context and other possibilities of Yin and Yang distinction.

The lower parts of the body, those closer to the Earth Yin Qi, are Yin. The Yin meridians are those that go upward, through the body, bringing out the Yin of the Earth Qi to Heaven. Conversely, the Yang meridians move downward, letting the Yang Qi of Heaven descend to Earth through the body. In the context of protecting the body from danger, the back of the torso is Yang. It can protect what is within. If something

were to fall on us, or an animal were to jump on us, we would naturally curl up into a ball, creating a kind of protective Yang armor with the back of our body.

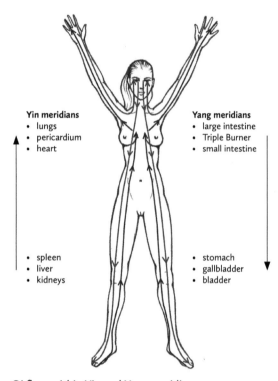

Yin meridians
• lungs
• pericardium
• heart

Yang meridians
• large intestine
• Triple Burner
• small intestine

• spleen
• liver
• kidneys

• stomach
• gallbladder
• bladder

Qi flow within Yin and Yang meridians

The front part of the torso is softer, more delicate, so it is Yin—it is hidden in the middle, inside, protected by Yang when we are curled up. So what is inside is Yin; what is outside is Yang. Thus, in the table we see the meridians divided into Yin and Yang. As such, however, we see the meridians simultaneously in the Yin column (fourth row from the top), but also in the Yang column (third row from the top). How is this possible? Here again, we have to take in consideration the whole context within which the division into Yin and Yang takes place. In the context of the organs, the meridians are Yang. Compared to the organs, there is more Yang activity in them, and they are located more on the surface, whereas the organs are at greater depth. Compared to the collaterals, however, the meridians are Yin because the collaterals—the tiny connecting branches between the meridians—are more on the surface than the meridians themselves.

The mass of the body is denser compared to Qi; it is slower and therefore Yin. At the same time, mass is able to store substances, which is also a Yin quality. Yin mass is dependent on the Yang of Qi because Qi is what sets mass in motion and also provides its functions. Conversely, Qi needs mass to make its action visible. As we have read, Qi also has a strong connection to blood, which is Yin, the more material component of the two. Qi thus appears twice in the table because its connection is more complex.

All the organs are inside the body. They are thus of Yin quality compared to the surface of the body and the meridians. However, according to their qualities and functional capabilities, we can divide them into Yin or Yang. The Yang organs are those in which movement is going on almost continuously. They are the hollow organs—that is, the various tubes such as the intestines and pouches like the bladder, stomach and gallbladder, where some matter is suspended for a while, where it is processed and moved on. So there is more movement, faster activity and also Qi. In the terminology of Chinese medicine, we call them *Fu* organs. On the other hand, organs that contain more mass—that is, a certain given tissue structure—are more designed for the storage of substances than for movement and transformation. And even if there is some movement going on in them, it is not as significant as in the hollow organs. These are the Yin organs, the so-called dense organs—the heart, lungs, kidneys, liver and spleen. In Chinese medicine terminology, we call them the *Zang* organs. Yin and Yang, however, are never absolute, but relative. The heart, for example, is clearly a Yin organ as described. Its pulsating contractions, however, carry within them a Yang quality. Here, Yang is found in Yin.

Every organ has some mass (Yin) and, of course, it also has some function (Yang). The function of an organ is Yang compared to its mass. The function of an organ is an important and inalienable part of the organ. Here, too, Yin and Yang create the whole. However, the organ is also connected to a meridian. A meridian functions as a kind of extended arm of the organ and its function. It connects the organ with other parts of the body and other organs, as well as with the surface of the body. Therefore, the meridian is Yang. In the context of the organ-meridian relationship, the organ has a Yin quality and the meridian has a Yang quality.

This multiple differentiation contains such elaborate details that we are left in awe of the fantastic matrix that governs the body. And especially how the Yin and Yang within it work beautifully together and take care of each other. We have stated that the front of the body is Yin and the back is Yang. If we were to "zoom in" on the lower limbs, for example, in terms of the structure, shape and functionality of the joints, we would notice that the back of the lower limbs is more of a Yin quality. The "architecture" of human joints is made up of two basic sides. When we bend the leg at the knee to 90 degrees, we notice that a kind of valley is formed at the back of the knee in flexion. That is a Yin shape. On this side of the knee joint, the skin is also of a softer Yin texture; this whole area is softer, and there is a condensation of Qi, or Yin. Conversely, on the other side of the knee, in front, the patella bone comes to the surface, pushes out and shows its sharpness. The skin is naturally rougher on that side of the knee, and there is an expansion of Qi into space. Thus, this side of the joint is Yang, and the projection of this side of the joint into space is also of a Yang quality. And if we want to push through something—that is, to exert Yang—we naturally involve this Yang side of the joint, which is sharper, firmer and harder.

When the knee is bent, its anterior Yang part is extended forward—that is, outwards. When the back of the knee joint contracts, it is softer, more vulnerable, receiving Qi inward. It is Yin in nature, and for better balance, the Yin principle needs to be developed on this side. So this zoom-in on the area of the knee joint has shown us how each part of our body can be divided into Yin and Yang sides and how they can work together in a complementary relationship to create balance in this way. I should point out, however, that not all parts are so obvious.

In connection with body protection, it has been written that the front of the body is Yin and the back is Yang. This is true, but only from this point of view. If we look at the body in relation to its more active and more passive sides, we realize that the front side of the body is more Yang. There we have the mouth with which we speak, the eyes with which we constantly register something; we perform all actions with our hands in front of the body, and usually we walk forward. So from that point of view, the front of the body is more Yang than the rear of the body. In the same way, from the perspective of light and darkness (seen and unseen), looking at the person in front of us, the front would be more Yang in nature compared to the back, which is not visible. The back of the body of this person would correspond to a more Yin quality from this point of view. So it is important to know the context and complementary relationship into which we are putting the world of Yin and Yang, and at the same time remembering that the two principles are not static in their complementarity, but constantly changing—where Yin increases and Yang decreases and vice versa. In the same way, every single part of the body, according to this point of view, can be once Yin and then Yang.

WHAT IS THIS DIVISION FOR?

It may sound too philosophical and theoretical, but I know from my own experience how the use of the principle of Yin and Yang helps in everyday practical ways in terms of the technical development of the mover and performer, as well as in creative work. In addition to the fact that the use of Yin and Yang principles leads us to respect the body's natural dispositions and possibilities of movement, it also develops much more detailed work in movement and spatial articulation or in the physio-dynamics of body movement. In Qigong, Taijiquan and other martial arts, this knowledge is used to cultivate inner strength and its use. We can now apply this knowledge to dance practice, contact improvisation or partnering. Yin yoga, for example, also works with the Yin and Yang principle.

The Yin parts and surfaces of the body have different potential movement possibilities compared to the Yang parts. Viewing the body through this concept, I often see when observing dancers how some use the opposite activity of the different parts of the body when moving. This way, there is more tension in the body, blockages of Qi, loss of balance and thus loss of energy and excess exhaustion. They work inefficiently with Qi because they impede its natural flow. When movers can use their body properly according to the principles of Yin and Yang, they can use Qi more efficiently in their performance.

In the context of Yin and Yang thinking about Qi, we can divide work with Qi into two basic complementary principles—*condensation* and *absorption* on one side and *expansion* and *projection* on the other side. Thus, the Qi in our body can either condense and absorb or it can work the other way around—expand and project. Condensing is Yin—it is about the inward direction, into the body; expanding is Yang—it happens in the opposite direction, out of the body and into space. We can relate these two qualities to the Yin and Yang surfaces of the body. The absorption and condensation of Qi takes place on the Yin surfaces of body parts. Here the body receives the Qi and lets it flow downward into the Lower Dantian (in the area of the center of gravity) and further into the Earth. On the Yang surfaces, projection and expansion take place. Through them, the Qi is projected into space, transmitted and expanded from the inside out. With such a conscious merging of Yin and Yang, we can feel how much Qi needs to be absorbed and how much needs to be expanded at any given moment. The body also somehow becomes better organized by this. A naturally correct alignment is created between the different body parts, and thus the body can use the structure that has been "designed" by evolution to the maximum extent. Movement becomes more pure and correct, and at the same time, through the body aligned in this way, Qi can flow continuously through the body while moving, but also generate additional Qi for the next impulse to movement. These principles are worked with, for example, in Qigong, Taijiquan and other martial arts, where, among other things, the control of the possibilities of the Yin and Yang surfaces and body parts is exceedingly effective.

These principles can also be used in terms of the correct use of the joints of the body. As mentioned, the joints have a Yin side and a Yang side. The Yin side is the inner one where the bending occurs; the Yang side is the outer one where the bone protrudes into space. If we use the Yang principle for the Yin side of the joint when moving, the joint will become overloaded and Qi can get blocked in it. An example might be a standing position where the mover stands on maximally stretched legs, pushing the knees back, so the kneecaps are unhealthily pushed into the joints for the sake of the stretched legs. The mover thus expands the Yin (inner, back) side of the knees, creating an unhealthy "X" shape of the legs, which is further deepened by this position. It means that the front side of the knees is being used in a completely opposite, ineffective way. This results in a blockage of Qi, weakening of the joint, weakening of stability and, of course, the gradual destruction of this joint. And this is, of course, undesirable. Conversely, when the Yin and Yang sides of the joints are properly engaged and working together, the Qi begins to flow through the joint, bringing the joint into its correct position. In addition, this flow of Qi nourishes the joint and a more effective cooperation between the physical and energetic levels of the body is created.

THE NECESSITY OF THE CRISIS

Understanding the principle of the nature of Yin and Yang transformations helps me personally to cope with difficult times in my life. Periods when I have a downturn and I am unable to work and create as productively as I am used to, or periods when my work is not as appreciated as I expected. Understanding Yin and Yang also makes it easier for me to cope with crises. Crisis is the opposite of a time when we are thriving, when we are in the spotlight or when we are loved. It is part of the Yin and Yang whole, and if, out of ignorance of its necessity, we accuse ourselves of failure, or try tooth and nail to remain in a state of well-being, or in a state of infinite creativity, we are hurting ourselves.

I admit that it is difficult nowadays. Today we do not even know what the natural flow of things is anymore. For example, in winter, when nature is restful and peaceful in the northern hemisphere, we buy fresh strawberries, spring onions or melons in the shops. We have no problem turning winter into summer within a few hours by flying to the other side of the planet because we do not want to respect the changes in nature and we have decided that winter does not suit us. We always want to have it our own way. I believe this is also due to the fact that we are taught to separate the "good" from the "bad," and the risk of black-and-white vision easily sets in. If we are able to see the crisis as part of the whole, we will realize that there is no such thing as "good" or "bad." There is only our ability to see both parts as part of the whole.

In the life of a mover, this is not easy to achieve either, because our work is constantly confronted with the outside world, with the opinions of the many people among whom we live, with whom we collaborate or in front of whom we present our work. We all need to share what we are. The problem, however, begins to appear when we try to make the results and success of our work come as quickly as possible and, most importantly, when we strive for permanent success. And when our ideas do not materialize, we get frustrated. Because we are used to looking more at what is going on around us, we are quick to be influenced by the opinions of others, forgetting what is going on within us. And we come under the pressure of circumstances. We are pressured by festivals, competitions, critics and colleagues. We are pressured to some extent by everyone we allow. But most of all we pressure ourselves.

Let us not be afraid of the moment when we feel that certain things are no longer going our way. Let us not be afraid to stop, to look ourselves honestly in the eye and admit to ourselves the tiredness and the emptiness and let it all out. Let us not force ourselves to be constantly productive and always in the spotlight at all costs. Let us know that it is in crisis that the beginning of our new strength and new breath is born. Only then can we do something that resonates with our inner self.

YIN AND YANG TRANSFORMATIONS OF THE NEEDS OF BODY AND MIND

Understanding the principles of Yin and Yang still helps me personally to cope with the transformations of the body's needs and the transformations of the body's capabilities. As we will read in the next chapter, Qi evolves throughout the year in the cycle of the seasons. Just as nature undergoes different stages of development and processes of transformation in each season, the human body also undergoes such transformations. To ask the body as well as the mind to be always equally productive is nonsense. If we try to do so, we suffer. We will deal with these needs in detail in the individual chapters on the Five Phases.

Health is also a matter of the harmonious connection of the body with the psyche. The body with its mass is the opposite of the subtle material psyche. Together they form a whole where one depends on the other. The state of one affects the state of the other. Our lifelong task is to learn to harmoniously reconcile our silent, inner, compact processes with our expansive action in the outer world. If we were only at home, thinking and planning, we would be disconnected from the world, and we would hardly carry out our plans. Conversely, if we acted only in the outer world, we would not be able to hear our inner wisdom and could not carefully plan our actions.

The constant striving for balance is one of the main principles of the cosmic law of Yin and Yang. Taoist philosophy does not force us to do anything, it does not teach us how to do things right, how to achieve the right rate between Yin and Yang. Taoist philosophy only encourages us to observe what happens naturally. To notice what naturally causes the alternation between Yin and Yang, what naturally creates the balance of life. It calls us not to contradict it, but to follow it.

CHAPTER 7

Five Phases of Transformation

Five Phases of development and cyclicality

About: development of Qi / cyclicality / relationships between the phases of Qi / the flow of Qi between the phases / the Creation Cycle and the Controlling Cycle / applying this principle in the creative process / table of basic correlations

I am fortunate to live and work in close proximity to nature and be able to observe the cyclical changes that take place in it. These are the transformations of the quality of Qi during the seasons—that is, the transformations of the Five Phases that we all more or less perceive. When one understands them, tunes in to and learns to respect them, one can make beneficial use of their typical qualities in one's life. For several years, I have been running year-round seminars for dance, Qigong or Shiatsu students called *Five Phases of Transformation*. We meet in each season and, in working together, we perceive the quality of each season and the changes that those seasons bring about—changes around us, but also in our own body, in our emotions or in the amount of Qi we have. We learn to listen to our body's needs, which are different in every season (every phase), and then apply this refined perception to our lives. In acupuncture, for example, different points are used in each season, Chinese dietetics adapts what we have on our plate to what the weather conditions are in that season and to what ingredients are naturally available in that season. This is actually the basis of prevention, so in this way we learn to avoid illness and also accidents.

The Yin and Yang transformations...of the seasons are the beginning and the end of all things and are the essence of life and death. Therefore to disturb them is to harm oneself; to live in accordance with them is to prevent the onset of serious illness. This is called understanding the right way, understanding the Tao. The wise man walks on that path, the foolish man turns his back on it.

THE YELLOW EMPEROR'S CLASSIC OF MEDICINE

YIN AND YANG IN A BROADER CONTEXT

According to the Taoist view of life, Qi is constantly evolving, but at the same time it repeats itself in cycles. This is the basis of its transformation but also its renewal. What rests in its depths in winter can manifest on the surface in spring, gaining strength that reaches its peak in mid-summer. During the late summer, the Qi gradually decreases and calms down, so that in the autumn it can sink back to the depths, where it finally rests in the stillness of winter. This cycle repeats itself every year, but it can also be seen in shorter or longer periods in different areas of our lives. If we take the day as an example, the morning is energetically similar to the fresh activity of spring, midday to the active summer, the afternoon is characterized by the descent of Qi, and then dusk and night are logically similar to the Qi of autumn and winter. The Taoists, who expressed themselves using images, related these seasons to the natural phenomena that characterize them. These are the phases of WATER, WOOD, FIRE, EARTH and METAL.

We are talking about the *Wuxing* theory, which is often mistranslated as "Five Elements" based on a narrow viewpoint. *Wu* does mean "five," but *Xing* cannot be translated as "an element." Rather, it is more accurately described as "to move, to transform." Therefore, a more apt name is the *Five Phases of Transformation*, or, in short, *Five Phases*. These phases are actually names for Qi in its various stages of transformation. Like the theory of Yin and Yang, the theory of the Five Phases of Transformation is based on the observation of natural cycles and the classification according to the interrelationship of the various phenomena.

The theory of the Five Phases is actually an extended model of the theory of Yin and Yang. It is a more subtle method of analyzing the individual phases of the transformation of Qi from Yin to Yang and, vice versa, from Yang to Yin. Examples are winter and summer. Winter is obviously dominated by Yin, summer by Yang. However, winter does not occur by nature turning on a switch when suddenly summer becomes winter. Winter comes gradually, evolving slowly. It starts as early as the FIRE phase—that is, in summer, when the Yin is quite minimal. It slowly builds up until it is really noticeable in autumn, and then it reaches its peak in winter. Conversely, Yang

weakens in late summer, it is felt very little in autumn, and it is at a minimum in winter. In fact, the theory of the Five Phases helps us to understand Yin and Yang itself to a greater extent.

WATER, WOOD, FIRE, EARTH and METAL were named by the Taoists not because nothing else occurred to them but because these phases behave similarly to the real natural phenomena of water, wood, fire, earth and metal. However, our translation is limited because the Western language works differently from Chinese. The word WOOD, for example, is a very imprecise expression. The WOOD phase works with the idea of the Qi of a living tree that is constantly growing into the sky, flexible but also solid. So it is not just any wood, such as a dead log for the fireplace.

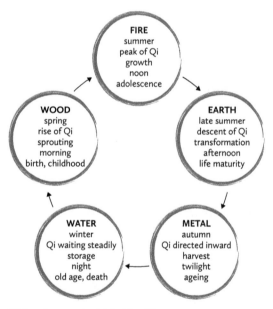

Qi development within Five Phases

The WOOD phase is characterized by expansive, upward energy. It is associated with the east, spring and wind; it is the time of sprouting, the beginning of growth, and it is therefore associated with birth and childhood in human development. Expansion in the sense of gaining a great deal of knowledge and experience is typical of the WOOD phase.

The FIRE phase is characterized by Qi radiating in all directions, a tremendous culmination of activity. It is associated with the south, summer and heat; it is the time of flowering and the beginning of maturation. Adolescence and, typically, liberation from one's parents, independence and the realization of everything learned in childhood are associated with it in the development of a person.

The EARTH phase is characterized by stabilizing and harmonizing Qi, gradually descending downward. It is associated with the center, late summer and humidity; it is a period of ripening and fruiting. Within human development, maturity and a time for grounding, stability, gentle quieting and more mature thinking and action are associated with it.

The METAL phase is characterized by a firming Qi, one that points inward. It is associated with the west, autumn and drought; it is a period of harvesting and processing, but it is also a period of withering. In the development of a human, therefore, it is associated with the beginning of ageing typical for going more inward, reviewing life and working more economically with one's Qi and its reserves.

The WATER phase is characterized by descending Qi and Qi calmly and steadily waiting; it is associated with north, cold, chill, passing away (death) or going into a latent state. Therefore, ageing and death (transformation into another state) are associated with it in human development; typical of them is the completion of the process and the use of acquired wisdom for a new cycle.

A CYCLE APPLICABLE IN ANY PROCESS

The Five Phases form a cycle in which each phase emerges from the previous one and is a prerequisite for the next one. Just as spring brings summer, summer ends with late summer, to be gradually transformed into autumn. The whole thing is brought to a close by winter, which is, in essence, a precondition for spring to begin.

Although it is a theory, it is richly applicable in every area of life— in work, in personal development, in the evolution of our relationships and, of course, in the art and practice of the mover. I will illustrate this by using the example of the creation of a piece of theater work. Choreographers or directors get an impulse, an idea, that they would like to create a work. The idea can come either from an inner impulse or from the outside; it does not matter. It is like a seed that begins to sprout inside them. The idea excites them, stirs them up, and the ascending WOOD Qi causes them to harness all the forces within and to begin to realize the first ideas. They reach out to co-creators and performers to "birth" the idea to the early stages of preparation. The FIRE in this

process is the subsequent intensive preparation of the performance—working with the actors, dancers, composer, designer, etc., an immensely expanding creative period when everyone is "burning" with the fire of creativity. This is followed by the premiere—the culmination of this period, but also the beginning of the calming of the overall energy of the process. This is typical of the EARTH phase. After the premiere, those involved may not rehearse as intensely, although time to maintain the quality of the performance obviously remains. Everyone is already enjoying a kind of "harvesting" of the fruits of their work; the show is being repeated, and it is making a profit, both material and immaterial—mental and spiritual profits such as appreciation, inner satisfaction, etc. This is followed by the Qi of the METAL phase—that is, the moving into oneself, which includes appreciation. The performance continues to present itself, the "harvest is gathered," and the creators state what worked and what did not work in it. They re-evaluate, they consider, so that they can benefit from this knowledge in the future. After a certain period of time, the performance has a final performance. When its mission is complete, the show "goes away" to make room for the birth of a new one. This is the WATER phase.

Every single thing we create or are a part of has such a process. The consistency in this process is evident in everything. Some of its individual phases may last longer, others will be shorter, they may be more or less intense, but they definitely follow one another in this order; one "gives birth" to the next—it is its prerequisite and its foundation. And this does not exclude the fact that the creation of different projects or activities by the same creator may overlap. The next project may emerge while the overall development of the Five Phases for the first project is still in progress.

We will discuss the specification of each phase in more detail in the following chapters.

RELATIONSHIPS BETWEEN PHASES

The theory of the Five Phases is constructed as a complete system. None of its parts can be removed from the whole, so if we want to look at an individual part of this system, we must look at it through the eyes of the whole. Even in life, it is not possible to separate the adulthood of an individual from her or his birth or ageing. It is crucial to understand each phase with all its connections and aspects, but it is also important to understand each phase in terms of the whole. The influence of the phases on each other has a given direction.

Let us look at the chart of the *Creation Cycle* or the *Generating Sequence* (creation, support), called *Sheng* in Chinese. We can see in it that the previous phase gives life to the next one. The cycle develops in a clockwise direction. In the terminology of Chinese medicine, this relationship is called *mother–child*, where the phase that nourishes the next one is the "mother" and the phase that follows is the "child." If the "mother" is well and nourishes her "child" sufficiently, "the child" can also flourish and enrich the whole. Thus, in full strength, "the child" becomes the "mother" nourishing the next "child"—the following phase.

In nature, wood supports or gives birth to fire by being a material for it. Fire supports the earth, the soil, by giving nourishment to the earth with its ashes. The earth gives birth to metal by creating in its depths the conditions for the formation and growth of minerals. Metal supports water by dissolving in it and providing the minerals for the water to subsequently give birth to and support wood. Wood needs water for its growth; without it, it could not exist. And we are at the beginning of a new cycle.

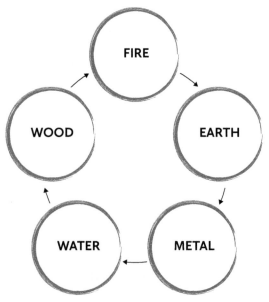

The Creation Cycle (*Sheng*)
WOOD supports fire by being a material for it.
FIRE supports the earth by giving nourishment to it with its ashes.
The EARTH supports metal by creating conditions for the formation and growth of minerals.
METAL supports water by dissolving in it and providing the minerals for the water.
WATER is needed for the growth of wood.

This means that in both the theory and the practice of the Five Phases, we do not see any phase in isolation from the others, but we consider them as joint forces and processes that energize and nourish the whole organism. The names of the phases describe movements, directions and functions, and are not strictly limited to their material aspect. They have been formulated to clarify the relationships between each other. The phases determine each other energetically. If one of them is weakened, the next one is weakened too. For the harmonious state of the whole, the Creation Cycle must function. However, sometimes it may happen that the "child" exceeds its "mother," that one of the Five Phases overflows and develops in excessive proportions. It can also damage the whole. In practice, we can think of this as excessive fear, for example. Fear is certainly important as a defense system, but if it grows to extreme or uncontrollable proportions, it is no longer beneficial for the person concerned. Instead of fear creating natural barriers and warning of potential danger, it begins to restrict the person and tie one's hands. This changes the quality of one's life. In this case, one has to intervene and, in terms of the relationships between the phases, begin to tame this "overgrown child." For these cases, we use the *Destruction Cycle* or the *Controlling Sequence* (in Chinese, *Ke*).

WOOD is controlled by METAL—excessive growth of a plant or tree (WOOD) is cut with a knife (METAL); METAL is tamed by FIRE—metal in the shape of a dangerous knife can be turned into jewelry by heating and remelting (FIRE); FIRE is tamed by WATER—here the example from life is quite clear: we extinguish fire with water; WATER is controlled by EARTH—waterways in nature need stable and solid channels to keep them from spilling out of their earthly banks; finally, EARTH is controlled by WOOD by the fact that the roots of plants and trees (WOOD) hold the earth together and thus prevent erosion. In our terminology,

we also call this relationship the mother-in-law–bride relationship.

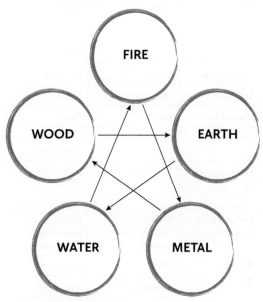

The Controlling Cycle (*Ke*)
WOOD *is controlled by metal by cutting an excessive growth of plants.*
FIRE *is tamed by water by extinguishing fire with water.*
EARTH *is controlled by wood by holding the earth with roots.*
METAL *is tamed by fire by heating and remelting.*
WATER *is controlled by earth by keeping the water channels from spilling out.*

The theory of the Five Phases contains two fundamental aspects. The flow of Qi between phases according to well-defined circles and sequences has been discussed so far. The second aspect is the fact that it groups things or phenomena with similar qualities of Qi into correlations with each other. To understand this information, it is useful to delve into the following table. We will discuss all the features and phenomena in detail in the following chapters, but the overall picture can be seen just in Table 7.1 on the next page. I remind you that the words in these should be taken with a grain of salt and with a certain amount of flexibility, because nothing is ever quite as definitive as our concepts would suggest.

Table 7.1 Basic correlations of the Five Transformations of Qi

Element	Wood	Fire	Earth	Metal	Water
Yin organ	Liver	Heart/pericardium	Spleen	Lungs	Kidneys
Yang organ	Gallbladder	Small intestine/Three Burners	Stomach	Large intestine	Urinary bladder
Year season	Spring	Summer	Late summer	Autumn	Winter
Day time	Morning	Noon	Afternoon	Twilight	Night
Direction	East	South	Center	West	North
Life cycle	Birth, childhood	Growth, adolescence	Life maturity	Appreciation of life, ageing	Old age, rest, death
Evolution of Qi	Rise of Qi	Peak of Qi	Descent of Qi	Qi directed inward from the outside	Qi waiting steadily
Growth cycle in nature	Sprouting, beginning of growth	Growth, flowering, ripening	Transformation, maturity, fruit	Harvest	Storage
Climate	Wind	Heat	Dampness	Dryness	Cold
Color	Green/blue	Red	Yellow/orange	White	Black/dark
Taste	Sour	Bitter	Sweet	Pungent	Salty
Sound	Screaming	Laughing	Singing	Weeping, crying	Groaning
Smell	Rancid	Scorched	Fragrant, sweet	Rotten	Putrid
Tissue	Tendons and ligaments	Blood vessels	Soft tissue, flesh, muscles	Skin	Bones, marrow, teeth
Body fluid	Tears	Blood, sweat	Saliva	Mucus	Urine, thick saliva
Indicator	Nails	Complexion	Lips	Body hair	Hair
Sense organ	Eyes	Tongue	Mouth	Nose, skin	Ears
Sense	Sight	Speech	Taste	Smell, touch	Hearing
Emotion	Anger	Joy	Pensiveness	Sadness, grief	Fear
Psychospiritual aspect	Hun	Shen	Yi	Po	Zhi

Our body is not a machine; it is a natural part of this process and development, and is naturally connected to the phases. In each phase, different organs of the body are more active or, on the other hand, more vulnerable, and so are the different structures of the body that are nourished by these organs. We obviously use individual structures such as bones, tendons, muscles, blood vessels and cartilage in our active life and profession, and we perceive in our own body whether they are fine or have problems. The problems are usually reported to us in the form of pain. We can feel in ourselves that, for example, in winter we do not want to move much; the body would rather rest and draw in strength. On the other hand, in the summer we need very little to awaken us to physical performance; we warm up our bodies faster, easier, and even the mind is more flexible.

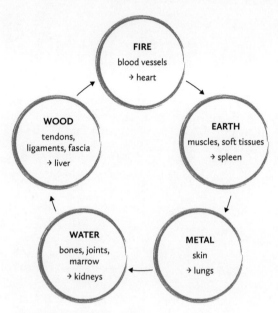

Five Phases and body tissues

Each of the phases has an effect on the manifestation of certain diseases. Some are stronger at certain times of the year, but at other times they lose their intensity. And if we can orientate ourselves in these interconnections, we can avoid these illnesses. There is, of course, also psychology involved. Each phase gives its Qi the prerequisite for the manifestation of a mood, mental activity or state of mind. Each of the phases differently affects our ability to be passionate about something, to pursue something, to persist in something, to have enough enthusiasm for something or even to let something just affect us. Thus, the phases affect not only our physical performance but also our creativity, perseverance and ability to overcome obstacles and difficulties that we experience in any area of life—for example, in the creative process, or in finding sponsors, or filling out grant applications. It is also important to realize that one phase influences the other. For example, if we do not give ourselves enough rest in the winter—the WATER phase—we will not have enough strength for the next WOOD phase, which comes in the spring and begins a new cycle of Qi, and we will suffer from spring fatigue.

So let us start diving deeper, reading the next chapters.

CHAPTER 8

The WATER phase

The human body in winter time

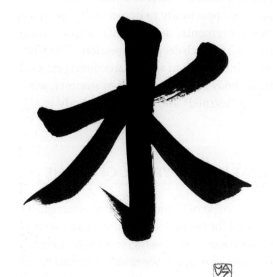

About: the prenatal source of Qi / bones, joints, cartilage and spine / fear / will-power / kidneys and urinary bladder / cold / depth, silence and rest / the Gate of Life / moxibustion / diet for winter and for the WATER phase organs

The three winter months are called "conservation and storage." Rivers are frozen and the earth cracks because of the cold. People should not disturb the Yang Qi. They should go to bed early and get up late, just like the rising and setting of the sun. Let the mind rest in peace as if you have a secret you don't want to divulge. It is also pleasant, as if someone told you a secret. Avoid the cold and keep warm. Don't let your skin perspire, otherwise the stored Yang Qi will be disturbed. This is why you must store Qi in winter. If you transgress this, you will harm your kidney Qi. You will suffer from flaccid paralysis in spring and your ability to suit spring will be weakened.

THE YELLOW EMPEROR'S CLASSIC OF MEDICINE

Chinese character for WATER

WHAT SHOULD A MOVER DO DURING THIS PERIOD?

Tune in to the energy of winter and relax. It does not mean switching off and stopping moving completely, but working less and more sensitively, avoiding exhausting the body in extreme performances, planning fewer performances and less mentally and physically demanding work.

Winter is an excellent time to immerse yourself inwards, both mentally and physically. Every year, winter is a time of death and rebirth at the same time. The mover should therefore also slow down, immerse oneself inward and draw strength in.

During my many years of teaching at various European dance schools, I have clearly observed changes in the needs and capabilities of students' bodies. In winter, they were slow and tired; during the morning training, their bodies and minds were still asleep, performances were weaker, and if the students or teachers pushed themselves to extremes, the result was rapid exhaustion and frequent injuries. On the other hand, if we changed the structure of the lessons by incorporating improvisation and conscious observation of their moving body, which penetrates more deeply, the results in the quality of movement were more visible. This process was, of course, slower, but it led to an understanding of the body, bringing students to a deeper understanding of the body's logic and needs. Winter is a time when movers have the opportunity to immerse themselves in their movements; during other seasons, there isn't time for such deep introspection. The results of this introspection appear later during states of higher body activity in spring or summer, when such a "learned" and "deepened" body is able to execute a better, clearer and more sensitive movement action.

Within the set structure of schools, it would probably be difficult to create a curriculum that would respect the energetic changes of the seasons and the related demands, possibilities and needs of the body, and to adapt teaching this in a truly comprehensive form. During winter, one small change could be to start with practical training at least an hour later and to finish school earlier. The number of performances could be lower and the "saved" time could be devoted to body awareness, anatomy, anatomy in movement and similar methods. I believe that if this happened, everyone would benefit—students, their bodies and achievements, teachers and their bodies and achievements.

My husband and I are both dance teachers and choreographers. Since we are freelancers, we can afford the so-called winter sleep. This means that we can take a break at least in January. We plan neither teaching nor demanding travel; we spend more time at home, practice Qigong and Neigong, and do some study of our own.

WHAT IS THE TYPICAL QI OF THE WATER PHASE?

In the context of Chinese medicine, water quality is typical for the period of winter. The energy of winter is slow, free-flowing, seemingly static and in a state of waiting. We notice it in nature—in the fields and mountains, the energy of trees and in the behavior of animals. In winter, night reigns, the daylight dims, temperatures keep falling; it seems as if the whole world has stopped moving. People who live in nature spend little time outside. There is nothing to sow, nothing to take care of in the garden, nothing to collect; no one even wants to leave the house. Animals also behave in this way in nature. And we make excuses such as "I am a human and I live in a city; it is not possible here. What will I gain by following nature?" Yes, in today's hyperactive, over-technological world of cities, such "hibernation" seems strange and unthinkable. We don't have the means to alleviate fatigue, because we have to go to work and we are forced to think that we are supposed to be as productive as in the spring or summer. We have the possibility to completely erase winter from the natural order of things by being able to fly to tropical countries on holiday in the winter months and return from them to the winter environment. Before Christmas, we operate at full speed, because we buy gifts, fill refrigerators, hand in year-end worksheets, play pre-holiday performances, etc. In winter, everything around is relaxing, but humans continue to make money, create and sweat... It's definitely possible, but then it is no surprise that we feel tired in the spring. According to Taoist philosophy, by doing this, we reach into our energy reserves.

If movers become aware of joint problems only through the pain, if their spine constantly hurts and they have to drink two to three coffees a day in order to function, and if they have problems waking up in the winter unless they take a hot shower, this might be a sign that there is something wrong. Bones, joints, having enough energy—basically, everything on which our profession depends—is related to the energy of the WATER phase. The organs in charge of all of this are the kidneys. Without exaggeration, I am stating that the kidneys are our foundation. Let's take a look at them.

KIDNEYS AS A PRECIOUS ROYAL TREASURY

Usually, people associate the kidneys with pain related to kidney stones, or they are able to imagine two organs somewhere in their back. At school, we learned something about how they filter blood, creating urine that we excrete from the body as a waste product. We also know that humans can live with only one kidney. However, few people associate our kidneys with something on which our lives stand and fall.

According to Chinese medicine, the kidneys are in charge of our "root," our beginning, without which there would be nothing. They preserve the power we received from our parents and in fact from all the generations of our ancestors. The kidneys are like a precious royal treasury, in which are hidden the most exquisite treasures that the "royal" family has stored, for generations. The quality of kidney Qi determines the amount of our life energy, how we perform, our talent and intelligence, our predisposition to diseases and ability to cope with them. Kidney Qi naturally determines the length and quality of our life, the joy of it, trust in it and the desire to live it. It is also in charge of our ability to pass it all on—that is, the ability to bear children and thus pass these treasures on to future generations.

This is what is called *Prenatal Qi* discussed in Chapter 3. Prenatal Qi resides in the kidneys. We have enough of it at birth, but unfortunately it is not renewable. As we go through our lives and the way we live our lives, we spend it. We can preserve it through Qigong or Taijiquan; only masters of these arts can restore it.

> **Functional circuit of the kidneys:** kidneys, bladder, bones, joints, cartilage, teeth, hair, ears, hearing, urine, thick saliva, the Will-Power Zhi, vitality, wisdom, emotion of fear.

WHAT EXHAUSTS THE QI OF THE KIDNEYS?

First and foremost, these are the daily metabolic activities of our body—digestion, natural nocturnal detoxification, cell regeneration, hormonal and sexual activity—and also thinking. However, if our body only used Qi for these actions, while living in a clean environment, we would live 120 years in good health. Taoists who consciously worked with their Qi lived to such an age. However, our way of life contributes greatly to its decline.

We rob our own treasury through several activities characteristic of humans. We live against the rhythm of nature, which includes staying up late, working night shifts, frequent traveling through time zones, and also frequent traveling without additional rest. We movers exhaust our kidneys with our profession itself, but mainly with its excessive demands and rhythm between work and rest. After all, our profession is sometimes similar to an endurance sport. The kidneys are also exhausted by disrespecting natural energy changes in nature, of which we are a part, by acting at the same pace in every season. From the point of view of Chinese medicine, it is illogical and unnatural to work in winter with as much effort as in spring or summer.

We destroy the kidneys with our fondness for extremes—excessive exhaustion of the body, extremely demanding physical and mental work, excessive sex, excessive fasting, diets, constant travel, frequent diving, movement at high altitudes, adrenaline and endurance sports, and exposure to excessive weather. The kidneys suffer from a permanent lack of sleep, which is the basis of their regeneration. They are depleted by a large number of pregnancies and abortions, and in the case of men, by a large number of ejaculations.

We can imagine the kidneys as batteries— more precisely, properly charged batteries. We received the Qi in them at our conception, when it was given to us as a gift. The way in which we spend it and the speed at which we spend it depend on our way of life. The kidneys are essentially full of Qi, but we often use it without renewing it, until it runs out. When the Qi runs out, it is no longer possible to "restart." In humans, such a condition is called burnout and ultimately death. While people are young, they function very well on this Qi, and they do not notice much loss of it, because the source is still quite plentiful. And even if they notice it, they can quickly overcome it and cover it with other activities. Few people consciously care for their kidneys; we do not realize the limit, volatility and fragility in their paradoxically enormous power.

COLD

Cold is typical for the WATER phase. When it is cold, all life processes are quiet and slowed down. Not everyone likes the cold. However, the positive side of this is that it forces us to fully rest in order not to exhaust our bodies and to conserve our warmth. We need the cold, but when we expose our body to it excessively, it harms our kidneys very much and deprives them of strength.

Cold can enter the body in various ways. The kidney meridian originates in the feet and rises up the lower limbs, and in the trunk it enters the kidneys. Walking barefoot on a cold floor causes the cold to get in very quickly via this meridian— through the feet directly into the kidneys—and this depletes and destroys them. The kidneys also do not tolerate the cold that enters them directly when a person walks in a short T-shirt with an exposed back in the area of the kidneys. The kidneys suffer when we drink chilled drinks in winter (but also in summer), when we do not cover our ears with a hat in winter because of our hairstyle or because we do not look good in the hat. The ears are connected to the kidneys, and our hearing itself depends very much on the kidney Qi. It is no coincidence that the ears resemble the kidneys in shape. Therefore, Chinese medicine advises us to cover the ears from wind and cold in winter. Cold can be stored in the body for many years and can turn into a chronic issue. It weakens the system, and the consequences can be constantly cold hands, feet, lower abdomen or buttocks. Some menstrual cramps are also very often caused by cold in the lower abdomen.

Hypothermia of the body causes stagnation in all areas of the body—on a physical and mental level. Hypothermia disables the activity of the kidneys and their ability to distribute heat throughout the body and to nourish the organs. The whole organism suffers, and its processes cannot be performed in full—from digestion through the locomotor (musculoskeletal) system to sexuality. Pain caused by cold is dull and deep-seated, and often arises completely unnecessarily, from our lack of awareness. In my therapeutic practice, we solved many chronic pains with dancers and athletes just by expelling the cold stored for years by the method of moxibustion. Moxibustion—heating acupuncture points and meridians—will be discussed later.

However, as movers, we often work on a cold floor, on which we rehearse all day and often barefoot. These are critical situations for the kidneys, in which they must fight and pump heat into the system from the rest of the body. We all can tell stories about the cold on an unheated stage during rehearsals, about working in a draft, about the unpleasant feeling when we have to stay in our cold sweaty training clothes for a long time. This coldness can then be felt even in the bones. No wonder that after such actions, movers easily get a cold or their knees, hips, lower back or the kidneys themselves start to hurt. And we feel more tired, because the cold consumes heat and therefore it also consumes Qi. The warmth in our body is actually Qi. Thus, the work of movers in a cold environment obviously requires more of their Qi. So, in addition to the energy invested in the work, these conditions also ask for energy to warm the body and to protect it from the cold.

However, the kidney area should not be overheated before entering a cold environment. The heat expands the pores of the skin, which acts as a kind of door from the surface to the inside. When the pores open wide due to heat, they stay open to the cold and wind. These weather factors can thus quickly and with no obstruction penetrate the body and weaken it. After a good workout, when the whole body is hot, we need to be careful, especially in winter, to cool our bodies a little before we return to the cold environment. Even a hot shower just before we are exposed to cold weather is not advisable. Therefore, it is necessary to finish such a shower with cold water to close the pores again, or allow the body to cool down a bit inside after the shower.

> The following tips may be a good way to eliminate the effects of cold:
>
> - For a rehearsal or training, use shoes which are conducive to our work but can also keep the kidneys warm.
> - Carry extra training clothes, especially underwear, and in a situation where you would have to stay in wet clothes for a longer time, change to dry and warm clothes instead.
> - Carry hot boiled water or hot tea in a thermos. Avoid drinking green tea in winter, because it cools.
> - Chinese medicine also does not recommend consuming milk and dairy products in the winter, because they cool, or citrus fruits for the same reason. Instead, we can find vitamins in root vegetables, fermented vegetables (pickles), parsley, broccoli, sea buckthorn juice, etc.
> - After a long time spent on the cold floor, it is advisable to warm the feet by soaking them in hot salt water when we return back home.
> - A "bath" in salt itself has a stronger effect: heat 2 kg of coarse sea salt either in a pan or in an oven and pour hot into a foot bath. When the salt cools down slightly, put your feet in it, cover the foot bath with a towel or a blanket until it radiates heat.
> - An excellent way to warm and energize Qi in the body is by practicing Qigong.
> - It is advisable to learn the basic techniques of moxibustion.

THE DEPTH OF WATER

In the autumn, everything moves inwards in order to be preserved and guarded during the winter. A wonderful example is a tree that loses its leaves from the surface because its Qi plunges into the deep structures of its body to find strength in resting. The same thing happens with the Qi of other living beings, including humans. A person's pulse is more difficult to feel in winter than in summer, because the Qi is deeper, and it takes some time for it to reach the surface. For this reason, it is easy to understand why it is more necessary to warm up in the winter. Qi needs time to "wake up" and emerge from the depths of our body to the surface. If we do it violently and quickly, we are subsequently more exhausted because we have reached into the deepest areas of our system.

From a psychological point of view, this depth is related to our deepest need—the will to live. The psychospiritual aspect, which is related to the will and resides in the kidneys themselves, is called the Zhi. The Zhi is responsible for our will to live, for the ability to enjoy life to the fullest, with or without obstacles. It helps us to accomplish all our plans and to turn our visions into a reality. It helps us to do whatever we aim for. We may have a lot of great ideas, but we need something that will help us bring them to completion. In a deeper sense, it is a force that helps us stand firm and trust the flow of life. It is the inner wisdom we have. And we really need that in our profession.

The kidneys, as the house of the will, are also a source of creativity and ingenuity, courage, artfulness, foresight, penetration and self-fulfillment. Lack of will in the kidneys leads to fear, lack of self-confidence and fear of the power of others. On the other hand, "hyperactive will" brings inner unrest, leading to workaholism which can result in exhaustion and "burnout."

In the mental sphere, there is another aspect that affects the WATER phase in us. The water itself does not have a shape, but it adapts perfectly to the situation in which it is inserted. In addition, it can overrun any boundaries and overflow any structure—it soaks, overflows, floods, etc. There is no obstacle to prevent water from moving. A person with good-quality WATER phase Qi is adaptable, able to "pour" into another, "flow into the sea," connect with the infinite, bring things to an end. Such a person is able to be devoted and attentive in conversation and really listen. Good kidney Qi is also associated with fluent, flexible and adaptable thinking. Strong kidneys are needed for self-confidence, high self-esteem, and the ability to realize goals and dreams. The imbalance of Qi in the kidneys is manifested by timidity, fear, hopelessness and even paranoia.

FEAR IS AN EMOTION ASSOCIATED WITH THE WATER PHASE

Fear is important in our lives. A certain amount of it can prevent us from becoming involved in life-threatening situations. However, excessive, exaggerated and frequent fear creates chaos in the flow of Qi in the body and weakens the kidneys. It also weakens their ability to protect our source. Fear, in its essence, has a connection with a reasonable usage of our reserves. When the water runs out, fear comes. Fear of death. Water is a guarantee of our survival and thus of our future. When it is missing or lacking, we feel the impending fatal consequences. The power of survival works in the form of the previously mentioned Prenatal Qi. We must always protect these innate reserves of ours; we must save them so that we can go far on our journey, and so that our journey may be full of enriching adventures and experiences. When we artificially dope with caffeine, tobacco, soft drugs, or other stimulants out of the need to go beyond our limits, or out of fear of losing strength, we have the misleading impression that we can go further and faster. This euphoric delusion results in drawing on our precious reserves and can completely obscure the real needs of the body. This usually leads to total exhaustion of the body. The feeling of exhaustion comes later at a younger age, because the young organism has enough internal reserves. The catch, however, is that after such a usage of the strength in youth, the organism registers exhaustion in old age after only little effort.

Fear is a state in which one feels scared of things and situations. This fearfulness can be on a conscious and unconscious level. Many movers live in latent but also quite obvious existential fear, because subconsciously we are worried that something might happen to our body, or if we will always have enough energy, enough work and an adequate salary. We also feel the ticking of the clock, so we want to do a lot at a relatively young age, and thus we harm ourselves many times unnecessarily. The ever-present fear that nests in our subconscious is also related to the fact that it is more difficult for movers to start families and have children, and even if we do, due to certain irregularities in the rhythm of our life, it is sometimes very difficult on all family members. So the fact that we exert the kidneys physically as well as mentally gives us clear information that the kidneys need to be cared for—literally, pampered. The kidneys love rest, as well as the joy of life and the zeal for what we do. Therefore, it destroys them when we work without joy or just for money. It is important that we care about the degree of joy in what we do. Last but not least, the kidneys suffer from disharmonious interpersonal relationships. They are energized by gentleness, tenderness, generosity and the will to live and let others live. Let's take care of them on all levels; in return, they will help us to devote ourselves to our profession for longer.

WHAT ARE THE KIDNEYS IN CHARGE OF IN THE BODY OF THE MOVER?

According to the philosophy of Chinese medicine, in addition to the role of blood filtration, separation of unused substances and impurities, and the storage of Qi, the kidneys are in charge of the most important constructional "movement tools"—bones, joints, cartilage and the spine. The kidneys use Qi to build their structure, nourish them and determine their strength and ability to regenerate. They are in charge of the so-called mineral economy of the body, so these body structures receive their nutrition precisely thanks to the kidneys and the circulation of nourishing blood and their Qi throughout the body through a network of energy pathways—meridians. As a result of the weakening of the kidneys, the bones lose their strength, joints lose their permeability and flexibility, the cartilage loses its compactness and protection ability, and the spine loses its elasticity, flexibility and supportive ability. Typical signs of kidney exhaustion are sore joints, especially knees and hips, osteoporosis, various bone deformities and growths, and lumbar spine pain. Mainly, the large joints belong to the kidneys. These stiffen due to the degeneration of the flexible cartilaginous layer that covers the bone parts of the joints to prevent excessive friction. About 70 percent of the body consists of water, which is also the basis of the fluids that lubricate the joints, allow us to move and, through this movement, connect us with the environment. Water is also part of the spine.

OUR HARDWARE IN THE BONES

In the Western view, the bones form the human skeleton. The skeleton is a kind of framework that protects the internal organs and at the same time acts as a support and structure to which other body structures are connected—tendons, ligaments, muscles, fascia—ensuring the movement of the human body. In everyday life, bones are not given much of our attention because they are hidden in the depths of our body and we tend to completely forget about them. We notice our bones only when we hit them, break them, when they hurt or when we begin to feel the problems caused by the loss of bone mass. We consider bones to be a dead mass that is somewhere inside of the body and holds us together. Taoists also perceive bones from their functional point of view, but the bones also mean something more to them. They are a basic substance where the physical dimension extends into energetic, even spiritual contexts. For Taoists, the bones are our deepest foundation; they are the matrix that will remain after the death of the body itself. Thanks to the bones, a trace of our soul remains after our death on Earth. Everything else decomposes, but the matrix stored in the bones remains.

However, Taoist wisdom is very close to ours. We are used to saying, "I feel it in my bones." This sentence explains that something really important is about to happen. We say this if we have a strong feeling, a premonition; we instinctively feel something—we are led by our intuition or our sixth sense. We feel it in our bones because the bones are connected to the fundamental source of Qi, which is stored in the kidneys and subsequently in the bones. By cultivating Qi through Qigong meditation exercises, it is stored even in the bone marrow.

The bones are dependent on the kidneys, and the kidneys are dependent on the bones. This relationship takes place at the level of the bone and bone marrow relationship. The marrow stored in the bones ensures their strength, firmness and flexibility; the bones, in return, prevent the essential richness of the marrow from shattering. And our whole organism depends on the marrow. Because the marrow produces blood, it is the basic nutrient substrate of our body.

In the Taoist tradition, bones work in the human body just as mountains work for the Earth. Just as a mountain naturally directs the flow and circulation of water and air, so bones naturally direct the circulation and movement of Qi, the Jing essence, the spirit, the blood, the marrow and body fluids—all the most important components of our body. In addition, the tradition believes that bones vibrate like hollow whistles, especially when Qi flows around and through them. These living whistles are responsible for the vibration of Heavenly Qi and Qi in the environment throughout the physical structure of the body. This philosophical view is confirmed by modern research that began in the middle of the last century. It proves that bones, as the body's only solid crystalline substance, are able to generate electricity. When the bones are pressed, they generate weak electric currents. These control the organization of bone cells and their arrangement into the supporting beams. This phenomenon is called the *piezoelectric effect* and has been documented by many studies. It is therefore possible to measure the electromagnetic field of bones, to measure how they receive and send electric currents to our organs, blood cells, nerves and meridians. At the same time, this delicate current in the bones works for the whole body as a kind of tuner. Taoists have long seen great importance in various exercises aimed at strengthening bones and bone marrow. Fortunately, these Qigong exercises still exist today. For example, the exercise called *Bone compression* is aimed at amplifying this current. With the help of an electromagnetic field, this exercise can regenerate bone tissue, which can be used, for example, in the treatment of bone fractures.

The respective bone cells mature faster in the corresponding electromagnetic field.

The bones are alive, constantly regenerating; even their shape is changeable. The skeletal structure is subject to a process of constant change during a person's life. Changes in children and adolescents are easily visible. Unlike an adult, a child has some bones that are not completely fused, and they have a much softer structure—some of them are even still cartilage. Children's bones gradually grow, lengthen and gain in density, volume and strength. However, the process of change does not stop even in adulthood, because bones are in a constant process of development during our lives. Even the bones of an adult are not unchangeable units. They are fed by small arteries that penetrate into the marrow and are connected to other structures—tendons, muscles and fascia. Therefore, the bones also change and adapt to the conditions and demands that their "owner" gives them. Conditions can be either destructive or constructive. Due to their plasticity, their balance can be destroyed or restored. I myself have experience with the change in the shape of my own bones after seven years of conscious work on their transformation. Conscious connection to one's own bones can fundamentally affect not only our health and the way we move but also the way we perceive our existence. Although the bones are in the depths of the body, almost every one of them can be sensed through touch or through meditation.

Every mover should feel obliged to take care of the bones and the kidneys. Caring for both is reflected in the whole body comprehensively. In one of my research studies, I asked dancers what dance brought them. The answer was: "Dance has brought me osteoarthritis." This is, in fact, not possible if the dancer or other mover knows that when we take, we must give. Especially to our own body. Dancing or other persistent movement requires more demands from the body than during its usual usage. When we drive on the highway at 150 kilometers per hour, the car consumes more fuel than if we drive at 90 kilometers per hour. We need to refuel more often, and that fuel should also be of good quality. Therefore, Qi needs to be replenished, regularly and with quality. One of the ways is food—information on the kidney diet and a few recipes can be found at the end of this chapter.

In my pedagogical work, I consider working with bones to be basic. In our seminars, working with bones represents the growth of our work. If we can consciously connect to our skeletal "hardware," our "software" (the movement expression) will also work more consciously. We call our work *Anatomy of Movement* or *Body Awareness*, in which people get to know their bodies through conscious work with the bones. We look at the bones in pictures, we get to know the connections between them thanks to three-dimensional models of the skeleton, but mainly we work with our own bones through movement—in pairs or individually. At first, we mostly improvise with a focus on the bones, the relationships between them, their movement possibilities or limitations. As students get deeper into their bones, we develop this work into more demanding movement patterns. Later, this perception becomes a kind of "autopilot" for movers, and they work with it automatically.

TUNE IN TO HOW IT SHOULD BE

One of the main things we bring to the attention of students is an awareness of the arrangement and alignment of the bones in their body. We live in a world where gravitational force acts on us. Our body is constantly exposed to this force and has to work with it so that we do not fall to the ground and surrender to it completely. When we lie down, we yield fully to gravity. However, we need to move and, in addition, we need to work in the vertical axis, so the body construction must be able to cope with this enormous force of gravity. Many structures are involved in this mechanism—bones, joints, muscles, fascia, tendons, ligaments, which hold everything together. However, bones play a major role in body statics. Each bone plays an important role here, so the body has fantastic support in this arrangement of bones. When the skeletal arrangement works well, the joints, ligaments, tendons, fascia and muscles also work well. If it does not work well, these parts of the body have to work excessively, and it makes them tired and can even deform them.

Nature "designed" us almost perfectly. When we start to look at our skeletal structure with the eye of functionally natural and therefore correct alignment, and we start to consciously use it in motion, we will avoid many health problems; we also save energy and our movement becomes more organic. This knowledge is priceless in partner work. We often do partner work with excessive muscle use. The muscles get tired and often deformed. However, if we learn to lift our partner with the energy which is led through the bones into the ground, and therefore not with the muscles, movement will be healthier, less energy-intensive and, of course, more natural. However, it is difficult to talk about all this, and students will understand the alignment of their skeletal structure only through personal experience and through practice. Anyone who has experienced it once does not want to do it otherwise.

Each bone of our body has its own story created by the way we use it. The story is logically affected by food, the use of the body in various physical situations, emotions and mental mood. A hunched spine, a curvature of the body to the side, flat feet, worn-out menisci, also chronic bone and joint pain, thinning bones and the like, all speak about the relationship we have with our lives. I read once that the height of most people's bodies does not correspond to the "original plan." The way we use our body makes it shorter. Our bones want to breathe, they want to live, they want to grow to Heaven, but we prevent them from doing so with our opinions, prejudices, routines or low self-confidence. Personally, I recommend working with the bones to every person, even an ordinary person who is not engaged in dance, sports or other physical activities. Discovering the essence of the bones in your body is like touching your intrinsic nature. When we feel them, we are aware of their shape and weight, and then we are more real. We do not deal with unnecessary things, we do not like to talk nonsense, we are true and clear. In conversations, we avoid indirectness and small talk; we easily see through manipulations, and we do not allow ourselves to be drawn into them. At the same time, we feel that what we say has value, we experience that we are heard and seen, and thus we trust ourselves. Our vibration is stronger, so we easily attract people with a similar focus. We can hear our inner voice or see the direction we are walking in. Bones are about our deepest reality.

SPINE—THE "FLOWING" VERTICAL COLUMN

The spine is the basic structural pillar of our body. Movers should be aware of their spine from the construction but also from the energetic point of view. It will help them make full use of its plasticity and become aware of its movement possibilities and structural connections with other parts of the body. However, they will also recognize its limitations, and when they respect them, they can avoid its destruction and pain.

From a purely practical anatomical point of view, the spine is a collection of vertebrae vertically arranged in a column, where this column is more like a snake, twice curved in an S-shape. This curvature ensures spine mobility, flexibility, functionality and a lively supporting ability. The construction of the spine allows a person to walk vertically and protects the spinal cord that "flows" through it. It is actually a kind of bone coat of the spinal cord, and it also functions as a distribution system, because nerves emerge from the spinal cord through the openings between the vertebrae to connect via their sensitive paths with the whole body.

At first glance, it does not look like it, but the spine actually "flows." The spaces between the vertebrae are filled with cartilaginous interverte- bral discs. These water-bearing disks allow spine mobility and flexibility. They are able to soften shocks and shakes with their liquid structure, and thus protect the spine. They also protect the flow of Qi that streams through the spine. We can also imagine the spinal cord as an extremely dense fluid in which Qi flows. All the informa- tion, all the data of our nervous system "flows" through the spinal cord and nerves. Movement of the spine can therefore have a very fluid, smooth and soft character.

Many of us limit our perception of the spine only to feelings of pain in some parts of it which we then tend to stress more and incorrectly. The tiny ligaments holding the vertebrae together often hurt; the muscles that have to hold this structure and balance incorrect posture of the body also ache. The culmination of our mis- understood opportunity to work with our own backbone is disk problems—displacement, ejec- tion and degeneration. Unfortunately, these are often the only times people realize that they have a spine. But the spine means much more for us.

In addition to the construction pillar, it is also a pillar of our overall personality—a "skele- ton of our identity." It's what we can rely on—a solid back, a support, a reinforcement, a refuge. The term *skeleton of our identity* means what we identify with in this life. The spine is a protective structure for our mission to be fulfilled here. No

wonder the nervous system, such a delicate part of our body, is connected to the spine. No won- der the fibers of the nervous system "flow" in the thick bundle of the spinal cord from the brain directly through our backbone, because there they have the necessary support and protection, and they use the spine as their distribution center. Taoists have discovered that there are Qi pathways in the spine area through which a very strong Qi stream flows. The spine thus creates a kind of Qi path that can flow through it and then spread throughout our organism, thus nourishing it. This life-giving Qi flows through these channels and is spread from them to the organs of the body, and in fact into each cell. It provides them with the nutrition they need for their growth, function and healing.

Let's have a look at these meridians. The *Gov- erning Vessel* leads Qi on the back of the spine and the *Conception Vessel* leads Qi on the front side of the body. Both of these channels start to activate shortly after the conception of a human being and develop completely in the prenatal stage. The Governing Vessel affects many health and psychospiritual issues. Its activity is closely linked to our original constitutional Qi and its source is in the kidneys. If Qi is lacking in this channel, one has a problem with identity. Such a person has "no back to lean on"—he or she might suffer from a lack of courage in life. In the belt area, opposite the navel, there is a place through which we "inhale" the rules and principles that we work with in our lives. This place is called the *Gate of Life* (in Chinese, *Mingmen*). Children without parents often have weakness in this channel; they have difficulty finding certain frames and princi- ples in their lives. The Governing Vessel springs from the depths of the pelvis, passes through the sexual organs, enters the back of the spine and through it enters the cranium, including the brain; then it continues through the top of the head, forehead, nose and ends in the mouth. Here it connects with the Conception Vessel. The Conception Vessel also rises from the perineum, passes along the front side of the spine upwards, ascends into the navel, leads through the solar plexus, the sternum and through the neck to the throat and the oral cavity. This channel has a strong influence on the ability to conceive a child but, in a psychospiritual context, on the ability to conceive anything, to become a creative person. These two channels are deliberately interconnected in the meditation techniques of the mouth by placing the tongue to the upper palate. The tongue is like a bridge that connects these two Qi channels and activates the common flow of Qi. This Qi circulation is the basis of Qigong or Taijiquan exercises, and Taoists say they link the *Microcosmic Orbit*.

Mingmen

The Gate of Life is a strong energy center that lies in the middle of the body, opposite the navel, in the area of the lumbar spine, between the kidneys at the level of the waist. It is the primary driving force of human life functions and the basis of our energy source. Mingmen is a part of the term *Kidney Qi*. It contains what is called *ministerial fire*, the fire that is needed for the activation of all the functions of the body. It is like a small, constantly burning fire in a gas boiler, always ready to ignite and to activate anything that is needed. This fire helps the digestive tract to digest food, but also takes care of the warmth throughout our body. It warms the organs to be able to function properly, but it also warms other parts of the body, including the peripheries.

The Mingmen is closely linked to reproductive function. Mingmen Qi in a man helps to produce sperm; in a woman, it is related to the uterus and ovaries and their functions. Also, the word *gate* refers to a passage, a kind of portal through which one can enter or exit. Taoists believe that at the moment of conception, it is through this gate that the man's energy deposit comes out and is received by the woman through her gate. When the fetus matures, it uses the power of the Mingmen to pass through the birth canal.

The Mingmen is also a place of our mental and emotional strength. It is a steady and strong place, a space of certainty on which we can rely in our lives. Therefore, caring for the Mingmen helps those who are frightened on a bolder journey through life. The entry point into this area is the point of the same name, Mingmen, the fourth point of the Governing Vessel (GV4), one of the eight extraordinary vessels. It is located in the space between the protrusion of the second and third lumbar vertebrae. You can find it in the picture of the Bladder channel later in the chapter. When we expose this area of our backs to cold, moisture or wind due to our passion for wearing short T-shirts and low-rise trousers, revealing not only a nice belly but also our Mingmen, we expose this source of Qi to "thieves." We allow this treasure to be robbed absolutely unnecessarily.

Another meridian related to the spine is the Bladder channel. It is the longest channel of the body, connecting our body from top to bottom, from the head through the torso to the feet. The acupuncture points of this channel on the area of the spine are connected with the nerves which are separated from the spinal cord and connected to the organs. They are known as transporting points (in Chinese, *Shuxue*) which, when stimulated, are able to nourish all the organs of the body through their connection to the nervous system. This is evidence that our nervous system is highly interconnected with the energy system. The Bladder channel is the only meridian in the body that has such an impact on all organs.

Daily care of the spine is extremely important. Proper posture, adequate movement, a smooth flow of Qi through the Microcosmic

Orbit and enough time to rest and sleep, that is what the spine loves. In my dance classes, I like working with the spine very much. I teach students to perceive and use its individual segments to discover its multifunctional plasticity through chain reactions and through the space in it. I also teach them to perceive the compact and nourishing stream of Qi that flows in it. In dance, we can work on activating the flow of Qi in the spine and direct it in different directions. Qigong, focused on Qi flow through the spine, is an appropriate preparation of the body for conscious dance. Dance is a suitable means of this care, but we must maintain a conscious focus when dancing and not overdo it. In addition to Qigong, I recommend to all dancers and movers methods such as Body-Mind Centering, Ideokinesis, Moving Anatomy, etc.

KNEES OF A MOVER

The knees are the most commonly injured joints of movers. But our profession really depends on them—on their health, strength and well-being. Indeed, when dancing, doing yoga or sport, we place significant stress upon them. They support almost our entire body weight. Our movement invention requires great adaptability, fast responses, stability and complete flexibility from them. With contemporary dance floor work techniques, the movements are performed on the floor and on the knees. It means that we demand an almost iron-like strength from our knees.

A complex mechanism

Despite its seemingly innocuous appearance, the knee belongs among the most complex of joints. The correct function of the knee joint is reliant upon the cooperation of several parts of a chain (the pelvis, hip, upper leg, lower leg, ankle and foot) that must all work together and depend on each other for function and movement.

The *knee bones* are one of the deepest structures; they provide strength, flexibility and stability by utilizing the entire skeletal system. The knee provides the connection of the femur with the bones of the lower leg (tibia) and a part of the patellofemoral groove and the kneecap (patella). The surfaces of the bones that are part of the hinge joint are covered with articular *cartilage*. Together with synovial fluid, cartilage allows the bones to move freely while reducing friction and protecting the bones from wear as the joint moves.

The function of the *knee ligaments* is to attach bones to bones and give strength and stability to the knee in the individual positions that movement requires; the menisci help the ligaments with that.

The *muscles* provide the source of movement. Thanks to their ability to shrink and release, the knee is able to bend, thus offering the body numerous possibilities for movement. The knees are at the same time interconnected by these connective tissues with the other parts of the body—primarily the hip and ankle joints. The condition of the knees thus affects them, and vice versa; the correct use of these joints, as well as the quality of the tendons connecting the muscles to the knees, affects the condition of the knees themselves.

Of course, *blood vessels* and *nerves* also pass through the knees. The knees are nourished by blood transported through blood vessels; nerves transfer brain impulses to trigger movement, and in return deliver information about the condition and movement of the knees to the brain. Such information includes pain, one of the warning signals that all is not well with the knee.

The *meridians* are also included. They pass Qi through the knees and thus link the knees to important organs and their systems. The knees are connected to the spleen and stomach, liver and gallbladder, kidneys and urinary bladder via their six meridians. The spleen provides the muscles with nutrition, while the liver is responsible for feeding the tendons and ligaments, their strength, elasticity, endurance and the ability to give muscles "drive." The kidneys are responsible for the health of bones, cartilage and menisci. In the professional realm of movement, we often encounter knee strains, stretching or tearing of the ligaments, meniscus damage or water on the knee. Each of these problems can restrict our plans and activities. And it's then up to us to ensure that we start listening to our knees to avoid more significant problems.

Meniscus—a unique tissue

The meniscus is a special crescent-shaped pad of cartilage. There are two menisci in each knee joint—medial and lateral, located one on each side of the knee—and they provide a cushion between the femur (thighbone) and tibia (shinbone). The natural weight and movement of a body can cause the bones to become very close to each other, reducing the area between the bones to such an extent that their surfaces could become damaged by friction. The main task of the menisci is to reduce friction while moving and to absorb shocks from jumping and landing. Because the menisci help to spread out the weight across the joint, they keep the bones from wearing away at friction points and keep the joint in its natural position.

Menisci are "intended" by nature to work in coordination with our body and not cause problems. It's not a fixed, rigid structure, but elastic and flexible, adaptable to individual conditions. The menisci can be likened to some kind of rubbery, moldable substance that constantly adapts to various conditions. While always retaining its crescent shape, it adjusts the thickness of its surface depending on the position of the bones within the knee at any given movement. It does this because of its constant "desire" to fulfill its most important function—the protection of the knee joint. And as the movement of a mover is often unexpected and quick, the menisci are able to respond unexpectedly and quickly. But there must be certain limits. This incredibly collaborative joint also needs our care. It needs anatomically healthy knee use, proper knee utilization, protection by using knee pads, to be warmed up and prepared sufficiently before performing or training and, last but not least, regeneration time and quality nutrition. If it receives these elements, it does not scream for help. If it does not receive these elements, then the pain from the knee will be heard. If this cry for help is ignored, the condition develops into gradual meniscus deterioration, followed by the deterioration of the bone cartilage and eventually the entire knee joint. Once in this state, the knee is like a car without wheels. Even though it still looks like a car, it will not carry us very far due to the friction of the road and the unpleasant screech.

With the above in mind, it is clear that meniscus damage indicates we have gone too far. We also process the theme of humble acceptance psychosomatically and symbolically through our knee joints. Nowadays, we don't have the need to bow down, be grateful, bend and humble ourselves. The ideal of today's times is a stubborn person keeping the head raised, a person who sometimes pushes the limits right to the edge. No wonder knee problems, and particularly meniscus damage, have gained considerable scope. The basis of meniscus injury is overload, and this disability throws light on some kind of pride and blindness. One should know one's limits and realize when one's efforts and performance are pushing beyond their boundaries. The inability to accept the real state, by suppressing modesty and ignoring the warning signals, especially in the form of pain, leads to the inevitable fact that we will have problems with the menisci.

Pushing our boundaries also leads to additional inconveniences—from over-stretching to even snapping of the ligaments. The knees are naturally protected against dislocation. The bones are connected and the knee joint is given strength and stability by ligaments. The anterior and posterior ligaments are the major joint stabilizers. The anterior ligament and the posterior ligament cross each other at the center of the knee. The anterior ligament limits rotation and forward motion of the tibia while the posterior ligament limits the backwards motion of the knee. There are also ligaments on the sides—medial collateral and lateral collateral ligaments. These fulfill the function of limiting sideways motion of the knee. So when they become damaged, the stabilizing function can be reduced, even lost, resulting in instability of the knee.

The ligaments must be firm and flexible at the same time. They have their limits and needs. If we want to execute excellent achievements with our knees, the knees must be fully warmed up and prepared before beginning training. Another suitable option is Qigong, which brings beneficial Qi to the knees. On the other hand, the knees are also tightened and strengthened by movement itself; the movement of the knee supports the ligaments and tendons, their strength and flexibility. However, movement must be executed anatomically correctly. The quality of the ligaments and tendons is also enhanced by diet, the harmonic energy of the liver and sufficient regeneration time; appropriate preparation prior to exercise and the proper anatomical movement of the knees are all necessary for knee health.

Energy flow

I have mentioned various organs of the body that to ordinary people do not seem to be related to the knees. According to Chinese medicine, the meridians that align the joints with these organs bring the organs into play. The menisci, cartilage and knee bones are, according to Chinese medicine, replenished by energy from the kidneys. If we wish to keep them healthy, it is advisable to look after the kidneys and nourish them with a good diet and Qi. The tendons and ligaments, as already mentioned, depend on the condition of the liver.

There are very strong acupuncture points located in the knee area, situated on the meridian pathways passing through the knees. This means that the knees are a kind of "meeting point" for the flow of Qi. This is another reason why ensuring they remain in good condition is so important—so Qi can flow naturally to where it's intended to go, but only on the condition that the knees are in a state of harmony. I will mention the most important points and their most important effects.

Zusanli (ST36) is a point located just below the knee, on its lateral side, along the Stomach channel. It is one of the strongest immunostimulatory points in the body; it supports the stomach and spleen in the processing of food and its transformation to Qi. In close proximity is the *Yanglingquan* point (GB34) located on the Gallbladder channel. It is, among other things, a master point for the tendons that nourishes, regenerates and cares for their continual healthy condition. On the medial side of the knee, the *Yinggu* point (KI10) is located on the Kidney channel. It is referred to as the biorhythm point and is responsible for acclimatizing our organism to changes in living conditions. It is often used, for example, for rapid adaptation of the body across time zones, thus helping with jet lag. At the midpoint of the transverse crease of the popliteal fossa, between the tendons of the biceps femoris and the semitendinosus, there is the *Weizhong* point (BL40) located on the Bladder channel, which, among other things, is often used for its ability to release blockages in the lumbar spine and sacrum, thereby eliminating pain in that area.

Psyche

In addition to caring for the knees with the proper anatomical use of the body, protecting them by using knee pads, allowing time for sufficient regeneration and good nutrition, relaxation of the psyche and awareness of certain life-linking events also helps the knees. Finally, in addition to the theme of humble acceptance that has already been mentioned, I will mention one more connection between the knees and our psyche. Symbolically, joints are a means of connecting one thing with another. They are crossroads for the circuits of Qi. Problems with joints occur when there is no natural interconnectedness of things, phenomena, situations, relationships, etc.—if the body doesn't connect with the soul, spirituality with materiality, and so on. At the same time, joints are also points where the Qi travels from one part of the body to another, so on the psychic level this is related to the ability of a human being to form connections and be able to use them in one's own life.

OTHER CONNECTIONS WITH THE FUNCTIONAL CIRCUIT OF THE KIDNEYS

We will return to the functional circuit of the kidneys, because we have not yet exhausted the summary of its effect on the organism. In the medical texts of Chinese medicine, we find information that:

The kidneys produce marrow, fill up the brain and control bones

From the Chinese medicine point of view, the marrow cannot be understood only as a bone filling. The marrow is a common matrix for the bones, bone marrow, brain and spinal cord. It is something that is our essence—the marrow, the pulp, the nucleus, the "substrate" for the nervous system. The marrow and bone marrow subsequently generate bones.

The kidneys control the reception of Qi from air

The kidneys attract and receive air inhaled through the lungs. Thanks to proper activity and sufficient kidney Qi, we receive Qi from the air and send it to our deepest structures. Taoists say that "the kidneys inhale and the lungs exhale." Therefore, for example, it is logical that Chinese medicine solves the treatment of asthma in two different ways, depending on whether the person has difficulty inhaling or exhaling. We can read more about this in Chapter 12 on the METAL phase.

The kidneys manifest through the hair

The kidneys, with their Qi, give the body a precondition for the perfect processing of nutrients from food and their transport into the blood, which, among other things, significantly nourishes the hair. The strength, color and also quantity of hair are decisive. Excessive hair loss indicates that there is something wrong with the kidney Qi. It is therefore logical that some women lose their hair more than usual after giving birth. Giving birth requires a large dose of Qi from the kidneys. If the kidney Qi of a mother was weak before giving birth, it will manifest itself after childbearing by further weakening or even emptiness. Another manifestation of kidney Qi weakness is graying of the hair. Taoist masters have their natural hair color even in old age. In contrast, many people turn gray at an early age. When replenishing Qi in the kidneys, we can, if we start in time, regain lost hair color.

The teeth are protrusions of bones

The deficiency of kidney Qi after giving birth can affect also the condition of the teeth. Teeth come from the same source as bones, and their quality depends on the condition of the kidneys. However, the condition of the teeth does not depend only on exhaustion from giving birth. Lack of Jing essence of the kidneys can also cause tooth problems in men at any age. At an older age, the loss of one's own teeth is therefore a common phenomenon. The term *tooth* in this context means a fixed part of the tooth—that is, the tooth itself, which has the same base as the bone. Gum problems are related to the spleen, which is in charge of the fleshy part of the teeth. When the Jing essence is weakened in childhood, it manifests itself in delayed tooth growth.

The kidneys open into the ears and control hearing

The ears are energetically connected to the kidneys. When you look at ears, you will notice that they look like kidneys. If the Jing essence is strong enough, it can ascend to the head and nourish the ears and clarify hearing. However, kidney Qi also has an impact on other dimensions of listening. When we are connected to our innermost selves, we are able to listen to others and really perceive what they want to tell us. There is a difference between hearing and listening.

The color of the WATER phase is black, dark

Dark colors—blue, dark blue, dark claret and even black—are naturally colors that evoke depth. The depth of kidney Qi and the WATER Qi phase is therefore supported by this color. If we need to support it, we can work with dark colors—for example, in what we wear. For food preparation, we choose dark to black foods, such as dark beans, black sesame and the like. However, the excess of dark color gradually begins to destroy the kidneys.

The taste of the WATER phase is a salty taste

The salty taste boosts kidney Qi. However, excess salt harms them and so it harms the heart. You can read more about salt and salty taste in the section below about diet in the WATER phase.

The kidneys control the lower orifices

Kidney Qi also controls the quality of the tonus of our perineum. By lower orifices, we mean the anus, the urethra and the vaginal opening. If their tonus is weak, there is a leakage of urine and stool, and premature opening of the birth canal during pregnancy. It is a sign that kidney Qi is not sufficient.

The assistant of the kidneys is the bladder

We mentioned this organ in connection with the flow of Qi through its meridian pathway along the spine. The bladder is directly subordinate to the kidneys, and its strength for fluid transformation depends on their Qi. The bladder leaves the clean part of the body's fluids in the form of steam in the body for irrigation, and the unnecessary turbid part is returned to the Earth in the form of urine. Its main task is to spread the transformed fluids into the body, to ensure the right degree of humidity, thus preventing excessive moisture or dryness.

PREGNANCY, CHILDBIRTH AND SUBSEQUENT CONVALESCENCE

Pregnancy is primarily about the development of the substantive existence of the fetus in the mother's womb. The fetus receives its primary charge from the Jing essence of the father and mother, but for its development in the womb, it receives the Jing essence from the mother's kidneys, as well as her Qi and nutrition from the blood. In the female body, energetic changes of astronomical dimensions take place during pregnancy. For the first three months of pregnancy, the flow of Qi is directed to the uterus to nourish the baby and the placenta. Qi and body fluids may therefore have difficulty flowing up and down the body; that is, Qi tends to be stagnated at the level of Three

Burners that were mentioned in the chapter on Qi. If Qi stagnates in the Middle Burner, digestive problems occur; if it is blocked in the Upper Burner, it affects breathing and Qi flow to the upper limbs; if the block prevents Qi flow in the Lower Burner, it affects the kidneys and bladder, but also Qi flow to the lower limbs. The growth of the child and the related increase in its weight affects the mother's spine and the meridians connected to the spine.

Another big change that happens during the process of pregnancy and birth is the transformation of a woman's blood into breast milk. The mother must therefore have enough essential substances such as blood, Jing essence and body fluids to nourish the fetus and ensure a smooth and free flow of Qi into her uterus. However, she must have enough of the substances for herself, because if she has little of it and gives the baby everything that the baby needs, naturally there will not be much left for herself. The result is a huge exhaustion of the Jing essence and blood substances after childbirth, which is manifested by great fatigue, hair loss or increased tooth decay. Energetically, it is natural for the mother to focus more inwards, to relax more during her pregnancy and to devote herself to the baby and her own needs. However, we currently live in a society that is set up to ignore a woman's pregnancy. Thus, at work, women must—and some women want to—perform the same activities and with the same intensity as if she were not pregnant. A woman is in a state of Yang, and she does not have suitable conditions for "yin-ing"; there is an internal tension in her, and an excessive consumption of substances that are to be stored for her and the baby.

Childbirth itself is extreme. It is a natural physiological matter, but it is extreme in that it requires a woman to outlay a lot of Qi. If there is an emotional tension added to this, because women are subjected by society to various prejudices that may block them from naturally preparing for childbirth, we have here the sum of energetic, physical and emotional expenditure. After giving birth, a woman needs to get her body back to its original state, but so too does her Qi need to get back to its previous state. It is necessary to rest, relax and switch off in order to regain lost strength. This is a very important period of childbearing (puerperium). After giving birth, many women rush to return to work or work at home around the baby. The result is fatigue and inhibition of the natural regeneration of the body and Qi. On the contrary, many new mothers, especially first-time mothers, feel full of energy and zest for life after giving birth. However, this surge of energy in the form of endorphins can be dangerous—a woman is not able to sense that her Qi can quickly become exhausted. This may manifest itself as a health problem in the future. So every female mover should think about how quickly she will return to intense physical activity. Six weeks is a period of convalescence, even if a woman does not feel it is necessary. During this period, a woman should "stay in her pajamas"—rest, take care of herself and the baby, and enjoy being taken care of. She should ensure that someone helps her with the baby during this period, because the diseases that can affect the mother at this time will be repeated throughout her life.

After giving birth, a woman's body needs time to restore the Jing essence. Taoists therefore recommend a break of at least two to three years between pregnancies. If the pregnancy and birth were difficult, an even longer break is needed. One that will ensure that the woman regains her strength. Last but not least, it is important to note that the energy and health status of a woman during pregnancy and after childbirth

Japanese cuisine has a fantastic vitalizing booster in its database—carp soup called *koikoku*. A powerful replenisher for Qi, blood and Jing, it is thus suitable also for exhausted mothers. You can find the recipe later in this chapter, in the section on diet for the WATER phase.

determines how much Qi and Jing essence her baby actually receives—what kind of constitutional basis she will give the baby. Therefore, Taoists advise both parents to consciously prepare for conception by improving their health at least two to three years before conception.

MOXIBUSTION (MOXA) IN THE MOVER'S FIRST-AID KIT

During my work in China, I encountered moxa sticks as a matter of course in the first-aid kit of the dance studios I visited. Chinese dancers have shown me how to use moxibustion for pain or fatigue. It is a traditional Chinese curative method of heating up acupuncture points to deliver warmth and Qi to the body. It represents a tremendously valuable and centuries-old summary of practical experience. It uses the knowledge of traditional Chinese acupuncture—the relationship between Yin and Yang, the knowledge of meridians, acupuncture points, and the system of the functioning of organs and the correlating body structures that each organ has to deal with.

In practice, it concerns the use of *Artemisia vulgaris*. It is either rolled into cigar-shaped sticks of varying sizes or small moxa cones are manually made from the dried "fluff" of this herb. The cone or moxa stick is ignited and smoldering (i.e. no longer burning), and it is then held a certain distance from a particular acupuncture point, or placed on the point itself through some kind of underlay—such as a slice of garlic or ginger, a sheet of paper or a coin. Moxibustion is also used on whole body surfaces (e.g. joints or longer sections of meridians). When using moxa, a substance that stimulates the nerve endings in the skin is released in the sweat duct of the skin. This stimulation triggers the activation of the brain and adrenal glands. They then release hormones that promote the effect of moxibustion in the body. The impact of the heat is not only local overheating, but it also increases thermal and electrical conductivity at the spot where the moxa was applied. This affects the energy exchange between the external and internal

For movers, I list a number of issues where moxibustion can be used:

- Filling heat and energy into the body exhausted by intense movement (which also concerns athletes or people working in cold environments).
- For prevent frequenting colds, for boosting immunity, for cold limbs or for excessive sensitivity to cold (during any given season), for local warming of the parts where coldness is felt (joints, tendons, muscles).
- Chronic exhaustion, weakness, chronic fatigue syndrome.
- Numb spots on the body.
- Arthritis, tendonitis, over-stretched muscles, injuries from dance or sports, osteoporosis.
- Back pain (also for lumbago), pain in the area of the hips, sciatic nerve, stiffening of the shoulders and neck, slipped discs.
- Depression.
- For internal heating for people who do not eat meat (Yang) but prefer raw vegetables (Yin) or dairy products (Yin).

environments of the body, activating the skin receptors and releasing the biologically active substances from the damaged cells. The heat, as well as the essence of the essential oil from the herb, passes deep into the body and, through the meridians, fills the body with Qi, promotes its circulation and eliminates coldness from the body. If the pain was caused by cold, the pain is removed too. In cases of a cold attack, without the use of moxibustion this problem cannot even be solved.

In some cases, moxibustion is simple to apply and therefore can easily be used with movers. The method also has the advantage that the person can apply it to him or herself. The only downside could be the smoke and intense smell that moxibustion produces. There are also carbon moxa sticks without the smell, which can be used indoors. From my own therapeutic practice, I have experienced that, for example, an affected sciatic nerve, Achilles tendon or shoulder cannot be healed without the use of moxibustion. These are the cases when cold or wind enters these parts of the body. It is my experience that, with such problems, neither yoga nor stretching of the affected parts will help. Even physiotherapy or osteopathic treatment does not solve the problem completely. When coldness nests down in the body structures, it cannot be taken out other than by using the moxibustion method. In this way, we have solved many chronic pains of my dance students simply by eliminating the cold that was kept in their bodies for years.

By overheating, one can excellently solve acute issues such as the penetration of harmful cold and wind from the air, which causes stagnation of Qi in the meridians and brings pain or numbness. Moxibustion is also excellent for long-term chronic diseases, digestive, respiratory or gynecological problems.

It is advisable to learn the basic techniques and methods and to learn about the contraindications of moxibustion. For this purpose, I have specially designed courses.

RELATIONSHIP OF THE WATER PHASE TO OTHER PHASES

According to the supporting *Sheng* cycle, which we discussed in Chapter 7 on the Five Phases of Transformations of Qi, it is clear that the "mother" of the kidneys is the lungs. Their quality consequently determines the quality of kidney Qi. This means that if we want to take care of the kidneys, we must also pay attention to the lungs. Smoking or living or working in an environment that damages the lungs also damages the kidneys. The EARTH phase, on the other hand, in the controlling Ke cycle, controls and limits the kidneys. With an excess of Qi in the WATER phase, the EARTH phase is able to limit it. In everyday life, however, kidney Qi does not suffer from excess. On the contrary, it is more likely to be deficient. This deficiency is caused by a lifestyle full of extremes, exhaustion, lack of rest, travel without subsequent regeneration, past diseases, etc. When kidney Qi is sufficient, the WATER phase can give birth to the WOOD phase and at the same time control the excess in the FIRE phase.

CONCLUSION TO THE WATER PHASE

Let's indulge in "hibernation" in winter. Let's rest more, focus on ourselves and not waste energy. When fatigue comes, try to respect it and lie down or at least slow down.

In winter, it is advisable to go to bed earlier and get up later. After excessive physical exertion or travel, take an adequately long rest. When a disease starts to "crawl" in, lie down under the quilt, have linden or elderflower tea with a tiny bit of spirits (e.g. peach brandy, plum brandy, applejack) and then sweat. In two to three days, you will be fine and will not have to spend two weeks recovering. Make sure you get enough fluids, but do not overdo it. Do not burden the kidneys with morning coffee or black tea, and treat yourselves to a warm breakfast. It is advisable to drink a glass of lukewarm or warmer boiled water on an empty stomach. Keep your feet and kidneys warm. Cover your ears with a hat so that the cold does not penetrate the body unnecessarily through them. During the winter, it is not good to push ourselves. It does not matter if in work or personal matters, our development has been slightly suspended or slowed down. Let things mature; give them the winter time to "ferment," vibrate and remain in relative stagnation.

Table 8.1 Main correspondences of WATER phase

Year season: winter	Yin and Yang stage: utmost Yin/Yin in Yin
Day time: night	Direction: north
Evolution of Qi: Qi waiting steadily	Growth cycle in nature: storage
Life cycle: old age, rest, death	Working cycle: termination, rest, charging
Yin organ: kidneys	Organ clock for kidneys: 5 to 7 p.m.
Yang organ: bladder	Organ clock for bladder: 3 to 5 p.m.
Psychospiritual aspect: Zhi	Virtue: wisdom
Emotion: fear	Climate: cold
Color: black, dark	Taste: salty
Smell: putrid	Number: 6
Tissue: bones, teeth	Body fluid: urine
Other body tissues: brain, marrow, spinal cord, inner ear, ovaries, testicles, genitalia, rectum, urethra	Other body fluid and excretion: sexual excretion, cerebrospinal fluid, hormones, thick saliva
Joints: knees, ankles, joints of the feet	Entry point of disease: ears, loins, feet, lower back
Sense organ: ears	Sense: hearing
Indicator: hair	Detrimental action: too much standing
Sound: groaning	Mental attitude: will, modesty

MERIDIANS

BLADDER CHANNEL (BL)/YANG

The Bladder channel is the body's longest meridian. It is a pair channel, with a Yang charge; Qi descends through it from top to bottom. In the image below, the channel is shown on both sides of the body. It begins in the inner corners of the eyes, emerges at the head, where Qi flows through the inner branch into the brain. It continues through the crown and nape to the neck, and under the 7th cervical vertebra it connects with other Yang channels. An immense field of its action takes place on the back, passing along the spine, in four streams of Qi flow. Here, Qi is connected to the nerve processes from the spinal cord, so it affects all organs that are connected to the nerves. It is also directly connected to the bladder and kidneys by the internal branches. It descends from the torso to the back of the lower limbs, continues through the back of the thighs,

below the knees and to the calves. In the ankle area, it meets the Achilles tendons, and on the outside of the feet, Qi flows to the little toes, where it ends and connects with the Qi of the Kidney channel. There are 67 active acupuncture points on this channel. The picture also shows the already mentioned point of *Mingmen* (the Gate of Life), GV4 on the Governing Vessel. Dashed lines indicate internal deep branches.

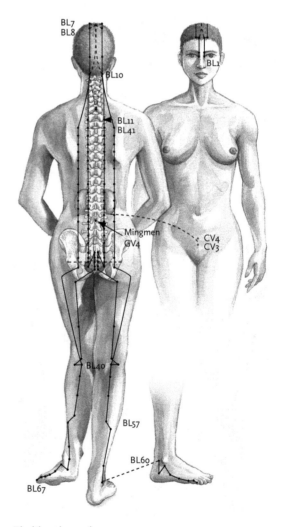

Bladder channel

The channel relates to the bladder itself and the problems associated with it—for example, urinary problems including incontinence and urinary retention. Thanks to the connection with the protrusions of the nerves from the spinal cord, it has an impact on all organs. In connection with the kidneys, it also has an effect on bone diseases including osteoporosis, some forms of arthritis, tooth decay, premature hair loss or graying, hearing loss and dizziness, lower back pain and weakness, and so on. No other channel has such a large number of acupuncture points through which it is possible to influence other channels and organs. Therefore, it is one of the most important channels of the body. At the mental level, it affects the ability to accurately perceive reality, the ability to integrate experiences and the will to live.

BLADDER CHANNEL IN MOVEMENT

Due to the length of this pathway and the number of areas of the body through which it passes, the channel offers us many possibilities for movement improvisation. As it passes along the spine, working with it has a significant effect on the entire paravertebral system and the nervous system. In movement, we can focus on working with the spine through various waving or flowing movements, imitating, for example, the movement of a snake or seaweed floating in gently moving water. We can even work specifically with the image of wakame seaweed which also resembles the shape of the spine. The gentle undulating movement of the spine from side to side helps to increase the spaces between the vertebrae, which revitalizes the vertebrae and intervertebral discs. It is advisable to rub the sacrum well with the palms, which will pleasantly warm it up.

Movement using the flow of Qi in this channel also affects the brain. It is an excellent stimulant. We can also involve the eyes, where the channel begins. We can either guide the movement with our eyes or we can actively observe everything around us as we move around the space. For movement improvisation, it is very interesting to connect the eyes with the little toes on the feet, where the channel ends. This way of using the channel in motion helps to realize the relationship between the eyes and the feet, between sight and walking. When we work with both ends of this channel at the same time, Qi is activated evenly throughout this long segment. Working with this channel in movement also helps to engage the back thigh muscles. We usually forget about these muscles in everyday life, which causes their permanent withdrawal. Activating Qi in these areas of the thigh during movement is a good way to pleasantly fill them with new fresh Qi. The result will be better elasticity.

The same applies to the back of the knees and the Achilles tendons. The Bladder channel is part of the chain of muscles that connect the Achilles tendons with the muscles of the thighs and spine. This chain is bound to the back of the skull. Working with it therefore affects the condition of the Achilles tendon, but also vice versa—the condition of the Achilles tendon will affect other segments of this chain, including the muscles of the back and the entire Bladder channel.

Let's also enjoy the connection of the Yang charge of the channel, advancing from top to bottom, with the Yin charge of the Earth.

KIDNEY CHANNEL (KI)/YIN

The Kidney channel is a Yin pair pathway that runs along the right and left sides of the body, from bottom to top. In the image below, only one side is shown. Qi from the Bladder channel flows into it in the foot, where this channel originates—specifically, in the middle of the foot at a point called the *Gushing Spring* (*Yongquan*), KI1. It is a strong energetic place of connection of our body to the Earth's Qi. At this point, we receive the Earth's Qi and transfer it to the lower abdomen, where we store it in the Lower Dantian. Qi then emerges internally to the groin. It enters the body, passes through the genitals and pours over the pubic bone into the Penetrating Vessel, one of the extraordinary channels. It passes through the entire torso and ends under the collarbones, right next to their articular connections to the sternum. Its main branch has 27 acupuncture points. In the trunk, it connects with its inner branches with the kidneys themselves, the lower part of the spine and the bladder. It protrudes through the diaphragm, liver and heart, and ends at the root of the tongue. In the area of the torso, it connects to the Pericardium channel. Dashed lines indicate internal deep branches.

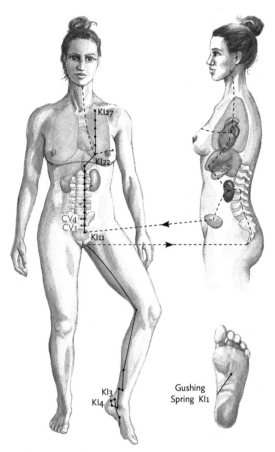

Kidney channel

The channel affects all kidney diseases, hormonal and endocrine disorders, all sexual problems, fertility disorders, disorders of normal physical development, growth disorders, the onset of puberty, premature ageing. It is also associated with chronic fatigue, exhaustion, fluid retention, water management disorders, hearing and balance disorders, increased tendency to injuries, brittle bones, tooth decay, feelings of cold or lower back pain, congenital and hereditary diseases. It acts as a filter for separating waste products from blood into the urine. It also has a relationship with the endocrine glands. At the mental level, it affects the handling of fear, the strength and harmonization of the will, the ability to progress in life, self-understanding, the ability to reach the wisdom of life and the ability to get things done.

KIDNEY CHANNEL IN MOVEMENT

This channel is not as dynamic as the Bladder channel. This is natural because it is located in the inner parts of the body and needs silence, calmness and Yin. However, it offers a deeper immersion in this Yin quality of Qi, but also a connection to the Qi of the Earth.

The channel itself requires calmer and slower movements. In movement improvisation, we use the inner sides of the lower limbs. We do not normally involve them much in motion, but when we consciously involve them, they repay us with a deeper feeling. If the movement comes from the inside of the feet, calves, knees and thighs, these areas will be filled with new Qi. At the same time, we will feel the entire lower limbs evenly nourished with fresh Qi. We can feel a smooth connection of the Qi of the lower limbs with the Qi of the torso. This will also help us to ground more consciously and deeply.

Due to this grounding aspect, we will, of course, also work with the feet, with the very source of the Kidney channel. Even in a static position, if we bring our awareness to the first points of the Kidney channel, the Gushing Spring, we will find these points really gush and bubble. We will perceive the ascending flow from the Earth upwards into our body through this channel. At the same time, our feet will open to the Earth and we will be able to root down in the Earth.

However, these roots have their source in the area of the Lower Dantian. When we connect the feet with the Qi of the Lower Dantian, we are like a massive tree. We can begin to use this physical sensation even when walking. We start with a very slow walk, which we can gradually accelerate. Even if the feet are physically disconnected from the Earth as we walk, our energy roots remain actively connected to the Earth.

Working with the Kidney channel in the Lower Dantian area also affects the uterus in women. Movement from the Lower Dantian is very vitalizing for this organ. In addition, if we draw the movement of Qi up the middle line of the body, the one that is most connected to our core, we will feel pleasant pulsations in the middle of the body. However, at the end, Qi must be sent back into the Lower Dantian, so that it does not get lost or scattered, or ascend excessively to the head area.

There are other interesting areas for movement in the torso area from which we can guide the movement of the whole body, or we can let the movement result there. These are the pubic bone, navel, sternum and sternoclavicular joints, which are those more raised joints under the neck connecting the inner ends of the collarbones with the sternum.

DIET IN WINTER AND FOR THE WATER PHASE ORGANS

Winter is a period of significant Yin energy. One needs more rest and peace in this season than in any other season. Therefore, the diet should also be simpler and should not contain extremes. Preparation should be simple, with an emphasis on protecting our internal organs from the cold. Therefore, it is advisable to limit raw vegetables, because they cool us internally. Raw fruit has the same cooling effect, so in winter it is better to consume it in a slightly stewed form, with cinnamon, cloves or star anise. We should mainly consume food from our latitude. If we do not live in tropical countries, we should avoid tropical fruit and fruit juices from them, because this fruit grows in the tropics and has a cooling effect. Raw vegetable juices and smoothies also have a cooling effect, so it is better to avoid them in winter. The priority should be long- and slow-cooked food to get the necessary amount of Yang that will warm and protect us at the same time.

Generally, cooking time should be long, definitely longer than in summer or late spring. Slow-cooked thick soups containing legumes are ideal. Soups containing root vegetables add natural sweetness and give the body a significant internal warmth. In winter, we can use a pressure cooker more than usual to prepare meals. Pressure cooking increases Yang through longer boiling and pressure in turn gives the body more Yang. We can also prepare our meals by stir-frying in a wok. Sunflower oil is more suitable because coconut fat and olive oil cool down. Don't worry about preparing meals using fat—in moderation, of course. We can get rid of the excess fat by cleansing in the spring. Consumption of seaweeds is also advisable for their rich mineral content. But do not use them so often, because they have a cooling effect on the body.

Root vegetables
Root vegetables (carrots, parsnip, celery, etc.) give us the necessary Qi. In addition to root vegetables, we can also include green leafy vegetables, and there should be no lack of fermented vegetables. Classic sauerkraut is advisable, and also other simple types of pickled vegetables. A more

complex pickling is kimchi (kimchee), originating in Korea, where not only vegetables but also rice, apple, ginger, seaweed, sesame seeds and shiitake mushrooms ferment together. Kimchi is considered one of the healthiest dishes, and in winter it is extremely suitable. When the vegetable is pickled, it is no longer raw; it has undergone a strong fermentation process which increases the Yang of the food, preserves all the vitamins and additionally supplies it with many enzymes.

Cereals

Cereals such as barley, wheat, rice and ideally natural rice are suitable in this period. Grains can also be cooked in a pressure cooker, ideally with kombu seaweed for its mineral content. It is advisable to consume pearl barley (*hatomugi*), because in winter people often have problems with inflammation of the bladder due to moisture. Pearl barley helps to eliminate moisture.

Legumes

Beans are ideal, especially adzuki, "kidney" beans, black beans, but also other legumes are suitable for the supply of protein. We choose the darker ones from other legumes, because the WATER phase includes dark color—brown lentils, dark beluga lentils, dark beans, etc.

Mushrooms

Mushrooms that support the kidneys are whole white mushrooms and shiitake. In addition, shiitake significantly supports immunity, and it is advised that they are consumed together with gelatin to solve joint problems. Chanterelle mushrooms or black trumpet mushrooms are excellent too. A risotto made of them is amazing.

Seed oils

All seeds and nuts are suitable, but kidney Qi is most complemented by black sesame. Walnuts support thinking and memory, because they have a strong effect on the brain, which also depends on the condition of the kidneys. It is also appropriate to use ginkgo biloba leaves to support brain activity, thinking during studying, etc. Very tasty and tonifying nuts for the kidneys are cashews. They are excellent as a base spread, cake filling, roasted in a pan with herbs or sprinkled with soy sauce.

Meat

Beef and beef broths with bones are also advisable for warming up the body. Broths with warming ingredients can be cooked for up to five to eight hours. Chicken soup is also excellent for this period. To support hematopoiesis and bone marrow, cut the chicken bones about halfway through the boiling of such a broth so that the bone essence boils into the broth. The bone marrow from a young grass-fed bull is also an excellent booster for the body. The calf-bone of such a bull, together with the marrow, is a potent tonic for the kidneys. This can be consumed after an illness and it is especially suitable for the elderly. Cook well for five hours.

Other advice

Add garlic, ginger or a shot of ginger and heating spices to meals—but not daily or in excess. When cold from the outside enters the body, sharp flavors are suitable for expelling cold, but otherwise we should handle them wisely, because a sharp taste opens pores, allowing wind and cold to easily penetrate the body.

Do not burden the kidneys in the morning with coffee or black tea on an empty stomach. It exhausts them!

It is advisable to drink a glass of lukewarm or warmer boiled water on an empty stomach. A bit of lemon squeezed in it will support digestion. Kukicha tea, which helps to de-acidify the body, with lemon or a teaspoon of soy sauce, is excellent. Sometimes we can also have ginger tea with honey, especially if we need to warm up. Grain coffee can be a substitute for classic coffee.

Cereal coffee is not only a good substitute for coffee, but due to its effect on our digestion, it is also a suitable medicine. More information about cereal coffee can be found in the section on diet for the summer, in Chapter 10 on the FIRE phase.

It is important to protect the internal organs from the cold, both inside and out!

Breakfast should be warm and cooked, such as porridge and soups. We can also try salted porridge, for example with soy sauce or cooked in vegetable broth with blanched vegetables. You can find several recipes in Chapter 11 on the EARTH phase.

If we suffer from the cold, we should omit green tea and mineral water, because they have a cooling effect. For the same reason, we do not consume chlorella or spirulina algae in winter, as they also cool us down. If you need to use them for another reason, because their positives attributes are many, do not forget to warm the body by adding heating spices and cooking for longer.

Strongly warming food

- **Meat:** mutton, lamb, goat, all kinds of grilled meat.
- **Spices:** cayenne pepper, chili, curry, ginger, garlic, pepper, fresh pepper.
- **Other:** blue cheese.
- **Drinks:** high percentage alcohol, yogi tea, mulled wine.

Warming food

- **Common dried herbs:** oregano, basil, satureja (savory), marjoram, red pepper, thyme, juniper, nutmeg, coriander, bay leaf, rosemary, chives, and also turmeric, masala, cocoa, poppy.
- **Vegetables:** Hokkaido pumpkin, fennel, sweet potatoes, raw and fried onions, brussels sprouts, spring onions, horseradish, leeks.
- **Cereals:** sweet rice, oats.
- **Fruits:** pomegranate, plum.
- **Drinks:** rice wine (sake).
- **Meat of the following animals:** chicken, pheasant, roe deer, wild hare, wild boar as well as ham, smoked meat, dried meat.
- **Fish and seafood:** eel, shrimp, prawns, lobster, cod, crawfish, tuna, plaice, smoked fish.

We can compensate for the lack of movement in the winter by consuming the so-called winter spices in tea or mulled wine—for example, yogi, ginger, cinnamon, chili, curry. They support the movement of Qi, which is slower in winter.

Drinking regime

Sufficient fluids are important at all times, although in winter, due to the cold weather, you need to drink less compared to summer. Excess fluid burdens the kidneys; with excessive drinking, the kidneys can even lose more minerals than they gain. So the need for fluids also depends on the composition of the diet and on how much exercise and subsequent sweat we expend. If we consume a lot of food that is dry, such as bread, biscuits or dried fruit, the need for fluids is greater. If we have soup and porridge, which are more liquid, on the menu every day, we do not have to drink in large quantities. The best indicator of whether we have enough fluids is the color of our urine: if it is pale, we drink excessively; if it is dark, our drinking regime is insufficient.

In winter, Japanese Kukicha tea is good to drink (see recipe below). It contains almost no caffeine, so it is also suitable for children. It has an alkalizing effect, thus strengthening the quality of the blood, and this in turn helps to strengthen and refresh us when we are tired. In other seasons throughout the year, bancha tea is suitable for daily consumption. However, pure spring water is the best. When it is boiled and prepared in a thermos for drinking throughout the day, it is an actual medicine.

Salt

The taste typical for the WATER phase is salty, so for the supply of Yang, we can salt a little more in winter than in other seasons. However, avoid consuming industrially produced salt and sodium glutamate. It is important to note that even sprinkling sea salt on already cooked food is not advisable. Adding salt to food directly on a plate is too aggressive for the blood. This way of adding salt to food allows the salt to dissolve very quickly and the reactions to this are not beneficial to the body. To add the salt flavor, it is preferable to use soy sauce (shoyu, tamari), miso paste or sesame salt gomashio (see recipe below). Salt and the salty taste can also be supplemented with miso paste and good-quality soy sauce, which also contains many enzymes. It is not advisable to cook with these sauces because boiling would kill the enzymes. Seaweed, white fish or seafood can also add salt to our meals. Sea salt should go through the boiling process, so we can add it to the meal about halfway through the cooking process, not after cooking. When cooking legumes, do not add salt at the beginning of cooking, because the salt would shrink the beans and close their surface, and we would have to cook them much longer.

Salt moisturizes, softens and dissolves blockages. It has laxative effects and helps to unblock mucus. It supports the kidneys in a reasonable amount, but damages them in sudden excess. Naturally salty food is appropriate—choose a slightly salty taste, but not overly salted foods. Excessive salt weakens the kidneys. Large amounts of salt are also found in low-quality cheeses, smoked and other semi-cooked products. Their insufficient taste is covered by an excessive amount of salt. Excess salt behaves the opposite way in the body—instead of softening, it shrinks and dries. This can lead to bone demineralization over time. In chronic excess, it damages the heart and increases blood pressure. A large amount of salty food causes blood to clot in the blood vessels and manifests itself in dull skin without luster. Excessive amounts of salt can also manifest in the mental sphere, causing withdrawal, irritability and emotional tension.

It should be pointed out that currently all industrially produced food is salted. However, if we consume one boiled parsnip a day, sliced and boiled in a little water for about ten minutes, we will significantly help the kidneys. It is best to eat it at 5 p.m., when it is kidney time according to the organ clock.

Seaweed

This sea vegetable is a rich source of minerals: calcium, phosphorus, magnesium, iron, iodine and sodium, and also a suitable supplier of vitamins A, B1, B12 and C. Seaweed also contains easily digestible proteins. Thanks to their mineral content, they balance the acidic effect of modern foods, thus creating a suitable alkaline blood quality for the body. They help to dissolve fat and mucus deposits that have been formed by excessive consumption of meat, dairy products and sugar. The most used include kombu, wakame, hijiki, nori and agar-agar.

Miso

Soy miso paste is a specialty of Japanese cuisine. It is excellent for creating a state of homeostasis. It is a fermented ripening soy puree, containing live bacteria and enzymes. It is helpful for healthy digestion and contains good bacteria that break down protein. It has well-balanced essential oils and vitamins and is alkaline. It also helps restore villi in the intestines; for this reason, it is advisable to consume it in larger quantities after treatment with antibiotics. There are several types of miso: soy miso, rice miso and barley miso. Do not cook miso! Cooking would degrade the enzymes in it, and therefore it is added to food only after it has been cooked. If heating the food afterwards, make sure that it does not boil. It is ideal to buy it only in glass jars because it usually tends to be pasteurized when packed in plastic bags. We also do not cook shoyu or tamari soy sauce, which are also full of enzymes obtained by fermentation that would be killed by boiling.

A FEW TIPS AND RECIPES

Broth from four sweet vegetables to strengthen the kidneys

Ingredients: Equal amounts of carrots, onions, cabbage and Hokkaido pumpkin; water, salt.

Method: Peel carrots and onions and cut them into pieces. Cut the cabbage and pumpkin too. Place all the cut vegetables in a sufficient amount of water in a large pot and boil for 20 minutes. Add salt and boil for another 20 minutes. Strain and drink this broth warm throughout the day.

Benefits: The broth warms from the inside, strengthens the kidneys and spleen.

Calcium supplement and kidney-strengthening formula

Ingredients: Black sesame and grated coconut in a 1:1 ratio.

Method: Roast both ingredients separately, then mix and eat 2 teaspoons every morning.

Benefits: This formula supplements calcium and strengthens kidneys.

Adzuki bean broth

Ingredients: ½ cup of adzuki beans, 5 cm kombu seaweed, 2½ cups water.

Method: Place the beans and the seaweed in unsalted water and bring to the boil; reduce the heat and simmer under a lid. Some of the water will evaporate, so add more water. Do not stir. Cook for about an hour until softened. Drink the broth as a beverage and eat the beans at the end, or add them to another other dish. You can add a pinch of sea salt, gomashio or soy sauce. Do not cook in a pressure cooker.

Benefits: Adzuki and kombu support urine production and strengthen the kidneys.

Sesame salt gomashio

Ingredients: Sesame seeds and sea salt in a ratio of 18:1.

Method: Roast the seeds and grind them in a suribashi bowl. This is a special bowl with indentations and a wooden stirring stick. Approximately 80 percent of the seeds should be crushed and 20 percent left whole. Roast the salt in a pan; while still warm, grind it in with the seeds to mix it in. Keep in the fridge. A well-made gomashio will last up to three weeks.

The ratio can also be 14:1 or 22:1 depending on the season and the person's condition. Children and the elderly should consume less salty gomashio.

Benefits: Gomashio neutralizes acids in the blood, thus relieving fatigue, nourishes and strengthens the nervous system, creates a stable ratio of Yin and Yang in the body and thus strengthens immunity. It can be consumed for morning pregnancy nausea or kidney problems. Daily consumption of 1 teaspoon of gomashio strengthens the body and helps to prevent diseases. It is ideal to consume it sprinkled on grains.

Kukicha tea

Ingredients: Kukicha tea, water.

Method: Kukicha needs to be boiled for at least 10 minutes. Put a handful of the tea in 1.5 liters of cold water, bring to a boil and let it simmer.

Benefits: Kukicha tea has an alkalizing effect, thereby strengthening the quality of the blood, and this in turn helps to strengthen and refresh when tired. It supports the kidneys—it is great for kidney inflammation and bladder infections. It calms, so it is suitable to drink before bedtime. It also soothes the digestive tract in gastritis and nausea, boosting vitality.

Miso soup for breakfast—basic recipe

Ingredients: Miso paste, water, kombu seaweed, shiitake mushrooms, onion or leek, greens and root vegetables (carrots, parsnip, celery, Hokkaido pumpkin, kohlrabi, cauliflower, broccoli, etc.), or some pre-cooked legumes.

Method: Soak a 6 cm long piece of kombu seaweed and dried shiitake mushrooms overnight. In the morning, take them out of the water, chop them and boil them for about 10–15 minutes. In the meantime, prepare any vegetables you have and cut them into equal-sized pieces. After the kombu and shiitake have boiled for 10–15 minutes, add the vegetables to the broth and cook for about 10 more minutes. Break the broccoli or cauliflower into small florets. Add them after the root vegetables; you can even add them at the end of cooking so that they are only slightly warmed, retaining their freshness and crunch. Once cooked, leave to cool. Meanwhile, dissolve 1 teaspoon of miso paste by stirring it in a small glass of cold water, then pour into the broth with the vegetables, gently stirring in.

If you have some pre-cooked legumes or cereals, add them too. You can also add some sprouts—for example, mungo beans or alfalfa. This soup has the greatest effect when fresh. If we want to reheat it, we should never bring it to a boil again, because boiling would kill the enzymes contained in the miso paste. If you do not have seaweed or shiitake, you can still make a good miso soup without them.

Benefits: The soup gives a pleasant start to the day, replenishes the life force, imparts a strong will to live, supplements glucose. In winter, it protects against cold, wind and damp, regulates the metabolism (burping, flatulence), supplies enzymes, nourishes the skin and blood (thus the skin cells get what they need), dissolves cholesterol in the arteries, veins, blood vessels and capillaries.

To replenish and restore energy, it is advisable to eat warm miso soup for breakfast throughout the week.

Koikoku—Japanese carp soup

Ingredients: Fresh carp (without bile but otherwise whole), equal weight of burdock root or carrots, cup of Kukicha twig tea, bancha tea, miso paste, ginger juice, onion.

Method: Cut the whole fish, including the bones and scales, into slices 5–7½ cm wide. You can take out the eyes if you do not want to cook them. Cut the same amount of burdock or carrots into thin strips. Put everything in a pressure cooker. Put the kukicha twigs in a thin linen bag and boil separately for a short time. Place the bag on top of the fish and vegetables in the pressure cooker, add enough liquid to cover the fish and vegetables, in a ratio of about one-third bancha tea and two-thirds water, and cook for about 1½ hours. The twigs of Kukicha tea will help everything to cook to mush, including the bones. Once cooked, remove the bag with twigs and blend the soup; if there are any solid larger bones left, remove them. Dilute with bancha tea as needed.

Add diluted miso paste to taste, but do not cook any further so that the enzymes of the miso do not degrade. Finally, add the juice of a small amount of grated ginger and garnish with chopped spring onions or herbs. Serve warm.

Benefits: It replenishes the essence of Jing, nourishes the blood and body fluids.

Delicious winter hen broth

Ingredients: Hen (ideally fresh, unfrozen), water, onion, root vegetables, ginger, Chinese blend of herbs, mushrooms and roots to replenish Qi: ginseng, lotus seeds, jujube, white jelly mushroom (*Tremella fuciformis—paj mu er*), goji, black sesame, *Angelica sinensis* root.

Method: Boil the hen in a large pot all submerged in water for about 3–4 hours. Halfway through boiling, add 2–3 large onions, quartered, chopped ginger and the herb mixture. Place the herbs in a cooking bag or large resealable herb strainer. Strain the broth. Add and cook the root vegetables for 20 minutes in this clear broth, adding salt in the last 10 minutes before the end.

Benefits: The soup nourishes Qi and blood, warms the stomach and spleen, thus supporting digestion. It replenishes the Jing essence in the kidneys, has a beneficial effect on the psyche and warms pleasantly in winter.

Recipe for regeneration of broken bones or worn-out cartilage

Ingredients: Six free-range organic eggs, 200 ml honey, juice of about 10 lemons, 200 ml cognac.

Method: Place the whole eggs in a glass jar. Pour enough lemon juice over the eggs to cover them. Leave to infuse for one week. The egg shells should dissolve, leaving only a soft membrane. Carefully remove the white and yolk, discarding the membrane, and strain through a sieve. Add honey and cognac and take 20 ml two times a day. Surprisingly, it tastes very good!

Benefits: This remedy replenishes the Jing essence in the kidneys and nourishes the bones.

CHAPTER 9

The WOOD phase

The ability to pass through and the elasticity of the human body and mind

About: creativity and vision / the liver and its ability to pass through / tendons, ligaments and bodily integrity / flexibility of the body and psyche / anger and the need to change what is dysfunctional / the gallbladder and its help in decision making / the ability to rest / wind and mobility / the eyes and the ability to see / diet for spring and for the WOOD phase organs

Humans are by nature created as very active and creative beings, ready to deliver a certain performance. At the same time, they are beings who desire to be able to express their activity and creativity in a concrete way, thus fulfilling their mission. In each of us sleeps an "atomic bomb of creativity" and that creativity wants to manifest itself—it wants to "flow." To do this, it needs an unobstructed path so that the flow can go its way. If creative beings are to maintain physical and mental health, they should carry out their ideas and the possibilities that are in them. If this does not happen, there is tension. The main topics of this chapter are the ability to pass through, smooth flow, performance, realization, flexibility, activity, imagination, creativity, growth and patience. It may occur to few people that all of this has to do with the organ under our right ribs—the liver and its functional circuit. The liver is the main organ of the WOOD phase, and it is responsible for our creativity and ability to realize it.

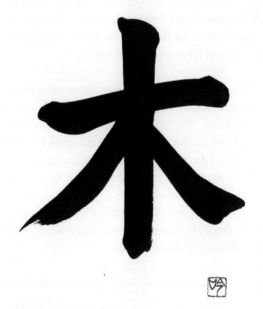

Chinese character for WOOD

Functional circuit of the liver: liver, gallbladder, tendons, ligaments, fascia, nails, eyes, eyesight, tears, bile, the Ethereal Soul Hun, emotion of anger and the need to break what is stagnant, flexibility of the body and mind, kindness.

THE wood PHASE AND SPRING WITH EVERYTHING THAT NEEDS TO MANIFEST

We will approach the "atomic bomb of creativity" with the example of the spring season. What happens in the spring never happens at such an intensity again during the year. After a long hibernation, everything in nature needs to manifest, revive, show itself—it needs to "explode." Everything grows at an incredible speed; everything blooms, smells, buzzes. The Qi of the Earth realizes its compulsive need for presentation and growth right in front of our eyes. It is a time when Qi, which was resting in the winter, is deployed with new strength. A force that is flexible and can overcome obstacles. If something stands in the way of the plant, it is able to twist in all sorts of ways, just to direct its Qi, its growth and development towards the sun. This is typical for the Qi of the wood phase; it is also typical for the energy of spring.

> *The three months of the spring season bring about the revitalization of all things in nature. It is time of birth. This is when Heaven and Earth are reborn. During this season it is advisable to retire early. Arise early also and go walking in order to absorb the fresh, invigorating energy. Since this is the season in which universal Qi begins anew and rejuvenates, one should attempt to correspond to it directly by being open and unsuppressed, both physically and emotionally.*

> THE YELLOW EMPEROR'S CLASSIC OF MEDICINE

Under the term wood, one should imagine living wood, a living tree that is strong but also flexible. It constantly longs for growth, which takes place continuously throughout the year, but intensively in the spring. The Qi of the wood phase is the life force that springs from the existence of the water phase. The forces that lay in the quiet darkness of winter (the water phase) are striving for their development. It is time for birth. In the human context, therefore, the wood phase is associated with our birth and the first period of our lives. It is childhood, our rapid early development, our urgent need to learn everything new, to try everything on our own, alone and straightaway. Therefore, the spring and the Qi of the wood phase are not only associated with the growth around us, but also the growth within us. However, this Qi accompanies us throughout our lives. It is our pursuit of sustainable development. Like a tree, we never stop growing throughout our life. This phase is therefore primarily associated with movement, motivation, development and the harmonious flow of life. If something stands in the way of this penetration, there is anger, annoyance, wrath, rage—emotions that try to break through obstacles.

AN EMOTION THAT BREAKS THROUGH

The emotion of anger is associated with the wood phase. In Chinese, they use term *Nù*. However, like many terms that come from Chinese thinking, Nù cannot be simply put into the one word of *anger*. Rather, it is a matter of *moving against*, a kind of *breaking through obstacles, breaking what is restrictive*, or even *moving against gravity*. This is the beginning of every new life and every new idea. The beginnings are difficult, accompanied by the limitation of common things—our own attitudes or the attitudes of the environment. Nù contains energy that can break through, so it can change. One change triggers a chain reaction of other changes, which most people perceive as a problem, and a force supported by the energy of WOOD is needed to handle this process. If it is held back, it transforms into a sense of anger and rage which seem to be the driving forces for breaking through obstacles. Around the second or third year of life, when we, as children, begin to become aware of ourselves, this is when the Qi of WOOD awakens very strongly. It really is a force! We research, expand, grow, and the problem begins when something stands in our way. Periods of defiance must be seen as part of this natural process, and boundaries must be created sensitively, albeit thoroughly. And it is Nù that is also characteristic of the liver and its entire functional circuit, and especially in the area of the psyche. We will clarify this more in the following lines.

LIVER, THE ABILITY TO PASS THROUGH, MOVEMENT AND THE REALIZATION OF OUR CREATIVITY

This piercing of the strong ability of Nù is inherent in the liver itself. The liver (in Chinese, *Gan*) is a relatively large organ with an even greater list of functions. It is located under the right lower ribs. It is anatomically connected to the digestive tract. The liver produces bile, which through the bile system goes from the liver into the small intestine through its first section—the duodenum—where it participates in the absorption and digestion of fats and fat-soluble vitamins (A, D, E, K). The liver thus provides complex metabolic functions such as the processing of simple sugars into complex sugars—the storehouse of our energy, glycogen. Most plasma proteins are produced and dissolved in the liver, and cholesterol and other fats are made in it; fats also decompose here; excess cholesterol is broken down into bile acids and excreted in the bile. The liver also has thermoregulatory functions, produces a large amount of heat, stores blood, glycogen, vitamins A, D, B12, and also metals—iron, copper and cobalt. It is associated with bilirubin, a waste product of the red blood pigment metabolism produced by the liver from extinct red blood cells. It also has a great influence on the detoxification of the body; it is in charge of the metabolism of alcohol, drugs and toxic substances.

The above is a list based on observations of Western medicine. However, few in the West would have thought that the liver is related to the well-being of our entire system, its physical as well as its mental side. In the Taoist context, we are talking about its Qi rather than the organ itself. The Taoists have observed that liver Qi is responsible for the flow of the Qi in the body. In the terminology of Chinese medicine, this task is called drainage and dispersion. Everything that has to move in the body, to flow, to fluctuate, to get into place, to nourish, etc., is under the administration of liver Qi. These are the movements of Qi in and between organs, the circulation of Qi in the meridians, the flow of blood in blood vessels, the movement of lymph, but also the routes of food in the digestive tract, the flow of body fluids and sufficient distribution of Defensive Qi, etc. It all depends on the even movement up and down, in and out, and the liver makes way for this by removing various obstructions. Our balanced digestion, regulation of bile secretion and excretion, regular breathing, fluid metabolism and regulation of menstrual blood depend on the quality of liver function. But also the ability to rest, and hence the ability to balance the state of tension and the state of relaxation. In this context, the liver is also in charge of regulating mental and emotional activities—the smooth flow of mental functions and emotions. Therefore, if people have harmonious liver Qi, nothing drives them mad very easily; on the contrary, they can express their disagreements in a moderate and clear way.

The big role of the liver is to let our emotions flow. Anger has a purpose in our lives. In its positive way, it is the driving force for change. It is therefore a question of the extent to which it manifests itself—whether its intensity will bring positive change or destroy, disrupt or block. To condemn anger does not help; it is more important to understand the intensity of anger and direct it. Anger occurs in the absence of the main virtues that form the healthy Qi of the WOOD phase in humans and are formed by WOOD Qi. These are kindness, benevolence, goodwill and compassion which are cultivated by harmonizing Qi in the liver itself.

However, in life, not everything we want and need to accomplish can actually be accomplished. In principle, two things tend to stand in our way—external circumstances and internal settings. A person has a plan, a certain idea, but the social environment does not always allow him or her to implement it. These are the external circumstances that we encounter in the profession of any mover. In order to accomplish our creative plans, we must overcome a mountain of obstacles. Since our work is often at the edge of the overall social interest, we must dig the path to its realization ourselves. We use a lot of effort to find space, money, systems, spectators, continuity and recognition for our work. It is possible, but not endlessly. If the obstacles are too great, or if it takes too long to overcome them, frustration and exhaustion occur. The result is that we are looking for other jobs, and talented artists often deliver pizza or sit in offices. From the point of view of Chinese medicine, this is quite a dangerous condition—a condition that a person cannot tolerate for a long time because one cannot accept the situation internally, which can eventually lead to illness. We can develop mental, psychosomatic but also organ diseases.

However, a person's internal setting is equally decisive. The smooth flow of emotions, the smooth flow of our inner happenings and accomplishment are ensured by the harmonious state of liver Qi. The state of Qi in our liver has formed throughout our lives, but the most decisive are the first years of life. The anger suppressed from childhood can develop into self-destruction; it can turn against us. The way of parenting as well as school education could, to a large extent, suppress our self-confidence. This can cause total mistrust in our abilities, and even the greatest talent can be blocked because of being afraid to manifest. Such stress inside must have some outlet. And so we can find ourselves at two extremes—either we tend to give up, let go of our plans and choose an easier way without realizing our own mission or we want to break through excessively, and this can result in compulsive tendencies to do everything at all costs. This condition is often accompanied by a tendency to explode quickly, because it pushes us excessively and we need to burst through. This also brings workaholism and the inability to switch off, to stop. These are the main psychic manifestations of disharmonious liver Qi. This condition also brings injuries. Injuries can break something with their energy, disrupt the routine, but on the other hand, and paradoxically, they hinder the realization again. In both cases, the smooth flow is blocked in us, resulting in frustration.

In harmonious liver Qi, the flow is smooth, and we are able to register what is possible and what is not. Harmonious internal adjustment can help us to perceive the correct timing. It is about accepting that not everything is supposed to happen right now. This is inner peace, acceptance and forgiveness. The Qi that we can turn into an activity while maintaining its flexibility is healthy Qi. And patience is also about flexibility.

THE HUN—THE ETHEREAL SOUL AND THE MENTAL WORLD

In Chapter 5, we mentioned various psychospiritual essences that reside in certain organs. The liver is the residence of the *Ethereal Soul Hun*. The Hun is the movement of our psyche in many directions—the movement of the soul out of the body in a dream, the movement towards other people and building relationships with them, the movement of the psyche related to our plans, projects, ideas, life dreams, creativity. It is decisive for our creativity; it represents the mental and spiritual world.

The Hun has a Yang nature, and its basic characteristic is penetration; it constantly invites us to move, to seek, to travel, to discover and to learn. This is generally typical of WOOD phase Qi. Thanks to it, we are full of visions and ideas that float out into our consciousness. When we create a work, our Hun is 100 percent part of this process. It brings us inspiration, creative ideas, sometimes very crazy ideas outside of reality, but also childish enthusiasm and the strength to implement them. In essence, the Hun is another degree of consciousness, the aspect of our soul that is most connected to the immaterial world. It does not hold much rational consciousness; it is more connected with intuition, impulsions, inspiration. Therefore, it is also associated with sleep and dreams. It takes care of our sleep, mainly because it is an opportunity for it to travel through a dream outside of ordinary reality. The Hun is therefore responsible for sleeping with a normal number of dreams. If it is oversized, we dream more than necessary because it does not want to get back to reality. However, it is also connected with our dreams in the waking state—that is, with what attracts us, visions that we would like to realize in everyday life. And it is the Hun that has the force that encourages us to go for our visions and accomplish them.

The Hun can be activated very quickly and dangerously when using drugs, albeit soft drugs. That is why people are more creative then, and the ideas that are produced then would be harder to find in the normal state. However, the need of the Hun to constantly travel and get into a different kind of perception is reaching the edge here. Yes, it wants to transport us to different worlds or dimensions, it wants to shape our elusive mental and spiritual world. But in order for our soul not to be lost in its unrestraint, yet be able to ground itself, it is influenced in our mental and spiritual world by other components of our soul, other psychospiritual essences that give it order and control and integrate its impulses into the mind. This role is performed mainly by the Shen Spirit, which resides in the heart, and by the Corporeal Soul Po, which is stored in the lungs. We will read more about them in the next chapters. A balance between them is essential for mental and spiritual health.

Thus, overall, the Hun creates space for us to grow, constantly learn and evolve. When we allow this natural WOOD Qi to grow, from this height, we are able to see into the distance, to observe, to look around. This opens up the ability to plan things for the future, hence into the distance, but it also cultivates our foresight. Without this ability, we would never be able to move from one place. If one has weakened WOOD Qi, they get used to standing still, cannot see ahead, plan or get excited about ideas—they stagnate. However, to realize ideas and plans, the liver needs the ability to implement them. Its strong partner here is its paired organ—the gallbladder.

THE GALLBLADDER MAKES DECISIONS

The gallbladder (in Chinese, *Dan*) is the partner Yang organ of the liver. Together, they are involved in the transport of bile to the digestive tract, but also in the smooth flow of Qi in the body. The channels of the liver and gallbladder are directly connected. There are several acupuncture points in the Gallbladder channel that help unblock liver Qi. In the old texts, the gallbladder is referred to as a *reliable faithful helper of the emperor* (heart), an *official of justice*, but the gallbladder also makes decisions. How to understand it? The gallbladder Qi helps to manage and control our judgment, estimation, balance, opinions and how we will enforce them; how we will accept other opinions, how to defend ourselves against new opinions. It controls what kind of decisions we make, gives energy and vigor to our actions. It provides the resilient strength of an imaginary tree, and thus the ability to orientate oneself in situations and make decisions accordingly. The gallbladder needs information from the liver, but also enough quietness to be able to consider all decisions. It is the organ which, with its Qi, either allows us or does not allow us to implement ideas. The unfettered liver brings plans and ideas; the gallbladder decides which of them to submit for approval to the emperor—the heart. To some extent, this brings security and trust to a person. At the same time, thanks to the gallbladder Qi, one is able to react more flexibly to unexpected situations by being able to get the most out of everything. The gallbladder Qi is also reflected in how flexibly and dynamically we can deal with our commitments, but also with our decisions. It also influences decisions regarding job offers.

Connecting gallbladder Qi to decision making also plays an important role in our practice of improvisation. Many movers practice improvisation in the form of performance. In fact, decision-making moments occur almost continuously in improvisation. When we learn to improvise, we are learning to make good decisions about when and how to enter the improvisation, what to do in the given moment, when to leave the improvisation and so on. Certainly, the ability to connect to the present moment plays an important role there, but decision making is the key. The gallbladder Qi is activated during improvisation and the ability to make the right decision depends on it as well.

MOVEMENT OF THE WIND

The wind is the most mobile of all the weather factors, so it naturally belongs to the WOOD phase and can easily distress the WOOD organs. The wind appears in every season, but it is the spring that uses it the most for spring cleaning. Without debate, it takes away everything that is not necessary, what is already weak and faded, which the winter has eliminated. As a weather element, the wind is very dangerous for us; it can attack us quickly, get under our skin and thus weaken our immunity. It is light and tends to rise; it is mobile and extremely variable. Taoists advise us to avoid the wind. One of the unfortunate features of the wind is that it enables the penetration of all other climatic injuries into the body. If the wind blows and it is cold, a big dose of cold enters the body with the wind. Conversely, if the wind blows and there is extreme heat, the extreme heat enters the body with this wind.

The way the wind penetrates the body from the outside is, of course, via the skin, while the fastest gateway to entry is the neck and the back of the neck. Diseases from the wind are extremely severe and the problems are unpredictable. It can be, for example, a sharp headache, a severe cold, a stuffy nose. If it gets into the eyes, it causes tearing, deterioration of vision, tics in the eyes; if it gets in the ears, it can cause various inflammations. It can even affect sleep, which will be very interrupted. Therefore, it is advisable during windy days, in drafts, but also in air-conditioned spaces, gyms, dance studios, offices, on an airplane, in the subway, etc., to cover the neck with a scarf or put a hood on the head to cover the ears as well. Nature has provided this weakness of our body with protection, there are several acupuncture points on the back of the neck, at the vertebrae of the upper thoracic spine and close to the ears, which can eliminate wind from the body. Moxibustion, mentioned in the previous chapter, is a good way to achieve this.

The wind is therefore said to be the cause of *100 diseases*. In the context of Chinese medicine, 100 diseases means all or many diseases. When the wind settles in our body, its excess causes restlessness, with which all diseases begin. For the wind, it is typical to move. If it is in the body, it is also manifested by traveling, and our pain or other physical worries move around the body. Today our knees hurt, tomorrow our shoulders, the day after tomorrow the small of our back, and we do not know what is really going on. The wind also causes various twitches, tics, shaking—movement of a different nature. Therefore, it is necessary to be careful of the draft during training, but also in everyday life. Be careful not to train in a draft or with an open window. A very unfortunate solution is an air-conditioned space in which we perform intense movement. In addition, we sweat, so the pores of the skin are open. This is an open entry for the wind, so it can harm us very quickly and deeply.

Wind can also enter us through food. Popular smoothies have a lot of wind in them. Where did it come from? Think about the process by which we prepare smoothies—mixing strong centrifugal energy without the possibility of grounding is a typical Qi of the wind. So in addition to the cold from raw foods, such a preparation method also absorbs this extremely mobile Qi. If a person consumes smoothies regularly, it will definitely have an effect on his or her health. The wind generated in this way can impair one's concentration or ability to ground oneself.

We also create wind with a modern online lifestyle. In the age of the Internet, non-stop online connections lead to the ability to handle in a short time and at once so many more issues than we would have dealt with all day in the past; the Qi of the wind has a wide scope. It is as if we were driven by that wind. Wind can be generated by work on a computer in which we have several windows open at once—we are working on something, and at the same time we have activated Facebook and are receiving comments, and we also have an open an email browser and are holding our phone to our ear. Simply put, we do not pay attention to one thing but several things at once, and we do not manage to pay attention to any of them properly. We fly like a leaf in the wind. Such wind will make us further unable to concentrate and we become distracted. And it is certainly reflected in today's communication between people, which is increasingly ceasing to be binding and stable, and does not offer room for real agreements.

The mechanism of wind formation inside us is strongly connected with the psyche. Emotions can cause a wind in our psyche that can significantly throw us off balance. We are not taught to deal with emotions economically. In addition to mental restlessness, the internal wind can cause problems with sleep, tics in the eyes, twitching of body parts, especially in the head and the face, because the wind tends to rise. The wind in a person is also manifested in one's speech. It is the case when someone is constantly running away from the topic; the listener has nothing to catch and so loses continuity in the sense of what is said. The result of all this can be volatility, instability, desultoriness, recklessness, inability to concentrate and so on. Ultimately, the wind can also affect memory, because with the great movement of everything around us and in us, we no longer have the capacity to remember many things. However, it also works the other way around. When we allow our emotions to "fly" without control, they will stimulate the formation of the inner wind.

MOVEMENT, TENDONS, BLOOD QUALITY AND PHYSICAL PERFORMANCE

So far, there has been talk of the Qi movement, which may sound too abstract. The movement of emotions or the way to realize one's visions is indeed an abstract depiction of movement. However, the functional circuit of the liver is also in charge of the physical movement of our body, and this is done through the tendons. The liver nourishes the tendons with its Qi and blood, thus ensuring the body's mobility, elasticity and softness. Let us go back to the idea of WOOD—as a young tree. Its body is soft, supple, full of vitality. When we lean on it, it elastically takes our weight. When we bend the branch, it does not break, but adapts. And when we release it, it will come back. So should our tendons, and by caring for them through caring for our liver Qi, we can maintain the quality of the tendons.

It could be assumed that movers naturally sufficiently protect their tendons. I do not dare to generalize, but in my view, it is not so. It is true that warm-ups before training are preparation of the tendons for exercise, and that if a tendon hurts, we apply some healing ointment. However, we do not know much about tendon health. We begin to be interested in them only when they hurt us, when we injure them or when we observe that they are contracted and that it is hard to loosen them up. We are only taught to use our body, yet we pay little attention to it. We take surgery for granted, although somewhere in our depths we feel that this is probably not quite right. A tendon injury can interrupt our dance career for a long time, and in extreme cases it can completely suspend it. I do not think any mover wants that. Unfortunately, few teachers or trainers teach us how to take care of our tendons or the rest of the body. Chinese medicine has brought me many possibilities into this gap of prevention. It not only teaches me what ointment to apply to the sore tendon, or which orthopedist to look for, but it teaches me how to take care of the tendons preventively so that there are minimal problems and maximum benefit.

Moreover, we are not used to consciously using the tendons when moving, and thus we do not use their real possibilities. We tend to manifest our physical strength with large muscles, which we think are also strong and capable of great performance. This Western-oriented notion of strength is often not true: a "masculine" man can easily be overcome by a more fragile-looking individual, who can work more with the Qi of bones and tendons. In dance, especially in partner work and contact improvisation, when often looking at how a relatively fragile woman lifts or shifts a man's weight, we encounter evidence that muscle strength is not decisive, often even less effective. If we use muscles to lift our partner's weight, we get them tired much faster than if we transferred the weight through the tendons to the skeletal structure and from there transformed it into the ground or space. The Taoist approach to the body teaches us that if we want to be truly physically strong—that is, strong in terms of flexibility and a kind of motor intelligence—we also need to pay attention to tendons in our practice. When we focus on muscle work, tendons remain unused, do not develop and remain weak. According to the experience of Taoists, healthy, nourished and strengthened tendons are essential for the development of physical strength and bodily comfort.

Tendons and ligaments are a type of connective tissue. Tendons connect bones to muscles, and ligaments connect bones to bones. The ligaments are located at greater depths, especially between the bones, and are usually short. Conversely, tendons can be very long and can run along several bones and on different parts of the body. We can imagine them as extremely strong rubber bands. They are elastic, which allows them to stretch and contract again. To maintain their flexibility requires paying attention to them through diet, proper preparation for performances, regeneration by relaxation, but also various Qigong exercises. Even the degree of mental resilience is reflected in the condition of the tendons. Tendons are essentially responsible for the mobility of the body, so they are extremely important for the mover. They contract and relax the muscles, thus moving the bones and joints, and the body as a whole. From the point of view of Chinese medicine, the condition of tendons and ligaments is subordinated to the nutrition of the liver, because they receive Qi and blood from it. The liver is responsible for movement, contraction and relaxation, and therefore the contraction and release of muscles and tendons. The "vehicle" of Qi for body movement is blood. The liver stores blood and distributes it to all parts of the body as needed. During the rest period, blood is collected in the liver, released during activity and sent to those parts of the body that are most involved in the activity. The liver therefore also supplies the tendons and ligaments with blood, thus controlling their quality. The quality of liver Qi is very important for tendons, because this Qi nourishes the blood, which then nourishes the tendons. Without this nutrition, the body loses its flexibility. If the liver is in good condition, it also affects the quality of its blood, and then the tendons, ligaments and membranes are sufficiently nourished. This is reflected in their strength, but also in flexibility, suppleness and sufficient moisture. This condition provides the body with active mobility, which is characterized by health and vitality in the tendons, then in the muscles and throughout the body. Conversely, if the liver and its blood are in a state of Qi deficit, this also affects the condition and function of the tendons. For example, if the liver does not have enough of its qualitative blood, the tendons and ligaments do not get the necessary nutrition. Then the body loses its flexibility, and the muscles lose the ability to stretch and contract. This manifests itself in all sorts of problems with tendons, membranes and ligaments. There is weakness, woodiness or fragility of the limbs, tremors in the muscles, shaking of the limbs, convulsions or convulsive seizures in the limbs. In extreme cases, there can be paralysis of the limbs.

A young mover who works with the tendons on a daily basis does not yet feel these extreme limitations. The fact that it is more difficult for a mover to warm up the tendons, but one may feel a strong and prolonged tension after training or after a performance, or pain or tremors, or the tendons quickly stiffen and shorten even after a short break; these may be warning signs that something worth thinking about is happening. An impaired state of liver Qi and blood will also affect joint mobility. The tendons are involved in the contraction and relaxation of muscles, and thus in the movement of bones and joints—that is, the overall movement of the body. Since the liver has the task not only of contracting the muscles but also of relaxing them, the imbalance can manifest itself in a stiff neck or such a small detail as clenching the jaw.

In addition, Chinese medicine, which includes Qigong exercises, has observed that tendons sufficiently nourished by the liver are a source of resistance to fatigue. The vitality of movement depends on a good condition of the tendons, which helps the body to achieve high motor performance and protect it from getting tired quickly. So it also depends on the intelligence with which we use the body in motion, in a way that does not require so much muscular energy, but rather the energy of tendons. We can clarify this in a simple test. Hang on to a bar with bent arms, using the muscles of the arms. How long will you last? You will definitely feel tired after a short while and you will be forced to stop. However, when you hang on the bar with your arms outstretched, you can hang longer without feeling much effort. In this position of the arms, the force is transferred from the muscles to the tendons and then to the bones. This mechanism can be advantageously used in dance partnering and in contact improvisation. It saves energy and also ensures a smooth flow of energy between partners.

This is not to say that the muscles should be forgotten and not involved at all. They get involved themselves at the stimulus of the tendons. We can grow muscles in a relatively short time, but when we stop paying attention to them, they quickly weaken. Tendons can maintain strength throughout our lives, and they can withstand much more before they are tired by physical exertion.

TENDON INJURIES AND THEIR TREATMENT

Tendon damage is many times more serious than bone damage. Bone can grow together faster than a tendon, and even the pain is stronger when the tendon is stretched or ruptured than with a broken bone or muscle disruption. In case of such damage, attention should be paid to the liver. Chinese medicine uses several herbal preparations to regenerate tendons through liver support, and the diet needs to be adapted to nourish the liver and to support tendon regeneration—for example, through Shiatsu or acupuncture treatments. In addition, it is possible to work with tendons and the liver through Qigong, which has in its "database" many exercises that support the nutrition and regeneration of tendons.

Tendons can also be treated mentally by changing the level of our consciousness towards the use of our body. Tendon injury can also suggest a mental correlation. Since everything is related to everything, our body tells us its worries about how we treat it, how we perceive ourselves and our surroundings, and so on. When movers stretch or tear a tendon, it is a sign that they are going over their limits. They tend to tear themselves, risking too much because of their ambition. Healthy ambition is stretched to a level that was no longer commensurate with the reality and capabilities of the body, and so the body responded in this way. Exaggerated ambition is mostly an image of a kind of emptiness inside the person concerned—the need to prove one's possibilities at all costs. Tendon failure is also the result of insufficient tendon preparation for performance, which also essentially reflects the person's access to the body. By tearing or stretching the tendon, the mover has the opportunity to get in touch with reality. The body thus took care of a kind of forced break. The person cannot move physically, but he or she can, figuratively speaking, move the brain. Such a pause is a space for thinking, for immersing oneself in oneself, where one can investigate, discover causes, and thus find out what he or she is doing against the body and why—to find out if it is really necessary and if it is worth it. A ruptured or torn tendon is probably not worth it, so this situation is a big challenge. It is an opportunity to change the current way of using the body and spirit. One can ask oneself questions like: "Where and why am I going over my limits? For what or for whom did I let myself be overwhelmed by unrealistic dreams? When does my ambition become a trap? What would I do if my body could not recover to its normal state?" My hope is that injuries can send us precious information that could help change the way we use our body.

However, there are ways to get the tendons in order. From my own practice during dance seminars, where we consciously work with tendons, I have experienced that intensive work with them through Qigong and conscious improvisations with the Liver and Gallbladder channels can bring great success even after relatively fresh tendon injuries. A student from Poland was at one of these seminars just a few months after rupturing her right knee tendons, and she was happy to tell me how she enjoyed dancing without pain—even more than ever before. Of course, she had to move differently than she was used to, and most of all she moved with an aware and attentive mind. This way of working gave her body the ability to know intuitively how to move so as not to hurt herself. She was surprised at how strong and at the same time how elastic her ligaments and tendons were and how much space she could feel between the bones in her joints.

During that seminar, we also worked with the method of detoxifying tendons with mung beans. This old Taoist method is a suitable method of regenerating or energetically strengthening tendons. Its main goal is to detoxify and it does so in a simple way—by tapping the tendons with bags filled with mung beans. Mung beans are generally good for health, and are commonly consumed, among other things, in cases of food poisoning. Their strength lies in the fact that they support the detoxification process. No wonder that they are part of many Chinese dishes in the form of sprouts. When used externally—tapping the skin—they have a great effect on detoxification as well. The result is the regeneration of damaged tissues, in this case tendons. Of course, it is advisable to work with this technique preventively, to cleanse and strengthen the healthy tendons, but also the joints, muscles, scalp, etc.

Tapping with mung bags shakes the fascial layers, thus separating them from each other, which relieves tension in the tissues and can subsequently lead to a detoxification process. Toxins are literally shaken from the fascia, muscles, tendons, bones, joint cavities and fluids, and subcutaneous tissue. In addition, tapping opens the pores of the skin, which significantly improves the absorption of healing Qi into the body. It is advisable to combine tapping with Qigong so that the accumulated Qi from exercise penetrates the meridians, where it can nourish the tissues with Qi and support treatment. However, Qigong is not essential, and tapping itself has a strong effect, so it can be practiced by a layperson. We tap hard, but not so hard as to cause pain. Rather, we focus on the feeling that the taps open the surface and at the same time act in the depths of the structures.

Making a mung bag is very simple. All you have to do is sew a narrow pocket from a sock-sized piece of fabric, into which you pour half a kilogram of beans and tie it with a string so that the beans do not fall out and the bag is compact. The simplest and fastest solution is to pour mung beans into a cotton sock. This variant does not look aesthetically pleasing, but as first aid it is sufficient. After a certain time, it is advisable to air the mung beans, clean them, let them be exposed to sunlight, or replace them with a new ones.

ACHILLES TENDON CONNECTS US WITH THE EARTH AND BUILDS OUR VERTICALITY

The Achilles tendon is the most important tendon for walking, running and jumping. It is also important in terms of overall posture and our personal stability. From an anatomical point of view, the Achilles tendon is our largest and strongest tendon. One has to strain it extremely in order to tear it. Its strength lies in its dense structure, but also in its cooperation with other parts of the body. So let us look at it from a Taoist point of view, which takes the individual parts of the body as part of the whole, where everything is connected to everything, and if something happens to one of them, the others react as well.

The Achilles tendon is part of a long chain of muscles that begins at the skull—the lower ridge of the nape of the neck. This chain includes the trapezius muscles (on the neck and back of the neck), sacrospinalis (erector spinae muscles), gluteus (gluteal muscle), hamstrings (posterior thigh muscles), gastrocnemius (superficial two-headed calf muscle) and soleus (deeper calf muscle). This chain of muscles is terminated by the Achilles tendon as it connects to the heel. The tendon and the heel are energetically and physically connected to the skull in this way. Our contact with the Earth, the "scanning" of the diversity of the surface we walk on, the ability to let our weight sink into the Earth, all connect from the heel to the brain through this chain. The Achilles tendon connects us to the Earth, and through this chain, it also builds our vertical axis.

Awareness of this chain is very helpful in healing practice. It is a whole in which every muscle, every part of the chain cooperates with the other parts. The injury of one of them affects the others; conversely, if when treating one part, we pay attention also to the other parts, it will help the whole, as well as the damaged part. All the muscles of this chain and their attachments to the bones (i.e. the tendons) together support the stability of the spine in its vertical axis and tune the symbiosis between the lower limbs and the spine during walking, running, dancing and other physical activities. The crest of the occipital bone is connected to the so-called proprioceptors. The proprioceptive system monitors the situation of the body, its organs and structures. It is related to the ability of the nervous system to register changes occurring in the muscles and inside the body through movement and muscle activity. It

is essential for proper coordination of movement, registering changes in body position, muscle tone and the progression of certain reflexes. In addition, this chain is a storehouse of emotional and psychological stress.

With the Taoist eye, we find that from the point of view of the flow of Qi in the acupuncture meridians, this chain is strikingly similar to the Bladder channel mentioned in the previous chapter. It is the longest meridian of the body through which Qi flows through the body from the head to the feet. In this pathway, Qi lines the entire chain of muscles, tendons, ligaments and fascia, and the meridian acts as a distributor between the individual parts of the chain, but also as an informant about the state of Qi. Qi passes the meridian through the Achilles tendon itself, so when there is some stress on the Achilles tendon, information about it spreads along the entire chain. Conversely, the condition of the other components of the chain will affect the condition of the Achilles tendon. Thus, it is advisable to relax the whole body as part of the therapy for Achilles tendon problems, which is what the Bladder channel is perfect for.

As already mentioned, we have to stretch the Achilles tendon extremely in order to tear it. If it breaks, it is a sign that we have overreached all our possibilities and we are literally tearing ourselves to pieces. From a psychosomatic point of view, this is a situation where we draw our weakness into the game. We overextend in order to accomplish some task, yet we risk too much for it. But by rupturing or tearing the tendon, we are suddenly brought back to reality. When the Achilles tendon lets go, it turns out that the activity, or some kind of record we are trying to achieve, is beyond our reach. The body serves a competitive mind, an ambitious or unconscious ego, which comes up with many unrealistic things. And so in time, it ensures a long break for us. Taking care of our tendons, and not only the Achilles, literally prolongs the career of a mover.

TENDONS AND GRACE OF MOVEMENT

Tendons have another important role, especially for movers. This is a kind of ability of overall coordination and interconnection of individual parts of the body into a graceful whole. With well-functioning and working tendons, the body is more compact, more flexible, and it acts as a coordinated whole, perfectly using the cooperation of all individual parts of the body into a whole. The more we cultivate awareness of our tendons, the more we give the body an interconnection, thanks to which the individual parts of the body cooperate with each other and together form a single, compact unit. When we talk about dancers, we come across different types. For some, the movement may be trained and the overall impression is more about dis-connection. These dancers do not seem to feel the compactness of their body; their movement expression is choppy and incoherent, and it can literally disturb us when looking at them. They are trained in terms of technique, but something bothers us there. In contrast, other dancers do not have to be trained in technique on a daily basis, but their movements are more complete, coordinated and connected. This unification of the body helps with smooth movement, when fluency and grace become, to some extent, the style of the dancer. Such a thing can be seen in an animal—an antelope or some feline beast, where the fluidity and balance of individual parts of the body is perfect, no part of the body is trained more than the other. Most fast-running animals do not have massive and muscular legs; on the contrary, they are slim and more sinewy. When we see an "antelope" or "tiger" on stage, it is a very pleasant and fascinating sight.

Everything moving in the body, but also the movement of the body itself, is significantly nourished by liver Qi. This is also related to our amount of capacity. Movement requires a certain amount of capacity, and we have it available if liver Qi flows harmoniously and evenly. Decreased capacity is a typical symp-tom of liver Qi imbalance—pay attention to it. Exaggerated activity and tension, the inability to stop and relax, and disrupted movement are also signs of imbalance. The liver is responsible for creating and maintaining a balanced relation-ship between tension and release, activity and relaxation.

OTHER CONNECTIONS WITH THE LIVER AND ITS FUNCTIONAL CIRCUIT

We will return to the functional circuit of the liver, because we have not yet exhausted the summary of its effect on the organism. In the medical texts of Chinese medicine, we find information that...

The liver stores blood

Blood has its source in the delicate substances of food and water. According to Chinese medicine, these are produced by the spleen and stored in the liver. The need for blood volume in particular parts of the body is different for diverse activities, and the liver is responsible for its distribution. For example, when we run, the liver sends blood to our muscles and tendons, and when resting, the blood returns to the liver. Insufficiency of this function can lead, for example, to impaired flexibility and pain in the joints, stiff limbs, muscle twitches—in these cases, the blood is not sufficiently supplied to these structures. Impaired or blurred vision, a dry feeling in the eyes and spots in front of the eyes indicate that the blood is not nourishing the eyes sufficiently. In case of dizziness, the blood is insufficiently distributed to the head area. Insufficient and irregular blood circulation also manifests itself as irregular and weak menstruation.

The liver opens into the eyes

The liver blood nourishes and moisturizes the eyes. Most eye and vision problems are related to liver problems, such as blurred vision, night blindness, eye floaters, eye inflammation, dry eyes, cuts, cataracts and glaucoma. The eyes are the most used sensory organ. Their use often pushes other sensory organs to the sidelines. The eyes therefore need sufficient regeneration and rest, especially nowadays, when working with a computer for several hours is the daily standard. We have never used the eyes so much in human history. A great remedy and relaxation for the eyes is looking into the distance, ideally at green hills or fields.

Liver Qi also affects our eyesight in a psychological context. Our strength also depends on our ability to see the invisible, to "read between the lines" or "see ahead"—that is, a kind of ability to anticipate, to see into the future. It has to do with the Hun.

The fact that in functional circuits things are really interrelated and mutually influenced is also evidenced by the experience of one student: we spent a long time in one seminar working with tendons, nourishing them through Qigong. After the seminar, she told me, "That's amazing, I can see better."

Liver Qi manifests in the nails

According to medical texts, nails are an extension of the tendons. Their nutrition depends on the quality of the blood and Qi of the liver. When adequately nourished, the nails have a natural pink color, a shiny and smooth surface. In the case of lack of Qi and liver blood, they suffer from weakness, fragility, various spots or scratches on them. The nails also symbolize our ability for the healthy aggression needed to assert ourselves, claw into something and, with their help, "climb up." This is indeed one of the attributes of the functional circuit of the liver.

Anger harms the liver and causes the rise of Qi

A few more words about anger. If anger is strong, it attacks the liver and Qi rises into the head. Then the blood follows Qi and causes dizziness, headaches, flushing, auditory delusions and fainting. The Qi of anger can also attack horizontally, attacking the spleen and stomach. It causes stagnation of food in the stomach, bloating, diarrhea with undigested food and the like. When the stomach is attacked, it can cause hiccups, vomiting and gurgling.

The green and turquoise color of the WOOD phase

The soothing green color also contains information about spring growth and, to a certain extent, freedom. It is good to take walks outside so that the eyes and soul can graze on the green, preferably with loose hair, which will help you enjoy more freedom, independence and a feeling of freedom.

How do we recognize a person with a disharmonious Qi of the WOOD phase?

A very typical example is a bile-like person—one who is angry with other people, but often also with themselves. This is connected with the fullness of Qi of the liver and gallbladder. The emptiness of Qi leads to disorder, the inability to have a system for things and quickly changing one's mind, leaving planning and decision making to others. To a large extent, it can also lead to disturbed self-confidence. Another typical feature is workaholism. Workaholics cannot switch off, cannot release tension and cannot naturally go from work mode to rest mode. They have disrupted this mechanism, and their Qi finds itself in prison—they are only on one side of the river. If there is too much wind in such people, then their speech is characterized by frequent deviations from the topic. Here, it is also evident that there is a weakness of gallbladder Qi, which cannot purify thoughts and express the words that are really important and essential. The fullness of the Qi of the liver and gallbladder leads to stubbornness, meticulousness, sometimes recklessness and silliness. Only evenly flowing Qi can allow us to rise above some of our requirements and to let things happen in a freer way. As for the movement of the body, the disharmony of these organs is reflected in problems with tendons and ligaments, but also with physical endurance of the muscles.

RELATIONSHIP OF THE wood PHASE TO OTHER PHASES

According to the Sheng cycle, which we discussed in Chapter 7 on the Five phases, it is clear that the "mother" of the liver is the kidneys. The wood phase has its source of life in WATER. The quality of the kidneys then determines the quality of liver Qi. This means that if we want to take care of the liver, we must also pay attention to the kidneys. In the psychological context, this means that if we refine and cultivate wisdom, which is the virtue of the kidneys, then anger cannot overwhelm us to excessive proportions, because wisdom nourishes generosity and kindness, which are the virtues of the liver. They can work more harmoniously with anger.

The liver is a strong organ, and its Qi quickly becomes excessive and easily gets out of control. It has an untamed nature; Qi is as fierce and restless as a general. The METAL phase controls the wood phase. If a tree grows excessively, we use some sharp metal to tame the growth. For example, when we become excessively angry, we are used to saying, "Calm down, breathe deeply." Activating Qi of the lungs can help tame excessive Qi of the liver based on this simple mechanism. Harmonious wood Qi can support the FIRE phase well and at the same time control the excess in the EARTH phase.

CONCLUSION TO THE wood PHASE

The liver and its entire functional circuit are harmed by long-term repressed emotions, the so-called pressure cooker, but also a long-term lack of warm human touch. When children are angry, they are actually asking for physical contact, love and proof that we accept them as they are. This is also true for adults. This deficit can lead to self-destruction or distrust in one's abilities. The liver also needs permeability in the form of expressing the opinions that are born in us, as well as the feelings that arise in us, whether it is feelings of fear, anxiety and worry or joy, affection and love. The liver is also harmed by long-term hypocrisy. This double life creates a conflict in us, a conflict in the smooth flow of Qi. The Qi of the liver is greatly affected if we say something that we do not agree with. The liver thrives when we laugh out loud. It also helps it if we allow ourselves to cry hard. It loves singing, it also needs to look someone in the eye when we talk to them. Children laugh and cry out loud, get angry, love, do not pretend, do not look away, require physical contact, sing loudly, yawn, say what they think. It is all medicine for the liver.

The spring sun will entice us to spend more time outside, but be careful of the cold and humidity that radiate from the cooled ground. Also protect yourselves from the wind. Add a lot of green to your diet, which will start the internal "photosynthetic" processes in the body and also help detoxify. Take the time for a suitable spring detoxification of the organism.

In the penetrating Qi of the wood phase, we feel an inner restlessness in us, the need to do something, to activate. The head is full of ideas, and the soul wants to realize them. This is natural for this phase and needs to be used. At the same time, however, we must be careful not to overdo it and exhaust our potential quickly and suddenly. We still have a whole year ahead of us.

Table 9.1 Main correspondences of WOOD phase

Year season: spring	Yin and Yang stage: Lesser Yang/Yang in Yin	Color: green, blue-green	Taste: sour
Day time: morning	Direction: east	Smell: rancid	Number: 8
Evolution of Qi: rise of Qi	Growth cycle in nature: sprouting, beginning of growth	Tissue: tendons, ligaments, fascia	Body fluid: tears
Life cycle: birth, childhood	Working cycle: idea	Other body tissues: nails, short muscles, peripheral nerves, irises, external genitals	Other body fluid and excretion: gall
Yin organ: liver	Organ clock for liver: 1 to 3 a.m.	Joints: shoulders	Entry point of disease: nape (back of the neck)
Yang organ: gallbladder	Organ clock for gallbladder: 11 p.m. to 1 a.m.	Sense organ: eyes	Sense: sight
Psychospiritual aspect: Hun	Virtue: kindness, generosity, compassion	Indicator: nails	Detrimental action: too much running (moving)
Emotion: anger (passing through)	Climate: wind	Sound: screaming	Mental attitude: flexibility, ability to establish

MERIDIANS

GALLBLADDER CHANNEL (GB)/YANG

The Gallbladder channel is a Yang pair channel, running along the right and left sides of the body, from top to bottom. In the image below, it is shown only on one side. It is specific because it is the only channel that leads through the sides of the body. Its Qi begins at the outer corners of the eyes. It continues to the ears, encircling them on the sides with three semicircular arches, thus covering almost the entire head. It continues along the lateral parts of the neck through the upper trapezius. It leads towards the shoulders and armpits. In the area of the trunk, it connects with the gallbladder and liver through its internal branches. It passes through the sides of the ribs towards the pelvis, where it penetrates deep into the hip joints. From there, the inner branch connects with the Bladder channel in the sacrum. It descends along the sides of the thighs, through the sides of the knees and calves, continues under the outer ankles and leads along the insteps to the fourth toes, where it ends at the nail beds on the outer sides of these toes. Its main branch has 44 acupuncture points. On the instep, Qi is poured from this channel into the Liver channel. Dashed lines indicate internal deep branches.

The Gallbladder channel affects all problems along its pathway, such as hip pain, pain in all the lower limb joints, rib pain, temple pain, headache, migraines, ear disorders, armpit swelling. It greatly helps the smooth flow of liver Qi and the smooth flow of emotions. It helps to permeate retained emotions, which are transformed into material formations in the bile ducts and gallbladder. In the psychological field, it is also related to the ability to make decisions.

GALLBLADDER CHANNEL IN MOVEMENT

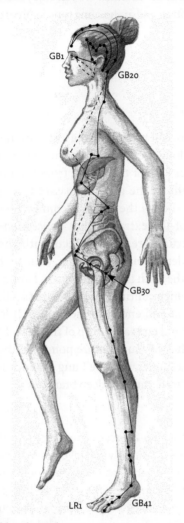

GB1

GB20

GB30

LR1   GB41

Gallbladder channel

The channel offers many possibilities for movement experiments, as it is one of the longest and the most diverting channels and runs from head to toe, leading mainly along the sides of the body. For movement improvisation, use the sides of the body—the sides of the head, temples, sides of the neck, ribs, outer upper ends of the femurs (large trochanters), iliotibial tracts, knees, calves and feet. Look for the movement possibilities of these parts of the body.

Conscious focus on the sides of the body will expand your entire body and at the same time your ability to see peripherally. Trust it and thus use less forward-looking movement. Gallbladder Qi is also related to the ability to see peripherally. The path begins at the outer corners of the eyes, hence supporting this ability. You can also play with copying the movement of someone else in the group with your peripheral vision.

An interesting feature of the channel for movement is its connection with the ears. In improvisation, let us be guided by sound: open the ears, sharpen the hearing and perceive how this work affects the movement of the whole body and how it activates the purity of hearing. Working with this channel really activates our hearing and thus purifies it so that we can use our hearing more and not leave most of our perception to the eyes.

When we work in movement with the ribs, the spaces between them open beautifully, the intercostal muscles relax, and Qi can flow better in this area. This movement also provides an internal massage to the organs and to the thoracic spine. As the channel penetrates into the depth of the hip joints, we intensively engage these joints in motion. Let the movement come from the hip joints and observe where in the body the impact of such movement will reach. Will it be the ribs, the neck or even the head? We can also focus on the hip joints and their energetic connection with the sacrum. Let us observe what perception such movement brings to the body.

The channel also passes through the iliotibial tract, on the sides of the thighs, which ensures the stability of the knees. We can improvise with the iliotibial tract, realize the stability of the knees and look for new possibilities of movement from the knees.

We can also work with the fourth toes—for example, by guiding the movement of the entire lower limbs from them.

The Gallbladder channel is connected to the

extraordinary *Belt Vessel*, which opens the way to the periphery and also to rotation. Let us improvise with rotation from the center of gravity of the body, realizing the connection with the Gallbladder channel.

After prolonged improvisation, Qi is strongly activated in the channel. We can enjoy this flow of Qi in motion and at the same time its Yang charge.

LIVER CHANNEL (LR)/YIN

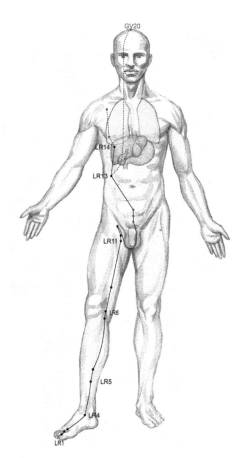

Liver channel

the nail bed. It runs along the insteps to the inner ankles along the calves, from the calf muscles to the inner side of the knees, from the inside of the thighs to the groin. It passes through the genitals. Below the navel, it connects with the points of the extraordinary *Conception Vessel*. In the trunk area, it connects with the liver, gallbladder, stomach and lungs. Its main branch ends in the sixth intercostal space. However, the inner branch continues upwards, passes through the throat and encircles the mouth. It leads to the eyes and ends at the top of the head. Its main branch has 14 acupuncture points. In the chest area, it connects with the Lung channel. Dashed lines indicate internal deep branches.

The channel affects detoxification, blood distribution, fluidity of movement, emotional harmony, ability to plan, tendons, muscle performance, ligaments, eyes, all liver problems, migraines, fatigue, stagnation, muscle pain and stiffness, menstrual cycle, erection, impulsivity, frustration, outbursts of anger or repressed emotions. Blocked Qi of the liver channel can manifest itself, for example, in the so-called lump in the throat—when we want to say something, but we cannot. Emotional tension also leads to stiffness of the mouth, which can result in vertical wrinkles above the upper lip. Pain on the temples also indicates disharmony in this channel.

The Liver channel is a Yin pair channel that runs from bottom to top, along the inner sides of the legs to the trunk. In the image above, it is shown only on one side. Its Qi springs on the outer (lateral) side of the big toes, right next to

LIVER CHANNEL IN MOVEMENT

The Liver channel is the Yin meridian, so its Qi leads from the bottom up. It is not as dynamic as the Gallbladder channel. However, in the area of the pelvis, it also connects with the points of the Conception Vessel and with the genitals, so that this section can be more dynamic in movement.

In the area of the feet, the Liver channel enables us to work with the big toes and insteps, when improvising in motion. Activation of this area of the body will help the feet to better root to Earth, and also to allow Qi to ascend from the bottom to the top smoothly and briskly. In movement, we focus on realizing its ascent to the top of the head. We can discover by movement the energetic force that brings Qi upwards.

The channel also offers sensitive work with the inner sides of the lower limbs. The perineal area can be released by a waving motion of the pelvis. With this movement, we also relax the lumbar-thigh muscle—the iliopsoas. Within the framework of various stretches, we will stretch the body pleasantly and give it more flow. When we focus our attention on the area of the groin and iliopsoas, we can release tension in this area, thus achieving the passage of Qi and then a better and more conscious connection of the upper body with the lower one. When moving, we can let Qi flow from top to bottom and vice versa, creating a smooth flow of Qi without obstacles.

The channel also opens the pathway to the ribs. We can involve the lower ribs in movement, specifically the 11th floating ribs, where the channel passes. Movement of this area will move the liver itself.

The inner branch connects the legs and the trunk with the top of the head. As part of movement improvisation, we can focus on connecting the feet with the top of the head.

At the same time, this branch allows us to actively involve the eyesight in our movement. As we move consciously with our eyes, let us perceive everything around us, and by so doing, open up more to our surroundings. This is also the role of the liver—to interact with the outside environment. Be sure to relax the mouth and lips as you move.

After longer improvisations, Qi is strongly activated in the channel. Let us enjoy this Yin flow of Qi in motion, but also in stillness.

DIET IN SPRING AND FOR THE wood PHASE ORGANS

In the spring, nature wakes up, Qi rises significantly upwards and a juicy, fresh, young green color appears all around. Young green leaves, shoots, nettles and other herbs, parsley, leeks, spring onions, chives, coriander, spinach, salad and various sprouts begin to grow. All this should also appear on the plate; it will give us a concentrated and fresh life force. In addition, these plants will help us wash out excess salt, which will then bring us the joy of movement through the revival of the tendons. Sprouted radish or young shoots of watercress can also help stimulate us out of laziness.

With increasing heat (Yang) around, the preparation of meals by cooking gradually shortens. Our body still needs Yang, but not as much as in winter. Therefore, the need for meat, baked food, salt and fats is also decreasing. Stewing and blanching are suitable methods of preparation. Blanching is a short boiling of vegetables in salty water, the principle of which is the heating of vegetables, but at the same time keeping their nutrients and crunchiness. We consume frozen food as little as possible, especially in the spring, when we need to start everything all over again.

Frozen food does not have information about a new beginning.

Green color

Since the color of the WOOD phase is green, all green vegetables should predominate—broccoli, kale, cabbage, celery stalks, Chinese cabbage, fennel, kohlrabi, cauliflower, chicory, etc. We don't need to be afraid of wild vegetables, such as nettle, dandelion, angelica, plantain, wild garlic, daisy flowers, violets and the like. However, let us not forget root vegetables, but choose young, new ones. With their mild sweet taste, root vegetables help to release liver Qi.

Food for releasing stagnated liver Qi

Garlic chives (Chinese garlic) can effectively stir up liver Qi, thus removing blockages. Stagnation of liver Qi creates warmth, even heat, in the body. Chives help eliminate heat and help Qi pass through easier. We should omit foods that produce heat and mucus. These are hardened edible fats and bitter or lower-quality oils. In contrast, cold-pressed oils—olive oil or oil from unroasted sesame seeds—are suitable, as well as ghee. An excellent oil for the liver is oil from black cumin or mustard oil. It even kills parasites.

Garlic chives also improve the digestibility of cereals and legumes. Stem celery has similar effects. It is recommended to eat basil leaves almost daily, as basil also warms us up, which is even more advantageous for us in the spring. However, in the case of excessive stagnation of liver Qi, it is not recommended to consume basil in its concentrated form, so we avoid pesto. Among the fresh herbs, bay leaf, watercress, rosemary, dill, mint, lemon balm and mustard leaves are also recommended.

Cereals

Wheat, rye, oats, spelt and barley are suitable for the liver, and the neutral base is rice, especially sweet rice.

Legumes

Lentils and mung beans are suitable, excellent even in the sprouted state. Sprouted legumes should be cooked; otherwise, they are very difficult to digest. Legumes contain lectins, which are difficult to digest and in the raw state are harmful to the body. They are eliminated by cooking, long-term soaking and the use of spices during cooking. We cook them with ingredients that reduce flatulence (marjoram, savory, cumin, basil, fennel). We also cook them together with seaweed, which also increases the digestibility of legumes.

Mushrooms

Most wood-destroying fungi are excellent, such as chicken of the woods, turban fungus, oyster mushrooms and the like.

Sour taste

The taste of the WOOD phase is a sour taste. We supply it in the form of fermented vegetables, so-called pickles, initially long-term fermented; later, we take pickles that have been fermented for a shorter period. In normal amounts, the sour taste is beneficial for the liver, but too much sour taste can have a counterproductive effect.

The sour taste is unsuitable for inflammation in terms of digestion, especially for the intestines. In the presence of celiac disease, Crohn's disease, ulcerative colitis, etc., it is very irritating and causes further chronic inflammation. You can read about the disservice of the sour taste during colds and flu in Chapter 12 dedicated to the METAL phase. For a healthy person, a sour taste is essential because it opens digestion, so it is given at the beginning of a meal. It is recommended to drink boiled water with a few drops of lemon in the morning to start up digestion and stir liver Qi.

Liver detoxification

The growing Yang is also associated with a greater need for fluids, which allow the body to get rid of toxins during this period. The liver is the largest detoxifying organ, and in the spring it has the best opportunity to cleanse the body. From what actually? How do toxins form and accumulate in us? Industrially produced foods with flavorings and colors are almost always oversalted. Toxins enter us through alcohol, tobacco, medications or other drugs, but also through the polluted environment in which we live. However, regular cleansing should also be done by people who eat a healthy diet, because their body also generates metabolic waste that needs to be removed from the body.

Even a small amount of honey has detoxifying effects, but it cannot be added to hot tea. However, there are two things to watch out for with honey: it can become toxic or lose enzymes if used incorrectly. Both cases depend on the temperature of the water, tea or food to which we add the honey. When added to tea or food with a temperature higher than 80°C (175°F), it becomes toxic. All its beneficial enzymes are destroyed at temperatures above 55°C (130°F). So it is all right if we prepare a drink or meal with honey up to 50°C (120°F). The greatest effect of honey is achieved in combination with fresh apple cider vinegar.

To support detoxification, it is advisable to take a celandine tincture in the spring, drink tea from the seeds of milk thistle (*Silybum marianum*) daily or take a teaspoon of oil from this plant. We can also use some tea mixture for the liver, which can be bought in the pharmacy.

In general, we should not eat fatty foods in the evening, including nuts and seeds, because the gallbladder and liver would not be able to process fats at night.

A FEW TIPS AND RECIPES

Spring cleansing green drink
Ingredients: Milfoil (Eurasian yarrow), dandelion, nettle, water.

Method: Soak equal amounts of herbs in cold water. Infuse for a few hours, then blend. Strain and drink 100 ml several times a day. To prevent overcooling, add warming spices such as ground cinnamon or ground cloves to the drink.

Benefits: This drink replenishes Qi, cools and detoxifies.

Smoothies
Ingredients: 1 tbsp almonds, 1 tbsp goji, 1 tbsp chia seeds, banana, apple, herbs (e.g. nettle, angelica, raspberry leaves) or grain sprouts (e.g. barley or wheat), pinch of warming spices (e.g. cinnamon, cardamom, cloves).

Method: Soak the almonds and goji ideally the night before. In the morning, prepare the chia gel by mixing 1 tbsp of chia seeds with 100 ml of water and leave to stand for 15 minutes. Blend the goji, almonds, chia gel, banana, apple, herbs and grain sprouts. Warm it up with a pinch of warming spices.

Benefits: This smoothy detoxifies and, with the warming spices, supports the spleen Qi. It has a slightly cooling effect. The blending adds wind to the body, which in spring, when the climate factor of wind reigns, can be excessive for us. Therefore, be more careful with smoothies in the spring.

Creamy cauliflower soup
Ingredients: 1 leek, cauliflower, soya (or oat or rice) cream, fresh basil, 1 tsp ume vinegar, water.

Method: Bring 750 ml of water to the boil, season with salt, add the sliced leek, a head of cauliflower, cut into florets. When the cauliflower has softened, blend or strain the soup until smooth, add the soya cream. Turn off the heat and season with ume vinegar. Sprinkle with chopped fresh basil.

Benefits: The soup supports the liver and the large intestine.

Nettle spinach
Ingredients: 4 large onions, 3 tbsp sunflower oil, 3 handfuls of fresh young nettle tops (top three rows of leaves), salt, 1 tbsp kuzu, water.

Method: Fry the finely chopped onions in oil, cover with water, add salt and bring to a boil. Throw in the rinsed nettles and cook for a maximum of 5 minutes. Blend. Bring back to a boil and thicken with kuzu dissolved in a small amount of cold water. Simmer briefly until thickened. Serve the spinach with rice sprinkled with gomashio or with mashed potatoes. (For more on kuzu, see Chapter 11 on the EARTH phase.)

Benefits: It detoxifies, purifies the blood, replenishes the blood and slightly cools.

Nettle soup
Ingredients: 4 large onions, 3 tbsp sunflower oil, 3 handfuls of fresh young nettle tops (top three rows of leaves), salt, water.

Method: Follow the same procedure as for the spinach, but add more water. You can add corn polenta or other grains to thicken. You can also add miso to vary the flavor.

Benefits: It detoxifies, purifies the blood, replenishes the blood and slightly cools.

Leek and kale pancakes with sauerkraut
Ingredients: Half a small leek, 1 cup chopped kale, 1 cup fine buckwheat or rye flour or fine oatmeal, 1 cup filtered water, 1 tsp salt, ½ tsp ground cumin, frying oil (organic sesame or sunflower).

Method: Slice the leeks lengthwise, then cut them into smaller pieces and place them together with the chopped kale in the water to boil for 10 minutes. Blend the vegetables with an immersion blender, add the buckwheat, flour or oatmeal, salt and cumin to the mixture to make a thicker batter. Place spoonfuls of the batter on the hot oil and shape into a pancake. The finished pancakes can be topped with raw sauerkraut, or the sauerkraut can be briefly fried in a little oil with the leeks.

Benefits: The buckwheat flour makes the pancakes soft and slightly cooling; it is gluten-free.

Green bread spread
Ingredients: Parsley (1 part), basil (1 part), pumpkin seeds (2 parts), olive oil, salt.

Method: Blend everything into a pesto-like paste. In spring, however, it is more energy-efficient not to blend but to chop. Although it is more work, blending adds wind to the body and we should keep this to a minimum in spring.

Benefits: It detoxifies, purifies the blood, replenishes the blood and slightly cools.

Green "bulguroto"
Ingredients: Bulgur, zucchini, peas, celery stems, salted stewed aubergine, red pepper, black pepper spice, mint or basil, spring onion.

Method: Boil the bulgur for 10 minutes and let it simmer for another 10 minutes. Add the chopped vegetables and garnish with mint or basil or the chopped green part of a spring onion.

Benefits: It detoxifies and replenishes blood and Qi.

CHAPTER 10

The FIRE phase

When the soul has joy in the body

About: the clarity of our intentions and actions / heart and the Shen Spirit / joy and the ability to handle success / enthusiasm and ability to put the whole heart into something / small intestine and clarity of the movement expression / ability to concentrate / openness and sincerity / speech / deception / sleeping / coffee / diet for summer and for the FIRE phase organs

"Put your whole heart into it!" We are used to saying this when we want someone to really perform well. And we are not talking only about body action. Above all, we want the outcome to be unique and real, full of energy coming from the heart, thus filled with our personality. When Julyen Hamilton teaches people to improvise, he always says, "You don't have to like what you do. You have to love it!" And that is exactly what this chapter will be about—about connecting to your heart and soul, about the flow of your soul outwards. About the fire quality in us, which radiates its energy around, which pleases, warms, gives life a spark. But if we do not tame it, it can also burn destructively.

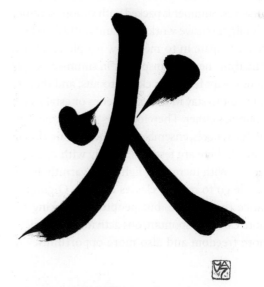

Chinese character for FIRE

THE FIRE PHASE AS AN ENERGY PEAK

The FIRE phase represents the Qi at its highest peak of the year. It is summer. Nature is in its highest activity—everything blooms, smells, flows with Qi; the colors around us are bright and radiant, attracting the attention of everything.

Fruits ripen and sweeten every day so that we can have a good harvest in the autumn. The young of animals become independent and begin to mature. Yang, which "slept" in the winter and actively woke up to life in the spring and gradually grew, reaches its highest point in the summer. The sun travels high in the sky, having the opportunity to shine long and intensely, and thus fill our Earth with its Yang. Days (Yang) are long, starting early in the morning and ending late in the evening. Nights (Yin), on the other hand, are short, starting late and ending early. Everything vibrates with life force; everything is active in the Yang phase. So summer is the culmination of Yang Qi—the ripening, maturing, joy of life, which is obviously the result of the effort of the WOOD phase that preceded the FIRE phase. From the point of view of human development, it is adulthood, a definitive separation from parents. In the FIRE phase, everything runs fast. What went slowly goes faster; what was inside radiates outwards.

OPENNESS

A typical aspect of this outward-looking quality is openness. After a relaxing winter and an impatient spring, we finally spend more time outside. We leave our homes to fully open ourselves to the world, and at the same time absorb the world into ourselves. Summer is packed with various summer schools, intensive workshops and festivals, which we participate in to meet new people and learn something new and inspiring. In summer, people do not want to stay in closed rooms, and they do not want to stay in closed societies or established groupings either. Therefore, it is natural and logical that schools, ensembles and theaters are closed; instead, there are festivals, mostly with open-air events. With increasing light and warmth, fewer people go to regular classes of yoga, Qigong or dance than before, but people are looking for more casual or spontaneous activities. They need more freedom and also more opportunities to experience new and unknown things. It is natural. Our body is also open; its Qi is more on the surface, and it wakes up to life faster compared to its activity in winter when it was deep inside. In summer, it is easier for us to warm up for training or prepare for performance. We gather Yang everywhere, which will keep us warm even later on in winter. However, if Yang, heat and openness do not watch over themselves, the opposite happens. Then such a person does not want to go anywhere, preferring to stay at home.

> **Functional circuit of the heart:** heart, small intestine, pericardium, Three Burners, blood, blood vessels, circulatory system, tongue, speech, sweat, the Shen Spirit, sleep, emotion of joy, openness, fairness, peace.

THE FIRE PHASE IN HUMANS

The Qi of the FIRE phase is adequately manifested in humans. It is an active, lush, expansive, radiant, expanding and warm Qi. It is a very attractive quality. In the human body, it is embodied in the organ of the heart and in the functional circuit of the heart. In general, people with balanced FIRE Qi like to actively participate in various sports or movement activities. They are basically open, and they usually love music, dance, entertainment and social events. They are cheerful, open, sociable, with a sense of humor; they are sensitive and stable. FIRE Qi gives us the ability to perform important tasks, to influence people, to convince them. The fire itself radiates, and so the FIRE phase in us is manifested by the degree of radiance of our spirit. It helps us put our soul into what we do. If we talk about dance, for example, then the FIRE in us helps us to become a dance itself and we do not just perform it. Thanks to FIRE Qi, we know what really fulfills us; we know our essence and mission. FIRE Qi is also the need to share what is inside us, our work or knowledge. It helps us impress students when we are teachers or fascinate audiences when we are performers. It also helps us to be fascinated by something or someone. It is shown in the expression of our personality; it is our individual character.

The FIRE phase is proud of the largest number of proverbs and phrases that help us clarify and understand the quality of its Qi. Among many, I will mention, for example: "to ignite," to "put one's whole heart into something," to "have your heart in your hand," to "take something to heart," to "be warm-hearted," there were "sparks between them." In fire, there is also the initial impulse— the spark, which, although initially small, has the ability to jump over at someone and ignite interest in them. We need FIRE Qi to be able to turn our plans into concrete actions. We need it not only so that can be passionate about something, but also so that we can realize that something with enthusiasm, overcome obstacles and see it to a successful conclusion. The active Yang of FIRE in us is a concrete act. The liver, driven by the Hun, designs, plans, brings forth visions and ideas, and the heart turns them into deeds.

BRIGHTNESS AND CLARITY

In addition to heat, openness and radiance outwards, fire is related to light and its associated brightness. The FIRE phase is largely related to our ability to brightly "shine" into our surroundings, to radiate our spirit. However, it also embodies the brightness of our inner purity. If we have a clear, unobscured consciousness, then we have the ability and need to think purposefully and express ourselves clearly. The ability and potentiality to concentrate also depends on our pure consciousness.

The FIRE phase is related to speech, the ability and the need to express, communicate, share. People with harmonious FIRE Qi express themselves clearly; they do not talk too much or too little, but they express themselves when it is really necessary. The imbalance in this circle creates overly talkative or nervous people, who tend to be overly cheerful and then very unhappy. They may also be over-performing or overly serious and shy.

The movers' language is mainly the language of movement, the world of non-verbal expression. This, like verbal expression, can be clear and concrete or vague, hazy and disorganized. It may be excessive or insufficient. This concerns the movement expression of the performers but also the ability of the choreographers or directors to clearly express what they want from the performers. They should also have a feeling for the degree of how much movement is really needed in the performance. Thus, the clarity of expression and the degree of movement in non-verbal expression show the quality of the FIRE phase in us. This clarity is supported by the balanced quality of the heart Qi. Its huge helper is the Yang partner organ of the small intestine. The small intestine has a role in the process of digesting food; it separates the pure from the impure. It leaves what is clean in the body and allows it to be processed further, and shifts the waste further to be eliminated from the body. Thus, compared to the heart, the small intestine is more connected to the physical, and therefore its Qi is decisive in the area of clarity of body movement. If the small intestine Qi is in disharmony, the movers cannot provide clear movement information. Their movement expression is confusing, not brought to an end; they pour one movement section into another and so on. The harmonious Qi of the small intestine is therefore important for movers, so this organ needs to be taken care of. An excellent means of learning movement clarity and measure are lessons of movement improvisation. Improvisation teaches the movers to fully perceive what their bodies are doing, what is happening *in* them, but also *around* them in the present moment. It teaches them to perceive the right moment to enter or leave the improvisation. Improvisation is also a reflection of whether the movers use unnecessary amounts movement or, conversely, too little in their expression. Improvisation is primarily about the inner state he*re and now*, which is an important "food" for our heart and soul. These exercises help the clarity of movement, but also energetically help the small intestine.

HEART—OUR INNER EMPEROR

The heart (in Chinese, *Xin*) is the main organ of the entire functional circuit. Its Qi is very similar to the Qi of fire—it radiates to the surroundings with its own beating, through which it distributes blood and Qi through the vessels into the whole body. Thus, by its nature, it evokes fiery expansion. Its Qi spreads quickly in all directions—just one beat and all the vessels perceive it. Although it is a Yin organ, it needs to have a Yang quality in it. It is the driving force of the blood circulation; it maintains the vital activities of the organism so that life does not end. It also ensures the warming of the whole body and its nutrition through the medium of blood. It is an amazingly powerful pump that pumps 200 million liters of blood during an average life. It is a typical image of the alternation of Yin and Yang Qi, the alternation of release and contraction—diastole and systole. It happens about 70 times a minute, about 100,000 times a day, 3 billion times in an average human life.

Throughout the organ system, Taoists perceive the heart as the governor, the emperor. It has a privileged position, but also important functions belonging to the governor. The heart is the master of other organs. Just as the emperor was, for the Chinese, the embodiment of the communication between Heaven and Earth and lived protected behind walls, so the heart is in the middle of the chest and is protected by the lungs and ribs. The heart even has its own "bodyguard." It is the pericardium, a saccate pouch similar to connective tissue. It has two layers filled with a small amount of pericardial fluid, which ensures the sliding movement of the pericardial membranes during the movements of the heart. The pericardium is a kind of barrier that is the first to stop disease factors that could attack the heart. These are, for example, heat, cold, emotions and the like. The pericardium thus protects the heart and faces the first attack of harmful Qi.

THE SHEN SPIRIT

The heart preserves the psychospiritual aspect of the soul—the Shen. Simply put, it is our mind, consciousness and feelings. The Shen cannot be translated in one word—it is our vitality, radiance, charisma, but also the mind in the sense of consciousness. For us, the Shen is a connection to Heaven and the source from which we come. The Shen is what makes us human. It is our consciousness that allows us to perceive all emotions. For example, anger is caused by the Hun of the liver, but the Shen of the heart feels it and knows we are angry. Therefore, one of the functions of the Shen is to control the emotional life and, as a result, it is permanently connected with mental and emotional states. Very often, emotional imbalance can be observed on the red tip of the tongue, which is the diagnostic zone of the heart. This does not necessarily indicate a problem related to the heart as an organ, but rather to the emotions that a person is dealing with. In addition to managing emotions, other main functions of the Shen are mental activity, consciousness, memory and sleep. When these functions are impaired, one suffers from limited sensitivity, sleep problems, impatience, inability to concentrate, hypersensitivity, forgetfulness or mania.

The Shen, also called *the vital force*, is reflected, among other things, in the gleam of the eyes. It is the spark that shines from the eyes, either from ours or from the eyes of somebody we are looking at. The phrase "the eyes are windows to the soul" describes this figuratively and precisely. The heart and its Qi, which presents itself with this spark in the eyes, also provides us with nourishment on a spiritual level. Only when we have a balanced soul can the Shen fully radiate from us and we feel complete. This is the Shen, which was also discussed in Chapter 3 on Qi in connection with the Jing essence and the Qi energy. Therefore, it connects us with the universe and the source from which we come.

LET US NOT DECEIVE OUR SOULS

For the harmonious Qi of the heart and the Shen, clarity in what we do is very important, but also clarity in how we think, what we feel and what we actualize. The heart needs to be convinced of what we do and to love it. Only in this way can we ignite ourselves for something appropriately and do it in accordance with our own soul. The heart is harmed by a lie—a lie to others, but also a lie to oneself. Many people have jobs that they do not enjoy, and there are people who even hate their jobs. In the life of performers, it happens that they do not like what they do and with whom they do it. They grumble and complain, yet they go on. We get used to justifying this by telling ourselves that this is probably how it is supposed to be, that it is not possible to do only what we enjoy, that life is a struggle, a suffering, and it is necessary to somehow push our way through. Alternatively, we tell ourselves that it is necessary to do what we do not enjoy, so that the time will finally come when we can do what we do enjoy. Yes, but only occasionally. Otherwise, it is a kind of excuse that significantly harms the Shen. Every organ perceives a lie, but the heart is most affected because it recognizes every lie and suffers from it. Every excuse or lie creates pathological changes in the heart Qi; it creates an obstacle to free communication with one's own spirit, but also to the free flow of Qi throughout the body. We suffer from various heart diseases, arrhythmias, anxiety, insomnia, tinnitus or migraines, and we feel that there is nothing we can do about it. It usually does not occur to us to relate it to what we do, what we devote our time, energy and soul to throughout our lives.

There can be several forms of lies towards oneself, but also towards others, and lies can also come in different shades, which we do not normally consider to be lies. It can be concealing, omitting information, pretending or presenting things in a false way, changing the value for either better or worse. A lie is also submissive flattery in order to gain some advantage, as well as self-centered action or manipulation of others. Even self-deception has a very strong impact on our heart and the Shen. Often, we either underestimate ourselves or overestimate ourselves and look for different paths to cover up the truth, and so we lie about our true nature. The mask we wear is also a lie, with which we live the other person's fictional life and not our own. All the lies and their different shades prevent the encounter with our true self, with our true spirit, and this weakens the Qi of the heart. On the other hand, the truth nourishes it.

ENTER-EXIT

As performers, we often portray different characters. We play roles, which are not really ours. It cannot be said that this is a real lie, but from an energy point of view, it certainly affects the flow of Qi in us. Can we separate ourselves from our role on stage? What do we actually do when the show ends?

Some of us are led to do some stretching after the performance to restore our muscles and tendons to their original biochemical state. Those who are less disciplined do not bother and immediately after the show they take a shower, get dressed and go home or to a restaurant for dinner. Few are devoted to how to consciously separate from life on stage mentally, how to separate from the character they portray, but also from the world of preparation and presentation of the performance, to which one gives 100 percent. We devote so much time and energy to creating the performance, modeling the character we play in the performance, and desperately little time to the process of stepping out of that character and separating from life on stage. In this way, we play with our emotional world, and we can remain trapped on some emotional level in specific performance for several months or even years. This definitely deprives us of Qi and often also of mental well-being and mental balance.

Usually, after the performance we go to sit somewhere together with our colleagues. We do it out of social need, but also because we subconsciously try to release internal tension by staying in the company with a little alcohol, a cigarette and maybe even marijuana. Such a solution is very common, but insufficient for mental stability and actually harmful to health. We forget about the psyche and emotions from a complex point of view, and the result can be chronic fatigue syndrome, emotional imbalance, digestive problems, various degrees of manic-depression, occasional or chronic depression, or partial loss of connection with the real world. It usually does not even occur to us that some conscious "exit" should be important. Performers start to think about it only when they find out first-hand that there is something wrong with them, that they are extremely exhausted not only physically but also mentally. When they find that they have problems communicating with others, that they have problems with their sleep, that they need to regenerate, but somehow they cannot, they very often take sleeping pills. Such a state is reflected in their creativity, and it starts slowing them down.

CONSCIOUS EXIT

While working with Qigong, I encountered an exercise that helps Qi and the psyche to get back. These are simple exercises, but they require conscious work with the mind and discipline. When you experience their effect, you will find that the relief you get from alcohol, cigarettes and the like is far from equal. In this case, it is internal Qigong—*Neidan*—which is the mental connection to the inner self after the performance and the anchoring of one's thoughts, feelings and

perceptual experiences back to oneself, to one's center. It is a kind of standstill, a short meditation in silence and solitude on how to call the soul back "home." A soul that traveled through the stage during the performance, but also through the auditorium. It even got inside the spectators' souls, or into other dimensions we have no idea about. This exercise is a kind of consciously performed ritual that acts as a psychological anchor. It is advisable if it is subsequently supplemented with some gentle physical activity. It is very helpful to shake the limbs, but also the torso, because it opens the body at the whole-cell level and so it is possible to comprehensively release tension from the muscle, tendon and fascial structures. This restores inner peace not only to the body but also to the soul. Ideally, such an exercise should be accompanied by a conscious intention to relax and separate from the performance. A sign can also be generated that symbolizes the moment of separation, such as a clap, a shout or a movement gesture. It is also necessary to massage and tap the face with your fingertips. The face is logically strongly connected with the character we played in the performance. Looking into the distant horizon helps to relax the eyes. We can relax our breath with a few bursts of exhalation from the depths of our lungs and chest, sending Qi from the lungs down to the area of our center of gravity, the Lower Dantian. I practice such Qigong after my own performances and I also teach it to my students.

PROPORTION IN EVERYTHING WE DO

Whatever we do, we need to know our required proportion. Any extreme weakens the heart Qi and the kidney Qi, and consequently the whole system. It can be an extreme in action, thinking or emotion. Any fieriness in anything affects our spirit, creates unrest in it and pulls a person out of the present. In general, we are naturally prone to extreme solutions and hasty decisions, or we overwhelm ourselves with things, information, activities and offers. This situation is normal, but our task is to filter, to learn to measure, and to refine a sensibility for it. Only this will bring us real satisfaction and joy. If we do not discover and cultivate these virtues in ourselves, nervousness, agitation, excitement and impatience accumulate in us. Excessive impatience is one of the symptoms of unbalanced heart Qi.

Due to the disproportionate amount of information that comes to us through the media and social networks, based on the many artificially nurtured reports of what would be good for us, we often suffer from desires that have nothing to do with our real needs. We desire something we do not really need, and we lose our Qi because we do not focus on the essence of what we really need. Thus, for example, it may happen that in the profession of a mover we accept many offers at once and then we do not manage anything properly, and we will certainly get extremely exhausted. Or we may lose track of our true abilities and begin to expose our own bodies to motion extremes. Everybody has different potentialities and different limitations. Our bodies have differing flexibility and are capable of different loads, so if we are not aware of our own potentialities, we can hurt our body a lot by moving. Failure to respect one's abilities naturally results in unpleasant injuries. On the other hand, if an injury already occurs, we often do not learn from it and impatience prevents us from thoroughly healing the injured area. This can destroy the body and consequently prevent us from using it actively. This is reflected in frequent knee surgeries, for example, or in allaying back pain by medications to cover the real cause of pain.

I often encounter impatience with students who feel that they have learned enough. They do not finish their studies and start practicing their profession without knowing everything about it. They do not go through important experiences, and they are not sufficiently prepared physically or mentally as they embark on their professional life. This is often counterproductive. They can throw themselves into several projects at once, which can totally exhaust not only their bodies but also their souls. In addition to injuries, inexperienced movers can go through unpleasant experiences with reality, strong disappointments due to their distorted expectations. This can create a great confusion in their souls, and many even come to hate this profession. Therefore, it is important to learn it and to build respect for these things, to cultivate a certain kind of correctness, inner satisfaction and patience. It is one thing to be activated by challenges, to overcome obstacles and to push one's boundaries so that one can develop. That is fine and to some extent necessary. But it is another thing to have a feeling for certain boundaries. When a person cultivates this sensibility, then there is no place for dissatisfaction, eagerness, a depressing desire for something or impatience. We are filled with inner joy, which does not need stimuli from outside.

FIRE NEEDS TO BE TAMED BY ITS OPPOSITE—WATER

Cooling our desires also helps to find the correct proportion. Fire ignites, blazes up and burns, but it can also digest "its food" quickly, burn everything around quickly and thus destroy it. With the culminating Yang, the Yang Qi of summer brings high temperatures, long-lasting light, activity, enthusiasm, but also excitement and restlessness. However, the maximum of one phase conceals the beginning of the opposite phase. It is depicted in the Taijitu symbol (the Yin and Yang symbol) as the small dot of the opposite color. In the greatest heat, the moment comes when nature seems to be silent for a moment. Every being surrenders to meditative silence and peace. The great heat forces everyone to escape again to the Yin (coldness, darkness, rest, calmness), so that we are not completely exhausted. Qi then necessarily drops—it is a siesta, so common and necessary in southern countries.

Yang and Yin are constantly related, and if we talk about Yang and the FIRE phase, we cannot explain it enough without its connection to the WATER phase—Yin. FIRE and WATER together form in the body the functional but also the spiritual axis of the human being. They are the most apt embodiment of the qualities and principle of cooperation between Yin and Yang. WATER is embodied by the kidneys, FIRE by the heart. The heart and kidneys are energetically connected in the body by a vertical axis. This basic relationship between WATER and FIRE is probably the most important aspect in creating balance in the human body and reflects the basic balance of Yin and Yang. Therefore, it is important to constantly think about the kidneys and work with them in the summer and at any time when we notice that the FIRE Qi in us is in imbalance. That is why it is also important to cool down. This will protect our body, but also our soul.

JOY BELONGS TO FIRE PHASE AND THE HEART

The connection of the heart with joy has been in our subconscious for ages. The phrase "the heart overflows with joy" also indicates this. Joy nourishes the Qi of the heart. It positively stimulates good functioning of the physiological activities of the heart and thus affects the entire system. When the emperor rejoices, the whole country rejoices. The joy we feel has two sources. It can come to us from the outside environment or from the inside. Under normal circumstances, joy soothes emotional tension, maintains a clear and pure spirit, and ensures that Qi and blood circulate regularly. However, we can somehow naturally get lost in what is offered from the outside, and therefore we can also get lost in the degree of our joy. We either suffer from a lack of it because we do not get what we desire, or we are overjoyed. And I would like to point out again, we often crave something we do not really need, but it offers itself to us and we forget to be in touch with our essence and our real needs. Then it easily happens that when we achieve what we have longed for, joy will not come. Or it will appear, but only for a moment; it will disappear too quickly, and another desire will fill us again.

However, joy is also able to be generated from our inner environment, without stimuli from outside. When we have the soul in balance, we naturally feel permanent joy within us. We do not have to make an extreme effort for joy to arise nor do we need to express it extremely. We just have it. It is ideal to feel joy with yourself, for how you are right here and now. It is the joy that evokes inner peace, and this peace strengthens the Qi of the heart. Then even all sorts of criticism of our work cannot disturb us significantly; furthermore, we are not dependent on the opinion of others, whether it is positive or negative. On the other hand, when we are not connected to our hearts, when we are overly dependent on the feedback and opinions of others, and when we are overly concerned about what other people think of us and our work, we lose contact with ourselves. Of course, feedback is important. It is also important to appreciate any well-done activity so that Qi can flow smoothly between people. However, if we cling too much to the opinions of others, we often adapt our work to them and cease to be ourselves. It may be that we then create performances for others to like and not those that we really want to do.

For the most part, of course, we only want to hear positive feedback. When we receive it, we are happy and we think it is a real reward. When we do not get it, or when there is a negative response, we are unhappy about it. But why? Why should we be unhappy that someone does not like something? Only we can truly appreciate ourselves. However, this requires a deep self-confidence, which is preceded by allowing ourselves to make contact with ourselves. Then we are behind our work, and we also have common sense about ourselves. Only self-confidence will bring us real inner joy that no one can take from us. Negative criticism is then a challenge for us to think constructively about our work, instead of letting it deeply hurt us.

Usually, joy is considered an exclusively positive emotion. But also the joy when coming out of balance has a negative effect. The phrase" after laughter, comes tears" declares it clearly. We do not say this phrase because we do not wish someone to rejoice; we say this because we are subconsciously striving for balance. The Shen is extremely distracted by excessive joy and ceases to be in its place. This hurts the heart and causes loss of Qi. This can be manifested by a lack of strength, fainting, lack of concentration, palpitations, depression, a tendency to deal with emotionally difficult situations by constant laughing or crying, or even hysteria. So even in matters of joy, balance is important. The opposite is a lack of joy, an inability to feel any joy in life. It is also a symptom of an imbalance of heart Qi. This usually happens in response to some previous disappointment in which the heart has closed or contracted so that no more pain could enter it. Compensation for this emptiness can take the form of cynicism, tyranny or addiction to entertainment.

HERE AND NOW

Joy is also strongly related to the state in which we are able to register and fully experience the present moment. The art of *here and now* can be learned through meditation. It is the time that we spend at home every day to calm down all the sensations around us during the day. However, meditation does not have to take the form of sitting in the lotus position. To meditate, in essence, is to be conscious, to be able to be in one's center, no matter what happens. It is therefore applicable in everything we do. Every activity in which we keep our consciousness alert and have contact with what we are doing right now is meditation. Then our work can also be meditation.

As a dancer, I have a lot of experience with cultivating the state of here and now—for example, in dance improvisations. When I know what I am doing, when I watchfully perceive what is happening on stage, I have an overview of my possibilities and abilities, and I am fully connected to a group of other performers. There is pure presence, which multiplies the power of stage performance. If improvisation is transferred from the studio to the stage and becomes a theatrical means of expression that is offered to the spectator, the state of the here and now is extremely important. An alert presence offers the viewer clear, legible information about what is happening on stage. It is the same with non-improvised performances. When we want the performance to be as good as yesterday and we try to repeat those successful moments there, we lose contact with the present and the result is forced, inauthentic. Relying on the power of the present moment is always our biggest asset.

SLEEP

We demand an incredible amount of activity from our body. In proportion to this, we need to regenerate. The ideal regeneration is a good night's sleep, which should be concentrated and last for several hours without interruption. We should wake up rested, feeling that we are looking forward to the coming day.

Our daily activity is a matter of Yang; rest and sleep are Yin. The relationship between Yin and Yang should also be balanced in this regard. In order for us to practice Yang, Yin is needed and there must enough of it in order for Yang to calm down. This will ensure a calmer regime, but also good-quality blood. Taoist poetics says that in order to fall asleep, our emperor, the Shen, must dive into the bath. By bath, we mean quality and sufficient blood—that is, quality Yin. If there is little of this Yin bath, then the blood is depleted by overwork, malnutrition, mental activity or emotions, and sleep problems arise. How do we get sufficient Yin Qi? It is not an easy task in our fast-paced life. Physical activities deplete Yang itself, but at the same time greatly weaken Yin. Another major eater of Yin Qi is mental activity and emotions. As a result, the functional circuit of the heart is depleted and the blood is also depleted of other substances, which are various body fluids. Therefore, our Yin is not a sufficient substrate for Yang to sink and calm down. We all have the experience that when we try to solve something during the day and we cannot let it go, we solve it even when we should be asleep. We cannot sleep, we wake up at night, or we solve it at night in a dream. Not to mention what it does to our sleep when we are mentally engaged with something just before going to bed. Emotions disrupt the flow of Qi and bring restlessness to the heart. This also depletes blood. In this context, too, the "exit" mentioned above is needed.

Here are some tips for building sufficient Yin that Yang can use to make sleep nourishing and regenerating:

- Do not work to exhaustion or long into the night, do not take things extremely seriously or stress because of little things, and do not stimulate your emotions more than necessary. In the evening, we should already be in a calmer rhythm. The computer in the evening is an extreme consumer of our Yin, as is regular television watching at bedtime. We should go to bed before midnight because the best sleep is before midnight.

- Consume more blood-nourishing foods—beets, red fruits, red wine, red meat and broths from it, black sesame, goji.

space for regeneration during the day and to plan your free days.

Good sleep nourishes the functional circuit of the heart. It brings us comfort and one can do a lot without burning the candle at both ends. Sleep duration is individual. For one who sleeps deeply and compactly enough, a few hours are sufficient, whereas for another who has interrupted sleep, even nine or ten hours are insufficient. If sleep problems persist and we feel that we have already done everything mentioned, it is still appropriate to find out if the place where we sleep is okay. Sleep can be disturbed by a geo-pathogenic zone in which the bed is located, the transmission of electrical appliances near our bed, or an unsuitable mattress or blanket, for example.

Most probably, some performers are now smiling, because it is not possible to fall asleep before midnight and ensure a calm evening rhythm in our profession. At least not regularly. It is all the more important to ensure sufficient rest and

OTHER CONNECTIONS WITH THE HEART AND ITS FUNCTIONAL CIRCUIT

We will return to the heart and its functional circuit because we have not yet exhausted its influence on the organism and other contexts. In medical texts, we find the following information.

The partner organ of the heart is the small intestine

The Yin quality of the heart is complemented by the Yang character of the small intestine. As we have already mentioned, one of its functions is to separate clean from waste. The small intestine (in Chinese, *Xiaochang*) has the ability to recognize what is essential, what the organism must absorb and what is unnecessary or even poisonous. That is why it is one of the most important organs. In Taoist terminology, it is the *court supplier of nutrients* to the body. As part of digestion and assimilation, it ingests, differentiates and transforms digested food so that it is possible to build quality blood from food components. So the small intestine determines how the food will be used, how much Qi from food will be transformed for us, how it will nourish us. This, naturally, strongly

affects our immunity. The whole process takes place on a section of 5–8 meters of its length, which fills most of the abdominal cavity. The inner walls of the intestine have a complex structure, consisting of thousands of microvilli, which form a kind of brush. It sorts and absorbs nutrients and sends unnecessary components further into the large intestine. If a flour diet predominates in our menu, we silt these villi up with a sticky paste, thus significantly reducing the absorption of nutrients.

The psychosomatic influence of the small intestine happens on a symbolically similar level—on our ability to receive, recognize and diagnose information that comes to us. It affects mental clarity and judgment. Thanks to the small intestine Qi and the Shen of the heart, we have a sense of justice and purity. If Qi is disharmonious, there is chaos in the information; we are not able to discern what to let go of and what not to solve, and we are not able to sense what is exhausting us. In a certain point of view, this also includes meticulousness.

Easy cleansing of the small intestine

Consume only pumpkin seeds all day. They must be roasted, peeled and slightly salted. You can usually buy them at the market. Take a maximum of two handfuls a day. It is necessary to chew them properly. However, the skin of the seeds remains rougher and becomes a kind of brush that "scrubs" the inner sides of the intestine. Drink enough fluids so that the waste can be more easily washed away from the intestine. This cleansing must not be used when one suffers from inflammation of the intestines; it is intended only for healthy people who want to cleanse themselves.

Pericardium and Triple Burner

The FIRE phase includes another couple of organs, in-between which is the Yin and Yang relationship. They are the pericardium and the Triple Burner. The Yin pericardium (in Chinese, *Xinbao*) protects the heart from harmful substances, creating a kind of barrier, which is the first to stop disease factors that could attack the heart. It also connects the heart with the WATER phase at the level of sexuality, and thus ensures the connection of the heart and love with the sexuality of the physical body. Its Yang partner is a system of three areas of the body, the Three Burners (in Chinese, *Sanjiao*) mentioned in Chapter 3 on Qi. Although it is classified as an organ and has its own meridian, it is not an organ in the true sense of the word. The quality of its Qi is decisive for the FIRE phase. It helps the heart by distributing a precious energy compound of the prenatal Jing essence with the postnatal essence obtained from food and inhaled air, which was also mentioned in Chapter 3. In classical Taoist texts, this process is described as *patient, conscientious refinement and purification*, which results in the precious, pure and subtle essences necessary for the harmonious life of humans. Today we would call

it *distillation*. The Triple Burner in this process includes all organs: the Lower Burner contains the intestines, the kidneys, the bladder; in the Middle Burner is the spleen, the stomach, the pancreas, the liver and the gallbladder; and in the Upper Burner are the lungs, the heart and the pericardium. All organs are involved in the metabolic process, and the Triple Burner is the administrator of the cooperation between them.

The heart opens at the tongue

Old medical texts state that the tongue is the *offshoot of the heart*. It is not for nothing that they say "what the heart thinks, the tongue speaks." Modern scientific research in the field of embryology confirms this connection. In embryonic development, it can be seen that the primitive tongue is formed in the area of the primitive heart, specifically of the pericardium. Thus, the tongue has been in contact with the heart since its inception; they even come from the same tissue lining—the mesoderm. The inner branch of the Heart channel protrudes into the tongue, and in this way Qi and the heart's blood travel through the vessels and pass through the tongue. The tongue, as an offshoot of the heart, is an external indicator of the state of the heart.

The tongue is also an important organ for speaking. The ability to speak, to express articulately, indicates the harmonious Qi of the heart, and we have already written about this clarity of expression. Speech is an important diagnostic alert for a disorder in the variable FIRE phase. To a large extent, it also results from the ability to listen and to hear in the sense of understanding and comprehension. The one who can listen can also refine the Shen. Perceptive listening is the deepest meditation. Only through real listening are we able to make real contact with others and with our real needs and our purpose. Incoherent, meaningless speech, constant repetition of the same topic, too many misused expressions or being closemouthed are manifestations of a disorder in the FIRE phase.

The heart governs blood and blood vessels

The vessels are the seat of blood and the paths where blood flows. The heart drives it with its beat, and thus distributes nutrition to all parts of the body. At the same time, the heart ensures that the blood circulates continuously. When the heart function is weakened, there is a lack of oxygenation and a lack of nutrition of other organs and tissues, which can be manifested by increased shortness of breath during physical strain or by pressure on the chest. In more serious cases, there may be flooding of the lungs, increasing swelling of the legs, abdomen and eventually of the whole body, and there may be life-threatening arrhythmias resulting in collapse or death. Weak heart function leads to chronic contraction of blood vessels in peripheral tissues and organs to "save" blood to keep other vital organs functioning.

In the previous two chapters, we focused on two phases—WATER and WOOD—and we also focused on the structures of the body that these phases and the organs associated with them are in charge of—bones, cartilage, joints and tendons. The movement of the human body depends on them. In the FIRE phase, the heart is in charge of the blood vessels. From the point of view of the mover's body, this is not a structure that we would obviously register, perceive and feel when moving. Blood vessels cannot even be strengthened or cultivated by movement, unlike the bones, muscles and tendons. However, the vessels move with us constantly during our movement and in all directions, and the bones, muscles and tendons are nourished by them.

The heart Qi manifests through the complexion

Blood circulation is also associated with the ability to carry blood up to the head. The blood vessels in the face are very numerous, so the skin and its glow reflect the state of the heart Qi. If the heart function is normal, the skin is not dull, but has a shiny glow. If the Qi of the heart is excessive, the face is red.

The heart controls perspiration

According to Chinese medicine, blood and body fluids have the same origin. Sweat therefore belongs to this circuit and has its source in the blood. Sweating is a form of cooling, but also a way for the heart to relieve our body of toxins. This is done 3 percent through the stool, 7 percent through the urine, 70 percent through the excretion of carbon dioxide by the lungs and 20 percent through sweat eliminated through the skin. The route for elimination is the lymphatic vessels, which are richly represented in the skin. Sweating is therefore normal and extremely important. It is natural that we sweat relatively more when we move, because the movement heats us up and we need to cool down more. We need to realize that in doing so, however, we are losing precious body fluids, which we must then replenish. A drinking regimen and a diet supplementing body fluids are therefore extremely important for movers. However, when sweating we also lose precious components in the blood, as blood and sweat have the same origin. Therefore, for example, people with poor blood quality are not recommended to stay long or to sweat frequently in a dry sauna, which causes a significant loss of body fluids.

Heat destroys the heart

Heat and fire are external harmful substances. The heat in the form of summer heat is extremely Yang in nature, so it destroys Yin. It rises and disperses, causing heavy sweating and thus damage to body fluids. Fire is different from heat because fire is not subject to seasonal weather changes. Fire burns, ignites, blazes up, attacks the upper parts of the body, consumes Qi, damages body fluids and causes blood turmoil. Fire causes the formation of abscesses and purulent rashes. Acne, for example, is the elimination of fire and moisture. Fire can enter our body from the outside through the weather, but it is most often generated by internal processes related to our emotional life, so it is largely dependent on the liver Qi. It can easily obscure the Shen when a person is unfocused, unable to concentrate or even mentally out of their normal context.

Red is the color of the FIRE phase

Red is a color that evokes love. Red was also associated with the emperor in China; in addition to yellow, it has a prominent position in temples and imperial buildings. We also mentioned it in connection with the mercury sulfide (vermilion) of the Three Dantians. And since the emperor of our empire is the heart, the color red is naturally assigned to the FIRE phase. This color therefore supports the heart circuit, yet, in excessive amounts, it can also destroy it.

THE RELATIONSHIP BETWEEN THE HEART AND OTHER ORGANS OF THE FIRE PHASE

Although the heart ranks among the Yin organs, it is the most Yang in nature of them all. This is caused by its fiery, expanding Qi, which also results in its ability to pump regularly and send blood throughout the body. The Heart channel has only nine points, which is the fewest of all channels, so it needs to transform the excess of its Qi in other channels. The small intestine helps by letting the heart release its accumulated heat into the Small Intestine channel. The small intestine therefore acts as a cooling assistant for the heart. For example, children's fever is solved by having the child drink fresh sour apple juice. It gets into the small intestine very quickly and cools it so much that the small intestine can then draw in the heat of the heart. The relationship to the kidneys, which eliminate the fire of the heart, is also important. The heart as a governor must also have a kind of guardian—the pericardium which creates a kind of barrier against the influence of disease factors.

RELATIONSHIP OF THE FIRE PHASE TO OTHER PHASES

According to the Sheng cycle, which we discussed in Chapter 7 on the five Qi transformation phases, it is clear that the "mother" of the heart is the liver. The quality of the liver Qi, then, also determines the quality of the heart Qi, which is evident, for example, in the smooth flow of emotions. The liver creates the necessary pathways for the flow of emotions so that the heart can connect with them and feel them. This means that if we want to take care of the heart, we must also pay attention to the liver Qi. The anger of the liver can be so strong that it reaches the heart so intensely that a person can have a heart attack after such an episode. The connection between these two organs is also at the blood level.

At the same time, the fire must be controlled so that it does not spread to excessive dimensions. This could be dangerous for a human being. Therefore, it is the kidneys in the WATER phase that regulate the intensity of FIRE with their Qi. We have written about this above. If the FIRE Qi is harmonious, it can nourish the EARTH phase well and at the same time limit the excess in the METAL phase.

CONCLUSION TO THE FIRE PHASE

In the summer, we should not overdo it with excessive exposure to the sun. It is advisable to cool with mint tea or green tea, both of which have a cooling effect. Iced drinks should be avoided, as they paradoxically generate even more heat in the body. The same applies to ice cream. We avoid frequent grilling. In summer, it is important to enjoy the feeling of freedom, to be outdoors more, in society, but we must not forget about our own anchoring, time for ourselves. Let us try to include more clarity in our lives by thinking, but also by communicating with others or with ourselves. Before we say anything, let us think about whether it is really important or whether it is true. Let us be honest with ourselves and others.

At the end of the summer, the days are colder, so it is advisable to have warmer clothes on hand so that the cold does not enter the body. We are slowly calming down and preparing for the harvest.

Table 10.1 Main correspondences of FIRE phase

Year season: summer	Yin and Yang stage: Utmost Yang/Yang in Yang
Day time: noon	Direction: south
Evolution of Qi: peak of Qi	Growth cycle in nature: growth, flowering, ripening
Life cycle: growth, adolescence	Working cycle: action, manifestation
Yin organ: heart	Organ clock for heart: 11 a.m. to 1 p.m.
Yang organ: small intestine	Organ clock for small intestine: 1 to 3 p.m.
Yin organ: pericardium	Organ clock for pericardium: 7 to 9 p.m
Yang organ: Triple Burner	Organ clock for Triple Burner: 9 to 11 p.m.
Psychospiritual aspect: Shen	Virtue: justice, uprightness
Emotion: joy	Climate: heat
Color: red	Taste: bitter
Smell: scorched	Number: 7
Tissue: blood vessels	Body fluid: sweat
Other body tissues: complexion, tongue	Other body fluid and excretion: blood, lymph
Joints: elbows	Entry point of disease: chest
Sense organ: tongue	Sense: speech
Indicator: complexion	Detrimental action: too much talking and loud reading
Sound: laughing	Mental attitude: love, openness, hopefulness

MERIDIANS

HEART CHANNEL (HT)/YIN

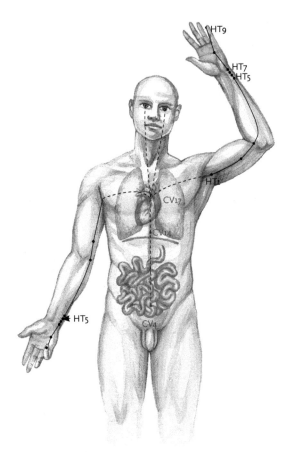

Heart channel

The Heart channel is a Yin pair channel, leading from the chest along the inside of the arms to the little fingers. In the image below, it is shown on both sides. It starts in the heart and is divided into three internal branches. The first passes through the diaphragm and connects the heart to the small intestine. The second protrudes through the esophagus and heads into the eyes, making way for the Shen to radiate through the eyes. The third branch leads to the armpit, where the main branch emerges to the surface of the skin at its first point. It runs along the inner backs of the upper arms through the elbows, forearms and wrists. It penetrates the palms and ends at the nail bed of the little fingers on the thumb side. In the area of the hands, it connects with the Small Intestine channel. The heart is also called the *lotus flower with nine gates*, which indicates that this path has nine acupuncture points.

The channel relates to the heart muscle itself. It affects heart disease and circulatory problems, palpitations, arrhythmias, etc. It also affects speech disorders, including stuttering. It also has an influence on excessive sweating, especially at night. It affects the spirit, helps to calm nervousness and affects sleep.

HEART CHANNEL IN MOVEMENT

The channel, with its Yin essence and shorter length, offers us immersion in subtlety. However, the lines of the little fingers on the inner sides of the arms offer an interesting, not very common use. When we work with them, it has an effect on the opening of the axillary area (armpits). The channel begins in the heart, at the depth of the chest, and leads to the arm. This deep source helps to integrate the arms with the center of the chest and, in fact, with the whole body, in addition to using the chest to move the arms and vice versa.

Interesting for movement is the use of the inner areas of the elbows, where the channel passes. Making the movement through these areas helps to fully open the flow in this channel, while physically feeling how Qi flows automatically from the elbows to the little fingers.

The track also passes through the palms and ulnar sides of the wrists (on the sides of the little fingers), which we can discover and activate in movement improvisation. It also includes the pectoral muscles and the sides of the upper ribs, which we can also consciously involve in movement. It will beautifully open our chest, helping us create more space for the heart and a little loosening of its grip in the chest, which happens during normal functioning.

The inner branch of the channel leads to the eyes, which gives us the possibility to engage the eyes, sight and conscious look in the movement. When we move with a conscious look for a while, the heart seems to be filled with this consciousness and the space which the movement creates for it.

After longer improvisation, Qi is strongly activated in the channel. Let us enjoy this flow of Qi in fast or slow motion, as well as in its Yin quality.

SMALL INTESTINE CHANNEL (SI)/YANG

The Small Intestine channel is a paired Yang channel, leading along the outer sides of the arms towards the neck and torso. In the image below, it is shown on one side only. It follows the Heart channel on the little fingers of the hands from their outer sides. It leads to the wrists along the outer sides of the little fingers and to the lower edge of the elbow bones. It continues along the outer side of the upper arms to the back of the shoulders, from where it zigzags through the shoulder blades and trapezius to the seventh cervical vertebra, where it connects with the Qi of the other Yang channels. From there, it sinks into pits above the collarbone, where it branches off. One branch leads down to connect the Qi of the small intestine with the Qi of the heart. It penetrates the diaphragm and stomach and plunges into the small intestine itself. This inner branch continues below the knees, to the Stomach channel. The second branch protrudes up the neck and continues through the lower jaw under the cheekbones. The inner branch connects with the Bladder channel at the inner corners of the eyes. It also passes to the outer corners of the eyes and from there ends its pathway at the ears and penetrates into them. Its main branch has 19 acupuncture points.

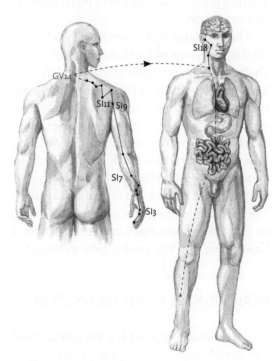

Small Intestine channel

The channel relates to the small intestine itself, affects the digestion and absorption of nutrients, stomach activity and abdominal pain, but also head and neck pain. As it leads through the shoulder, it also affects the pain and tension of the neck and muscles of the shoulders, as well as problems with the scapulas. It also has an effect on problems with the ears and nape, and rheumatic and nerve diseases of the upper limbs. It also influences the upper parts of the neck and face, eyes, temples, ears and larynx.

SMALL INTESTINE CHANNEL IN MOVEMENT

This channel is more dynamic than its paired Heart channel. Its little finger line, leading along the outside of the arms, enables us to use the arms and body more to the sides and back, thus helping the body to open up more into space. The movement can be led by the entire back line of the arms, or by a very specific place on the elbows between the ends of the radius and ulna bones, on the so-called *funny bone*. This will turn it into a huge source of inspiration for arm movement.

The channel also offers work with the back of the shoulder joints and with the shoulder blades. The human body is capable of relatively large and interesting movement of the blade bones, but we are not used to using them when moving. If we work consciously through the movement with the blades, they will come to life a great deal. Our back will seem to have "back eyes." We will be more sensitive and receptive to what is happening behind us, and we can respond adequately. The back is no longer a zone of unconsciousness; on the contrary, with this work we can develop a huge feeling in it. The Small Intestine channel is, after all, connected to the eyes themselves by the inner branch, but also by the connection to the Bladder channel, which begins in close proximity to the eyes and leads to the back of the body. It is therefore natural for this channel to "see" what is behind us.

By working with the shoulder blades and shoulder joints, we activate the entire shoulder girdle. And as the channel passes through it, working with it provides a kind of energetic nutrition for the area.

On the face, we can enliven the cheekbones in motion, where the channel passes, and also move the head and then the whole body from the temples. The inner branch leads below the knee, and we can use it to connect the top of the body with the knees. This will also pleasantly ground us.

After longer improvisations, Qi is strongly activated in the channel. We can really enjoy this flow of Qi in motion, but also in the stillness that takes place after it and enjoy its Yang character.

PERICARDIUM CHANNEL (PC)/YIN

The Pericardium channel is a Yin pair channel that runs through the inner side of the arms. In the image below, it is shown on one side only. It starts in the middle of the chest in the area of the heart and pericardium. One inner branch passes through the diaphragm all the way down to the Lower Dantian, thus connecting all Three Burners. The superficial, main branch starts at the nipples from the outside, turns upwards towards the shoulders and leads down along the shoulder bones (humerus) along the biceps between the Lung channel and Heart channel. It passes through the elbow joints, then through the inner sides of the forearms between their two tendons. It runs through the wrists into the palms and from there to the top of the middle fingers. In the palm area, one flow line separates to the ring fingers, where it connects to the path of the Triple Burner. The Pericardium channel, like the Heart channel, has nine acupuncture points.

The channel affects heart disease, circulatory disorders, hardening of the arteries, varicose veins, poor blood circulation, circulatory disorders, angina pectoris, palpitations. It has an impact on the psyche because it calms the mind. It also has an effect on the stomach and can harmonize it.

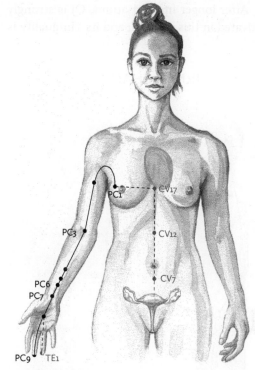

Pericardium channel

PERICARDIUM CHANNEL IN MOVEMENT

The channel, with its Yin essence and shorter length, offers us immersion in subtlety. Its origin in the chest helps to integrate the arms with the whole body in movement and, in addition, to use the chest to move the arms and vice versa. The center line of the inside of the arms offers an unusual use of the center of the elbows and the center of the forearms. When consciously working with this area, Qi will be pleasantly opened and this area will be revived. Likewise, the center of the inner sides of the wrists can be invigorating for our movement vocabulary. In addition, working your wrists in motion helps energize Qi in the palms. The Qi in the channel passes through the center of the palms and it spreads to the entire palms and hands. This gives us great support

ability. The palms can also be used in motion to carry the weight of the body—that is, to transfer the weight when leaning against a wall, the ground or a moving partner, for example. They can also be used for walking on all fours. In this case, we can play with being some kind of animal, and perceive what the contact with the floor does with the Qi in our palms. We can still develop this perception in upside-down positions—that is, in handstands. Can we use our palms as soles and have feet as sensitive as palms? Yes, it works.

In the palms, the channel branches into middle fingers and ring fingers. So we can also use these two pairs of fingers to move the hands. We realize how little we normally use them in life, and moving them will help activate Qi in our hands.

After longer improvisations, Qi is strongly activated in this channel, and its Yin quality is physically felt. Let us enjoy this flow of Qi in motion, but also in stillness.

TRIPLE BURNER CHANNEL (TB)/YANG

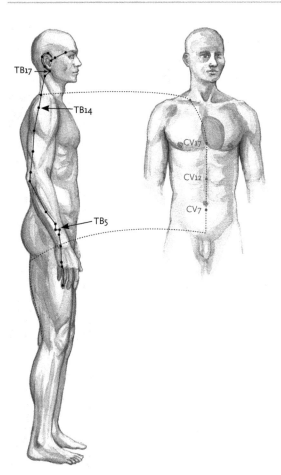

Triple Burner channel

outer sides between the Large Intestine channel and Small Intestine channel, between the radius and the ulna to the elbows. It ascends from the upper arms to the shoulders, and from there its inner branch leads Qi under the seventh cervical vertebra to connect this Yang channel with the other Yang channels. From there, it runs forward through the trapezius muscle to the pits above the collarbones. It splits here. One inner branch penetrates the chest; on the sternum, it connects with the heart and the pericardium. It passes through the diaphragm down to the pubic bone and from there to the back of the knee joints (popliteal fossa). The second branch, directed towards the ears, encircles them from back to front. It ends on the face next to the eyebrows, but with the inner branch it connects with the eyes and by another flow line with the Gallbladder channel. Its main branch has 23 acupuncture points.

The Triple Burner channel is a paired Yang channel, shown in the image above on one side only. It follows the Pericardium channel. It starts on the outer sides of the ring fingers at the root of the nails and continues along the outer side of the hands between the ring fingers and the little fingers. On the forearms, it leads through the

The channel affects the harmonization of the connection of all Three Burners. It is also responsible for protecting the body's immunity through the lymphatic system, regulation of urinary tract patency, thermoregulatory disorders, circulatory disorders, general cold or overheating, lymphatic disorders, fluid and toxin retention in the body, immune disorders, lack of resistance to infections and diseases, and allergies. On the emotional level, it supports the care of oneself and loved ones.

TRIPLE BURNER CHANNEL IN MOVEMENT

The section of the channel on the arms is relatively uninteresting for movement, but we can work with the outer sides of the wrist, elbow and shoulder bones. The outer sharp sides of the elbows provide interesting material for movement. At the shoulders, the channel becomes more interesting. It hits the upper trapezius and the top of the shoulder blades. We do not normally use this part in motion, so we can revive it by working with the channel. Let us discover what it is like to move the top of the shoulder blades and what effect it has on trapezius, neck or upper limbs. This area is naturally connected to the neck. Through movement, we can perceive the connection of the top of the shoulder blades with the neck and use the softness of this connection. Under the ears, the channel enters the cavity between the jaw and the sternocleidomastoid muscle, which brings interesting possibilities for movement. As it passes around the ears, we can involve the ears and hearing, as well as peripheral sensations. In movement improvisation, we can work with the hollow under the earlobe. We can perceive how this affects the movement of the head and neck, but also the whole spine.

The end of the channel at the outer ends of the eyebrows helps to relax and widen the face, activating sight and thus refreshing the perception of space.

The inner branch leads backwards below the knee pits. In motion, we can realize the connection of the arms with the torso and with the back of the lower limbs.

DIET IN SUMMER AND FOR THE FIRE PHASE ORGANS

In summer, Yang typically dominates, radiating in all directions. It is hot and dry, so you need to add more Yin to your diet for hydrating and gentle refreshment. It is advisable to increase the intake of vegetables, especially green and leafy types. Raw vegetables have cooling effects and help create body fluids that need to be expanded in the summer. Raw and fresh guarantees a new replenishment of Yin substances, which are washed out of the body by sweating. However, a lot of raw vegetables may not benefit a weaker spleen—those people with poor digestion due to the weakness of the spleen Qi. If a lot of raw vegetables are consumed, cold also occurs in the stomach, which can manifest itself in loss of appetite. In this case, you should add a little ginger to your rice in order to restore the Yang of digestion.

Therefore, we also cook vegetables in the summer, but for a shorter time. We blanch, simmer briefly, cook for less time—vegetables can be crunchier. Soups should not be thick, but should contain a lot of water. In addition to salads from raw vegetables, there are excellent salads from short-fermented vegetables or pressed vegetables. This is a salted vegetable, fermented under a weight for only a few hours. From the leafy vegetables, fresh vegetables with large leaves are best, such as lettuce, iceberg lettuce or Chinese cabbage and, of course, other vegetables that are ripening at that time—zucchini/courgette, cucumbers, tomatoes, artichokes, chicory, all vegetable tops and small salad herbs such as arugula/rocket, radicchio and the like. We use less of the root vegetables, yet thanks to the red color of FIRE, the beetroot is an excellent vegetable.

Grilled vegetables have more Yang in them, so it is better to avoid them. This is even more true for grilled meat. Although barbecue is very popular nowadays, it should be handled with care in the summer, and really only used occasionally. Grilling is one of the most Yang, hence the most warming food preparation, which in the strongest Yang of the summer can be dangerous for Qi of the functional circuit of the heart. Various grain sprouts will help us cool the organism, and we can add these to almost everything—soups, cereals, porridge, vegetables, meat, etc. The best are sprouts from small seeds—mustard, watercress, arugula/rocket, alfalfa, radish, etc. Sprouts of grain and legumes are not easily digested.

Meat

Meat is Yang itself, so in summer it is advisable to limit consumption of meat. Salt less, use fats, but in small amounts.

Fruit

Friut is suitable, because it is ripe and it offers itself for consumption. In cases of internal cold, cook the fruit lightly. In summer, tropical fruit is suitable, which cools significantly.

Cereals

From cereals, more Yin kinds are suitable—corn, couscous and bulgur, which are cooked for short times. But also amaranth, quinoa, buckwheat and rice.

Bitter taste

The bitter taste supports the Qi of the heart, pericardium and small intestine. People usually neglect it in their diet, which is a pity. Definitely do not avoid it in summer. From herbs, we can add to salads, for example, ribgrass, celandine, dandelion and nettle. Arugula/rocket and chicory have an ideal bitter taste.

Red color

Indulge in red fruits. The color of the FIRE phase is red, so we consume everything that is red and edible. For example, cherries are ideal, especially the big heart-shaped ones that are literally made for the heart. Furthermore, strawberries, raspberries, chokeberry and other red berries. Red grape juice is also delicious. The overall color of the summer should be reflected in summer meals. Use a lot of fresh herbs that have a positive effect on physical activity. Do not be afraid to include something unusual in the dishes, such as flowers. On the plate can appear marigolds, lavender, hoary cress, rose, clover flowers, dead nettle, mallow, wild thyme, chamomile flowers, dandelion flower, daisy, but also pumpkin flowers, zucchini and the like.

> **Cooling and refreshing foods:** Cereal and legume sprouts, mung sprouts, tomatoes, zucchini/courgettes, eggplant/aubergine, cucumbers, peppers, olives, umeboshi plum, pineapple, kiwi, citrus fruits, mango, papaya, watermelon and yellow honeydew melon, raw fruits in general, yogurt, dairy products, mineral waters, herbal teas, green tea, mint tea, beer, seaweed, salt, soy sauce, tofu, soy milk, buckwheat.

Fluids

In summer, the need for fluids increases. The heat makes our pores open and ventilate. We sweat more and thus lose fluids. On warm summer days, however, we should not quench thirst with extremely cold or iced drinks. It is an extreme shock primarily to the stomach, which, as we know, needs heat to digest food sufficiently. Intake of very cold fluids will cause a second shock to the kidneys. In both cases, the body cools down, which in turn requires harmonization and the associated higher consumption of Qi. In China, in the summer, even in the greatest heat, we found large public thermoses with hot boiled water almost everywhere. Even in the Middle East, they quench thirst with hot tea—however, it is mint tea, which in itself has a cooling effect on the body. Green tea, herbal teas, corn silk tea, fresh fruit juices and even mineral water are cooling too. People with an internal cold and a weaker spleen, and therefore poor digestion, should be more careful with their drinking. Suitable is pu-erh tea, which pulls Qi down and has a beneficial effect on emotions.

Coffee

Coffee is healthy in small doses, but it can harm in big ones. We know this—even the fact that it can be an addictive drug. Having coffee from time to time with friends for a feeling of well-being is nice. Native Americans consider coffee to be a shamanic herb, thus intended for shamans on special occasions, and not for daily consumption and not for everyone. Coffee has a naturally bitter taste, so it benefits the heart's functional circuit to a reasonable degree. However, having coffee to stop feeling drowsy is not the best solution. We reach for coffee when we suffer from fatigue, drowsiness or lack of concentration, or when we need to overwhelm our body with the conviction that we are still able to continue for a while. However, fatigue and lack of concentration have a reason, and that is the lack of Qi in the spleen and the lack of Yang in the kidneys. Coffee helps us to overcome these alarming signals of the body for a while, but it does not eliminate the cause. On the contrary, coffee deepens this condition, plunders these organs even more, pulls the Jing essence out of the kidneys. Fatigue and drowsiness are actually a kind of instinct for the body's self-preservation, which limits us and invites us to rest. Therefore, if we suffer from an excessive need for coffee, it should be taken as a warning signal to put the kidneys and spleen energetically in order. The easy way, which we do not even need a doctor for, is to take more rest, take breaks at work, go for walks, and thus revitalize our brain. If our fatigue is associated with low blood pressure, chewing *Schisandra chinensis* will help instead of coffee. In addition, caffeine is a kind of blocker. This means that with a large amount or regular consumption, it blocks the absorption of necessary nutrients into the body.

Some tips to help you when you have a need for coffee

If during long-term study or exhaustion we need to reach for a cup of coffee, and since our kidney Qi is precious for us, we should try to walk instead. If there is no time for it, a simple self-massage technique will also help. There are two acupuncture points on our head. The first is located at the top of the head on the Governing Vessel; it is the point *One Hundred Meetings* (in Chinese, *Bahui*, GV20). Tap the point or the entire top of the head with the fingers of one hand at least 100 times. On the same channel, in the groove between the upper lip and the nose (philtrum), there is a point *Man's Middle* (in Chinese, *Renzhong*, GV26). Dig your nails into it so intensely that drops of tears come out of your eye canals. The massage of the earlobes is also excellent, especially pulling them down. It activates the brain and our attention. At the same time, however, I would like to point out that even this advice should not be misused either. If we are really exhausted, choose sleep or a moment of rest in a horizontal position.

Grain coffee

For a "coffee treat," there is an excellent substitute of grain coffee. It does not contain caffeine and, with its delicate taste, will satisfy even the most demanding "tongues." Grain coffee complements the Qi of the spleen, and if its Qi is in order, we also have enough Qi for everyday use. In addition, it is also suitable for lack of heart Qi and kidney Yang. It is made from roasted grain, most often from barley, spelt or rice, and it can also contain chestnuts, figs or chicory. The kind of Slavic coffee is the so-called *acorn coffee*, made from roasted oak fruits—acorns. It tastes very good and is very nutritious. If a little almond or rice milk is added to it, it tastes delicious.

Grain coffees warm the spleen and stomach, which our digestion needs. At the same time, they help carry moisture away from the body and also encourage intestinal peristalsis. However, they are not recommended for high blood pressure and general irritation associated with liver Qi stagnation.

Three reflections on smoothies

- **Excess of Yin.** Almost all smoothies are cooling because they are made from uncooked ingredients. Excessive consumption of smoothies can cause a deep cool-down of the digestive organs. If we cannot give up smoothies, we need to add at least a pinch of heating spices (cinnamon, chili, curry, etc.). Smoothies are therefore extremely Yin in quality and should not be consumed by people with Yin pathology, people who, for example, have problems with fibroids or fluid-filled cysts or are overweight from water retention, or people with poor digestion who need a cure by warming up.
- **Wind.** In addition to the cold, we also bring wind to the digestive tract and the whole organism with smoothies which are prepared by blending. If there is a lot of wind, it brings restlessness, distraction, inability to concentrate. For this reason, smoothies are unsuitable for children and adults with attention deficit hyperactivity disorder (ADHD).
- **Extreme.** Blending food in a blender offers a thin mushy drink that can contain up to 600–700 grams of vegetables or fruits. This is extreme—we would not normally consume that much. We would normally have to chew fruit or vegetables properly for consumption. However, such a liquid form of food does not encourage us to sufficiently chew and mix it with saliva. This way we do not supply the necessary alkaline component from saliva to digestion.

I recommend looking at smoothies from several points of view. One is the nutrients in fruits and vegetables, which is undoubtedly true, but on the other hand are the factors mentioned above. It is necessary to test, compare, feel and perceive its impact on the long run, and not just to be led by unilateral reports on their effects. Everything in the world, including smoothies, has two sides of the coin.

A FEW TIPS AND RECIPES

Cooling rice dish with grapefruit
Ingredients: Arborio rice, hazelnuts, raisins, agave syrup, yogurt, grapefruit, butter, salt or coconut oil.

Method: Cook the rinsed rice in water in a ratio of 1:2, together with a pinch of salt, raisins and chopped nuts soaked overnight. Once cooked, stir in a little agave syrup, add the yogurt, finely chopped grapefruit and stir. Serve with a knob of butter or coconut oil.

Benefits: It is refreshing, creates juices, keeps the Qi down.

Quick pickles
Ingredients: Any vegetable, ume vinegar.

Method: Thinly slice any vegetable and toss with ume vinegar instead of salt. Let it ferment for a few hours.

Benefits: Pickles pleasantly cool down and produce enzymes. Do not add salt as it would burden the kidneys.

Beetroot soup with goat cheese and rucola

Ingredients: 2 or 3 beetroots, 1 onion, sunflower oil, soy cream, salt, fresh arugula/rocket, goat cheese, water,

Method: Fry the chopped onion in the oil, add the chopped beetroot, cover with water, season lightly with salt and cook for about 15 minutes. Once cooled, blend, add the soy cream and bring to the boil again, but only briefly, so that the beetroot is combined with the cream. Serve topped with goat cheese and fresh arugula/rocket.

Benefits: This soup replenishes the blood, supports the heart, spleen and pancreas. The beetroot, onion and sunflower oil warms, making this soup more suitable for cooler summer days.

Creamy tofu dessert

Ingredients: 2 blocks of white tofu, salt, ground cinnamon to taste, 100g dried raisins (or other dried fruit—e.g. cranberries, apricots, dates, figs, mulberries), rice or maple syrup, 2–3 tbsp soy cream, water, pure cocoa or carob powder. (Cocoa can also be replaced by molasses mixed with tahini sesame paste.)

Method: Soak the dried fruit in advance for a few hours. Mix water and syrup and put two-thirds of this mixture in a saucepan, add the tofu crumbled into small pieces, a pinch of salt, the soaked fruit and cinnamon. Simmer for about 5 minutes on a low heat. Once cooled, blend, gradually adding the rest of the liquid mixture and soy cream until you get a smooth cream. Serve in bowls garnished with fresh mint or other herbs or edible flowers. If desired, you can add more flavor and garnish with maple or rice syrup, or pure cocoa powder.

Benefits: The dessert lightly cools on warm days, supports the spleen, the pancreas and the heart, and generates juices.

Cooling mungo beans with tofu

Ingredients: Smoked tofu or seaweed tofu, 3 tomatoes, salt, onion, marjoram, oil, some sprouted mung beans.

Method: Put the tomatoes in boiling water and let them steam, then place them in cold water. Fry the finely chopped onion in the oil, add the tofu cut into small cubes, fry together briefly. Add the tomatoes, which have been peeled, the marjoram and the mung beans, season with salt. Simmer for 15 minutes, stirring occasionally, adding water if necessary.

The skin of the mung bean is quite difficult to digest, so it is ideal to remove it after cooking.

Benefits: Cools and detoxifies.

Peppermint tea

Ingredients: 200 ml hot water, 2–5 fresh mint leaves.

Method: Pour hot water over the mint in a glass and leave to infuse for 3–5 minutes.

Benefits: The tea expels heat from the body, cleanses and cools the liver.

Watermelon cocktail

Ingredients: Watermelon, pinch of ground cinnamon, fresh mint.

Method: Put the melon and cinnamon in a container and blend. The seeds can be removed in advance if you do not want them. Serve garnished with mint.

Benefits: The cocktail strengthens the heart and small intestine; it has a cooling effect. It is also good for heatstroke. We can also boil the green rind of the melon in the water and drink the water.

Salty watermelon

In Asia, watermelon with Himalayan or black salt is popular. It is eaten to replenish the missing minerals and trace elements that we sweat out in the summer. Of course, salt must be used in moderation, not only for reasons of taste, but also for unwanted excess salt.

Benefits: It strengthens the heart and small intestine, has a cooling effect and replenishes Qi.

CHAPTER 11

The EARTH phase

Returning to the center

About: the human center / stability / regularity / stomach and spleen and their ability to transform / digestion of food as well as of life situations / ability to think constructively / muscles and muscle care / master point Zusanli / dampness / pensiveness / the Intellect Yi / traveling and ability to adapt / sugar / diet for late summer and for the EARTH phase organs

Everything that is created of the universe meets in the center (between Yin and Yang) and is absorbed by the Earth.

THE YELLOW EMPEROR'S CLASSIC OF MEDICINE

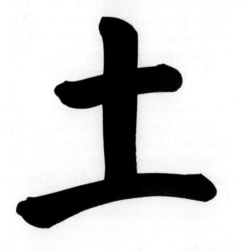

Chinese character for EARTH

The WOOD phase was an active increase upwards, an effort to manifest, to break through. Yang Qi gradually rose to reach its energetic peak in the FIRE phase. In summer, all processes in nature were in peak activity (Yang). The sun reached its highest position (Yang), the colors around us were bright and glaring (Yang), we spent a lot of time outside (Yang), because in the summer it was warm (Yang). Days (Yang) were long, and nights (Yin) were short. In order to maintain balance in nature and in ourselves, Qi must begin to fall (Yin), calm down (Yin) and gradually prepare for the rest of winter (Yin). During the autumn METAL phase, Qi will concentrate into itself; it will shrink, so that in the winter WATER phase, it can attain its maximum winter rest. The transition from Yang to Yin is the late summer and the EARTH phase.

EARTH CENTER

Late summer is a time of return, an attractive time of transition. It is a milestone between what has not yet completely left and what has not yet come. It is the center. The EARTH phase has a special position among all phases. It is the source of all phases, the center from which they arise. In the original texts, EARTH is shown in the middle position, in contrast to the pentagram shape that we have encountered so far. In this older representation, EARTH forms the center, the fifth direction. Four directions, four points of the compass—east, west, north and south—are, according to the Taoists, anchored in the middle, which guarantees a balance between them. The image of the phase distribution in the pentagram developed from this theory.

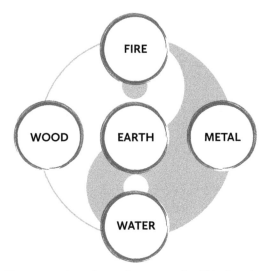

The EARTH phase forms the center, the fifth direction

NECESSITY OF RETURNING TO THE CENTER

Whatever we experience, no matter what project we do, what event we organize, what we study, how we raise children or experience a relationship, it always has the same course. After the ascent, we reach the top, and it is naturally followed by the descent. Of course, it does not have to be a total fall, but the downward direction is a condition in the development of everything. We cannot be at the peak of our careers all our lives; we cannot flourish all the time just as intensely. The dynamics of our work commitments or the circumstances that affect us are formed by life, so that everything has an ascending and then a descending direction of development. Return is a condition for development. Every time we get from the top to the bottom, something new starts. However, it is human nature to cling like a limpet to what we consider ideal at any given moment, and to feel frustrated when it ends. Since no one has taught us this, we are not able to easily accept the ends and more demanding periods. The summer is over, with everything pleasant and carefree, and many of us do not want to enter the next stage. But even the end of summer and what comes after it is important, and you can develop a great love for it.

QI OF THE EARTH PHASE BUILDS UP STABILITY

The transition between Yin and Yang is essentially an effort to consolidate stability. Late summer still offers pleasant warm days, but at the same time it prepares us for the cold, the damp, the dark. Its great privilege is the fact that it is a period associated with nutrition. From the diversity of summer, fruits have developed that store the energy of summer—warmth, light, love—the basic preconditions for feeding ourselves and providing sustenance to others. The rich harvest is a gift from our planet, and this harvest culminates in the period of late summer, in the EARTH phase. The symbol of the Earth is the image of a nursing mother who does not deny food to any of her children. It is therefore natural to associate the EARTH phase with food intake, with the digestion and processing of nutrients, with the transformation of food into Qi, and thus with the organs of the stomach and spleen. Mentally, however, we also digest life situations, process what we do and reap the rewards of our work.

Another feature of the EARTH phase is the fact that it can ground us. Strengthening the center—the organs of the stomach and spleen—but also strengthening the Qi in the center of gravity of the Lower Dantian through various Qigong exercises helps us to "sink the roots" into the ground under our feet. It helps us to strengthen physical and mental stability. When the stomach Qi is weakened, it can cause, for example, stagnation of food in the stomach. However, stomach stagnation can be caused by an unpleasant life situation or by a person we are uncomfortable or annoyed with. If the stomach Qi is strong enough, nothing will easily upset us; we can flexibly adapt to changes or pressure on us, although perhaps not immediately. We feel stable. At the same time, the Qi of the EARTH phase can ground a person who has "their head in the clouds" and does not have "their feet on the ground." Stability is therefore one of the basic aspects of the harmonious EARTH phase in us, and strengthening its aspects will also strengthen our stability. It is the ability to anchor, to root, but also to adapt quickly when the environment or life situation changes. Roots are important, but a certain dose of flexibility is also needed; otherwise, rooting can bring us restrictions, ossification and non-freedom. Meditation or peaceful contemplation is a good way to ground yourself healthily and to find one's center, the state of *here and now* in everything we do. Qigong and Taijiquan are also appropriate means for grounding. Of course, the physical experience of grounding will also help mental grounding, anchoring in one's own center, in oneself.

In terms of physical stability, using our center in motion is very important. If we want to maintain balance, we must be able to connect the feet with the Earth itself, but also with our center—the center of gravity. The exercises in which we learn how to root ourselves into the Earth are very effective. The degree of connection with the Earth—that is, the level of stability—is visible during movement performance quite markedly in everything that the mover does on stage or in the studio. Trembling or shaking in the legs, tripping, loss of balance, falling and so on are all signs of weak rooting, a weak connection to the Earth underfoot, but also to the Earth center of gravity. In contrast, movers who are confident in their connection with the Earth, and who have a sufficiently developed quality of the EARTH phase, radiate physical as well as mental stability in their performance. The ability to connect to the ground (floor) and use its support is extremely necessary in dance—for example, in partnering and contact improvisations. The floor is another partner to the dancer, who uses its support to support his or her dance partner.

TRANSITIONS BETWEEN PERIODS AND SEASONS

The EARTH phase is thus the center; it is the central stability and strength that allows a peaceful transition from one quality of Qi to another. There are several such transitions in our lives. They are caused by our constant development and the development of nature around us. Transitions from one phase of life to another can sometimes be gradual, smooth and pleasant; other life changes can take a very dramatic turn. It can be a change of job, starting a new school, a change in family circumstances, a change of partner, a change of residence, travel, etc.

Changes that cannot be avoided—and we experience them several times a year—are changes in the seasons. It would seem that this is not radical, but what happens in nature during the transition from one season to another is quite a force. The wildest transition is between winter and spring, accompanied by strong winds and storms with thunder and lightning. When one day it is beautiful and warm, we feel like wearing a T-shirt, and the next day we pull the winter jackets out of the closet again. Even the transition from summer to autumn through the late summer is no weaker in its intensity. During the day, strong sun still shines, but mornings and evenings can be unexpectedly cold. This period is also characterized by the fact that the weather of all four seasons can be shown during just a few days. Weather with really high temperatures appears for a few hours, but then the air temperature is able to drop by more than 10°C.

In a few hours, everything is completely calm, as if the beginning of spring, but suddenly strong winds come and in the higher areas even snow. Late summer can remind us of the whole range of weather conditions, and then everything returns to normal. So unless we are sufficiently armored with internal Qi or good clothing, cold and damp pathogens will easily enter us. These transitions are difficult for the human body, and therefore rhinitis, influenza, infections and sometimes epidemics spread more easily during these periods.

The EARTH phase in this context is not a real time of year. However, it is able to show its strength in the transitions between the four seasons. Each season lasts 73 days, and the transition time to the next period—18 days—belongs to the EARTH phase. EARTH seems to hold all the seasons together. These transition periods are constant, with a deviation of one or two days depending on the specific year.

This cycle can be better understood in the image below.

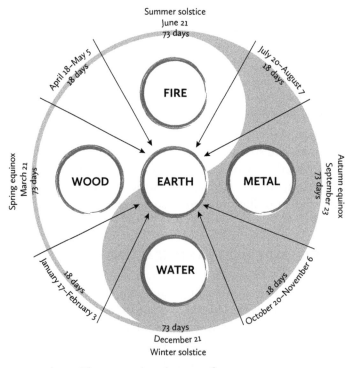

The EARTH phase between four seasons

According to the Chinese calendar, there are four transitions:

- From winter to spring between January 17 and February 2.
- From spring to summer between April 18 and May 5.
- From summer to autumn between July 20 and August 7.
- From autumn to winter between October 20 and November 6.

In all transition periods, it is extremely appropriate to work with the EARTH phase in us. If, for these 18 days, we support the organs of the EARTH phase with diet and support through the so-called EARTH points on certain meridians, we ensure that we are healthier, more stable and more adaptable. If we cannot support and stabilize them ourselves, it is advisable to look for an experienced practitioner of acupuncture, medical Qigong or Shiatsu, who can harmonize us during this period through the stabilization of the EARTH phase and help our adaptation.

SOURCE OF QI FROM FOOD

We already know that the Qi we have in our lives has two sources—prenatal and postnatal. Prenatal Qi, inherited from our parents, is a very powerful resource, but it should rather be seen as a reserve; it should be protected and disposed of carefully, so that it will last us a long time. Therefore, we need a second, postnatal source, and we get it from food, water and air, which we receive in our everyday life. The masters of the food component of Postnatal Qi are mainly the stomach and spleen. Thanks to them, food is transformed into Qi, which flows through the blood and through the meridians and thus nourishes the whole organism. Blood quality and Postnatal Qi quality depend on the quality and regularity of the diet and on the quality of the air. Together with Prenatal Qi, Postnatal Qi builds vitality and immunity—it is a source for us to have enough Qi for life and to enjoy it

adequately. Good-quality and healthy blood is the basis of our health. The spleen and stomach are therefore key organs of our Qi. In everyday life, we spend an enormous amount of Qi on physical and mental activities. It is important to realize that if we spend, we must also refill. Therefore, it is alarming in this context that some people resist normal food intake for fear of gaining weight. By their actions, they do not replenish Qi resources and use up their reserves. Unfortunately, this is common in the world of movers.

Functional circuit of the spleen: spleen, stomach, pancreas, digestion, mouth, lips, taste, saliva, muscles, the Intellect Yi, emotion of thoughtfulness and worry, pensiveness, sincerity, stability.

SPLEEN—TRANSPORT AND TRANSFORMATION

The spleen is the source of life for other organs. The five viscera long for the breath of life that comes from the spleen. The spleen is the basis of the existence of the five viscera.

THE YELLOW EMPEROR'S CLASSIC OF MEDICINE

According to Chinese medicine, the spleen is one of the most important organs of our system because of its close connection with Postnatal Qi. The term *spleen* (in Chinese, *Pi*), from the Taoist point of view of the human body, means the cooperation of two organs, the spleen and the pancreas. Both organs are involved in the transformation of food into Qi. Western medicine has observed that the pancreas produces pancreatic juices that contain important enzymes needed to break down macronutrients, the basic energy sources of sugars, fats and proteins. In addition, it contains specific cells, the islets of Langerhans, which produce insulin, a hormone that ensures that glucose enters the cell and is converted into energy. Western medicine does not give much importance to the spleen, the small organ behind the stomach on the left side of the trunk. But the Taoists do. They know that food enters the stomach, which digests it and sends it to the small intestine to process and extract the necessary nutrients. At the same time, however, they are convinced that the spleen "pulls" from food and water the subtle essences, the energetic part of the nutrition, and transports it to the lungs and heart. In the lungs, this food Qi is enriched with air Qi, and the Postnatal Qi produced in this way

is transported in the form of blood, thanks to the pulsing of the heart, throughout the body via the blood vessels—the pathways of the bloodstream. Of course, the spleen is also closely related to the kidneys, the source of Prenatal Qi. It is the main organ responsible for digestion and assimilation of nutrients. At the same time, it transmits and transforms water and moisture in the body, and participates in the regulation of fluid metabolism. Thus, it transports the delicate essence of food and at the same time transports the fluids needed for each tissue to be nourished and moisturized. Fluids that have not been used are immediately sent to the kidneys.

Old medical texts call the spleen a *blood producer*. The spleen controls blood production through food processing and at the same time preserves it. By preservation, we mean that the spleen can use its Qi to keep things in place. If it has strong Qi, it keeps organs and other parts of the body in place and prevents them from falling. These include a drop of the stomach, uterus, bladder and also the "slipping" of the intervertebral discs. In this context, it is also responsible for keeping the blood in place—in the blood vessels—so that it does not spill over the body. If we bruise excessively and often, and we do not even know how it happened, or we have more cracked veins than usual, it is a sign that the spleen Qi is weak. Of course, bruises may be the result of a bump or a fall. Even in this case, the rate of regeneration of cracked capillaries and veins indicates the quality of the spleen Qi.

MUSCLES—THEIR CAPACITY, BUT ALSO THEIR SHAPE

The spleen is of great importance for the mover. The quality of the spleen Qi depends on how much Qi we process from the food needed for our proper functioning, and determines the quality

of the muscles. Abundance and harvest, which are the themes of the EARTH phase, are embodied in the human body in the form of muscle mass. I am amazed at how generously nature has shaped our muscle mass. With great imagination and generosity, it gave us about 640 muscles of various sizes, widths, lengths, strengths and abilities. Our muscles are fine, short, narrow, small, long, dense, wide, coarse, flat or even round or spindle-shaped. The smallest muscle measures only 1 mm; the longest muscle of an adult can measure up to 50—60 cm. We have more than 40 mimic muscles, and we need ten of them to smile. We can control some muscles with our will, and with that same will, we can also work on their strength, flexibility or volume. These are the skeletal muscles that we control during movement and on which our movement depends. However, nature controls certain muscles itself and does not let us interfere. These include the heart muscle and smooth muscle—for example, the muscles of the inner walls of the intestines that help transport food, or the muscles of the uterus that help expel the baby at birth. Muscles also participate in matters that we are not even aware of—pupil size changes, bladder enlargement, swallowing or breathing. The vocal cords, which we do not normally perceive as muscles, are one of the most perfect muscles in our body. They can oscillate in different directions and with different intensities.

Muscles are truly fantastic, and every mover and performer should feel obliged to take adequate care of them. Thanks to them, we can move, often in an unusual and persistent way. We have the strength to lift, push or pull, and we can also sing or use the face in acting. However, in addition to their performance, muscles are also protectors of the internal organs and bones and at the same time an energy shield against the penetration of external pathogens into our interior. And they are also the "sculptor" of our body—they shape our figure. And when we realize that our muscle mass makes up about 35 percent of our body weight, we realize that it is something that deserves our attention and care.

The care of our muscles can be divided into several levels. The first is diet—that is, the care of the spleen, which provides the muscles with nutritional and energetic nutrition. The second is the level of physical use of the muscles, which includes appropriate and sufficient preparation of the muscles for physical performance, proper care of the muscles after physical exercise and maintenance of the muscles during breaks. By this, I mean, for example, a holiday when a person does not have daily training, but also the period after an injury or childbirth, when a person cannot move with such intensity as before. The third level is our relationship to the muscles—this includes conscious work with our own body during training, rehearsals or performances, which ensures that we do not abuse the muscles during movement excessively.

Nutrition and energy for muscles

The diversity of the muscular world naturally requires a large dose of quality nutrition. Chinese medicine says that the condition of the muscles depends not only on the movement itself but also on the state of Qi in the spleen and stomach. These two organs are most responsible for food processing and its transformation into Qi and blood. In Chinese medicine terminology, we would say that the muscles are nourished by the subtle essences in the blood, produced and transported to the body by the spleen. Muscles are naturally very vascularized, so they are conditioned by the state of the blood. The spleen, of course, works with the stomach to digest food, so the muscles also depend on the quality of the stomach Qi. In other words, what we eat and how we eat is reflected in the quality of our muscles. And as soon as we neglect these two organs, we also neglect the muscles.

Normally, we are in a hurry to eat, so we gulp the food and do not chew it properly. Consequently, we cannot digest food thoroughly—that is, take everything important from it. In addition, we expose the stomach to stress, which results in fermentation in the gastrointestinal tract and subsequent acidification of the body.

Acidification is perceived today as an important cause of many diseases. In terms of muscle, the body's acidification is noticeable, for example, because the muscles become sensitive and painful when pressed. However, under normal circumstances, it is possible to compress a muscle almost to the bone without hurting it. The concentration of acid in the muscle causes fatigue, so over-acidified people are always tired even without physical exertion, sleep poorly and have a very difficult time recovering.

Muscles need a regular intake of a variety of foods, especially protein, carbohydrates and healthy fats, ideally in their natural form. Vitamins, especially A, C and E, which help muscles reduce pain after exertion and accelerate their regeneration, cannot be missed. During physical activity, vitamins C and B are the most consumed. Iron is undoubtedly important for the formation of red blood cells. Other minerals such as calcium, iron, zinc and magnesium are also needed. From the point of view of Chinese medicine, it is naturally those foods that support the spleen and the entire EARTH phase. You will find them at the end of this chapter in the section on diet. In addition, a muscle cannot function well if it is malnourished, dehydrated or non-oxygenated. So plenty of fluids and a supply of clean air are just as important for the muscles as all the food components mentioned. Smoking reduces the level of oxygen in the blood, thus damaging the muscles. Alcohol, in turn, dehydrates the muscles and prevents the absorption of the necessary nutrients for the muscles. Thus, both of these activities weaken the spleen, and the muscles cannot give sufficient performance. When I see my colleagues or students smoking during training breaks or before or after a performance, a chill runs down my spine.

Nourishing muscles by movement

Muscles love movement; it provides them with Qi and nutrition. Only when the body moves can Qi circulate in it, and organs, muscles, tendons, bones, skin or body fluids be revitalized. This minimizes blockages, pain and other problems. Of course, movement must have its limits. Yoga, Qigong, dance and various recreational sports are ideal for the average person. In the world of the mover, this rate is often exceeded.

It is important to prepare the muscles for exercise, to warm them up and to cool them down after exercise and restore them to their original state. It is something that every teacher of dance, yoga, sports or any physical activity should teach their students and devote time to. If I have students who do not know how to take care of themselves, I recommend they come to the class at least 15 minutes before the start so that they can prepare their bodies for the performance with various stretches and warm-ups. At the beginning, it is the *warm-up*. At the same time, I design classes so that we have time together to calm the muscles and tendons and to *cool them down*. But how? For this purpose, in addition to the basic yoga asanas, I also teach students Qigong. One small thing is also important—after training or after a performance, take off your sweaty clothes, which are in direct contact with the muscles, as soon as possible. Why? Because the spleen does not like moisture, and therefore moisture also destroys muscles.

Dampness and muscles

In the context of Chinese medicine, dampness is a pathogen that harms the spleen more than all the other organs because it prevents it from performing the function of transforming food into Qi. It can enter the body in two ways. Internally, we get dampness into the body by consuming moisture-forming foods, which weaken the spleen and the entire digestion system. With respect to the spleen, we should avoid them. They are listed later in this chapter.

Dampness from the outside can enter the body during a longer stay in a humid environment—for example, during a long stay in a swimming pool, greenhouse, steam sauna or a damp home. As for the muscles, the most tangible and closest moisture we can expose them to is staying in sweaty clothes after physical activity. If we believe that "it will dry on me," we can weaken the muscles with a long and regular exposure to moisture. Dampness, which acts on the muscles for a long time, causes them to gradually weaken and weaken, and penetrates deeper through the muscles into the spleen itself. The spleen then does not have enough Qi for good digestion, nutrition does not get into the muscles, and we are in a vicious circle. Therefore, let us make sure that we carry spare clothes with us and change our clothes as soon as possible after sweating.

In addition to problems with the spleen and muscles, dampness can also manifest itself in various smaller or larger edemas, especially in the lower part of the torso or body, because moisture as such is naturally heavy and therefore falls. Furthermore, it can manifest by various degrees of weakness of the limbs, a lot of mucus in the lungs, but also in the genitals (discharge), diarrhea, heaviness in the head, sticky saliva and the like. Dampness accumulated in the body into the mucus is heavy; it does not want to move much, and therefore one can feel heavy, numb and clumsy. At the mental level, a person is not able to think clearly or constructively and has a clouded, dull mind. This can even develop into depression. Dampness is also eliminated through the skin—acne is a typical example of moisture in the body, also associated with heat.

Muscle fever

In connection with the conscious care of muscles, it is also necessary to mention muscle fever, which every mover certainly knows. Muscle fever always occurs when we expose muscles to excessive physical exertion without prior preparation, when we do not devote enough time to warming up the muscles and tendons for exercise, and when we do not take enough care of the muscles after exercise. Muscle fever is a natural reaction of the body, which is basically a kind of manifestation of the instinct of self-preservation of our muscles. They do not want further ill-treatment, and therefore they use pain to prevent us from inflicting it. Some sources say that lactic acid is excreted during muscle strain, causing muscle fever pain. Modern research, however, claims that if we load unheated muscles suddenly and in excessive amounts, small muscle fibers literally break. These are, of course, micro-cracks. These cause small inflammations that induce a different biochemical state in the muscles, and we feel it as pain and an inability to move the muscles as we would like. However, I know from personal experience that persistent extreme muscle fever does not have to happen. I am a professional dancer who gives performances in a studio or on stage. I am also a freelancer, so I do not have a completely regular workout, which means that my body also experiences longer breaks. I really know what muscle fever is. In recent years, however, I have found that the longer I practice Qigong, the less my body suffers from muscle fever. In addition to various stretches in preparation for physical performance, I involve Qigong in my warm-up. Qigong distributes Qi in a wonderful way to every cell of every muscle fiber or tendon. Where there is Qi, there is warmth, so Qigong also warms up the muscles, even if we do not really move very intensely with it. At the same time, by clearing the Qi flow, Qigong allows the muscles to receive the nutrition from the organs that belong to them. Qigong is also suitable after exercise. It definitely regenerates the muscles better than a hot shower, which can hurt them even more.

Relation to one's own figure

In addition to movement activity, muscles are also involved in building the shape of the body. They shape our body contours. People who struggle with their weight usually feel the need to get rid of fat. But that is only one part of the whole. The second is that our figure is conditioned by the shape of the skeleton. On the surface, however, it is shaped by muscles, and we can work with them. When neglected, they are flaccid, and any weight loss and fat loss under the skin will not help them to look good. In the whole process of a nice body shape, the most important thing is the good quality of Qi of the spleen and stomach. People with impaired Qi of these organs can either fight with being overweight or, conversely, be too skinny. Many slimming diets go unnoticed if the person consumes food that disrupts the Qi of the spleen. These are mainly cold, raw foods and mucus-producing foods. And common diets are mainly about raw vegetable salads, fruits and fruit juices, yogurts and cheeses. Weight problems can only be meaningfully solved if we harmonize the spleen. The spleen likes warmth—that is, cooked food. This does not always mean that we have to cook the food for a long time; sometimes just quick cooking (blanching) or steaming, which leaves the necessary nutrients in the vegetables, is enough.

Muscle abuse during movement

The last level of muscle care is their conscious use in movement. As a trained dancer, I know a lot about body abuse in dance and for dance. During my eight years of study at the conservatory, I accumulated a number of health problems because I only learned to use my body and not to understand it. Unfortunately, many educational institutions do not offer information on how to work with the body consciously. By consciously, I mean respecting the anatomy, the natural mechanics of movement and the healthy physio-dynamics of the body in order for the body to stay healthy in this profession for as long as possible. When completely sore after study at the conservatory, I came to approaches such as the Release technique, Body-Mind Centering, Feldenkrais Method, Alexander Technique and Ideokinesis. I was excited. My body could not wait to be consciously used, reprogrammed and healed in these ways.

By abusing muscles, I mean using them excessively. In normal dance practice, which has not gone through the process of being aware of movement, we use muscles more than necessary. And often we engage muscles in a movement that we do not need to engage at all. This is because they often teach us to dance in such a way that we just repeat the movement blindly without understanding the mechanism by which the body should perform it. Some things we have to learn very quickly; we are required to be as good and efficient as the best student in the class, which leads to some kind of "racing." Respect for individual anatomical possibilities is often forgotten. Therefore, in my pedagogical practice I do not focus on the form, but on the principles of anatomically satisfactory performance of movement. However, this takes longer. We can learn to do some things with the body in a minute, but learning to do something with the body correctly can take several days or weeks. And many people do not want to invest the time or they do not know that they can. All this is not to say that I do not work my muscles when I dance. I do work them, but I try to do it economically and efficiently.

Psychic connections and symbolism

In schools, we are burdened with a huge amount of information that we do not manage to process. We are required to deliver a great amount of physical activity which we often do till we are drained. As professionals, we perform at a lot of shows and we are part of many projects because we think that if we did less, we would be less valuable. This naturally prevents us from devoting adequate time to the things we do, and thus from doing them truthfully. However, the truth requires more time and attention.

Muscles carry the symbolism of the state of "being seen" and, of course, the symbolism of "strength"—the ability to use force to be seen. Bones, as we mentioned, carry the symbolism of "being true." They are more in our depth, core, essence, and therefore it takes longer to work with them. Muscles are more on the surface, and if we work only with them, they lead us to superficiality, to a state in which, due to lack of time and the need to devote ourselves to the truth, we remain naturally more superficial. People working in this way show this by the state of their muscles. Their muscles are extreme, strong, firm, tense, enlarged, protruding.

Why are many female dancers, so to speak, masculine, muscular and sinewy? I believe that is because they consciously or unconsciously try to match their dances with men. Female dancers have fewer opportunities than male dancers because there are so many more of them than there are men. They must therefore fight to be seen. They often choose male, Yang approaches for this. For fear of rejection, they try to fit into a more Yang-oriented environment in which strength, the ability to break through, quantity, speed and action reign. If we are to go even deeper into this topic, then someone who wants to be seen has a reason for it. This usually conceals the need to compensate for something. From a psychological point of view, this is about compensating for a deficit—perhaps a deficit of attention in childhood from parents and the people closest to us, and by those who taught us at school.

SUPPORT IN REGULARITY

Regularity is one of the prerequisites for our stability, and the spleen urgently needs it. Regularity gives us the possibility of order, a certain system that helps us to function even without us perceiving it. The rhythm of life, the rhythm of some important organ functions and also the rhythm of our activities are extremely important for the balance of the EARTH phase in us. Our planet is subject to regular rhythms, and therefore life on it is stable. The rhythm of the Earth is like a heartbeat that does not need to be influenced, but it still ensures that we live in peace and harmony.

Certain fluctuations in rhythm are fine in our lives. A trip for a vacation, from time to time a party or an overnight stay or a fasting, all make our lives more colorful. But disrupting and disrespecting certain fundamental rhythms can affect our health. Regularity in food intake, regularity in defecation, regularity in the phase of activity and rest, alternation of day and night, repetition of seasons, women's menstrual cycle and the like are all rhythms maintaining the harmonious state of the EARTH phase in us, which affects our whole life. Only an innocent deviation from regularity, such as traveling on vacation, can disrupt a person's regularity of defecation. If the spleen and stomach of the person are in order, the consequences are not so unpleasant and long-lasting.

Another disruption of regularity many of us encounter twice a year. It is about the time change in spring and autumn. We all know very well that we need some time to adapt. If the EARTH phase organs are in order, adaptation will take place quickly and without any difficulties. However, if their Qi is weaker, one takes longer to adapt to the change of time and becomes more tired.

One of the worst ways to disrupt regularity is through work shifts. When someone works a few days in the morning, a few days in the afternoon and a few days at night, it completely disrupts the biorhythm. The result is digestive problems, sleep problems and, in women, disruption of the menstrual cycle, which can ultimately lead to infertility. A significant change in rhythm occurs when traveling across time zones. We will get to the topic of travel in more detail in the following pages.

When adapting, it is appropriate to support the EARTH with diet, but also by supporting Qi through acupuncture points. One of the strongest is the point of *Zusanli*, on the Stomach channel, which you can read about below. Select from foods that support the EARTH phase; they are included at the end of this chapter.

All cycles of our lives are conditioned by regularity.

The birth of a sense of confidence in the internal course of affairs also depends to some extent on regularity. And so trust, honesty, openness, composure, balance and tranquility of the mind are related to the EARTH phase. Other virtues of the EARTH phase are fairness, balance, equilibrium, impartiality and fair-mindedness or non-judgmental acceptance. If these virtues are not of good quality, worries, anxiety, compulsive thoughts, doubts and excessive thinking do arise.

THE SPLEEN AND OUR MENTAL POTENTIAL

The power of stability also affects us on a mental level. The EARTH phase is related to thinking. The psychospiritual aspect of the spleen is the Yi. It could be defined as thinking, as the ability to give a concrete form to an idea, that comes from the soul of the liver aspect, the Hun. The role of the spleen is the ability to concentrate and organize thinking, to neaten the thoughts in order to realize an idea. Here again, stability and the ability of the spleen to keep us centered is needed. But it is also a mindset capable of self-reflection. This thinking is manifested outwardly in a person through speech and through words that should be in accordance with what we have in the soul (heart)—simply to be honest. Words (thoughts) that we drop from the inside out must be filtered beforehand. It is about cultivating, even an "alchemical filtration" of internal "gusts" and carrying out careful self-reflection. The healthy Yi creates a kind of filter or supervision of our thoughts and enables the maturation and absorption of our experience. So it is about being true to one's self in the creative process and as creators or performers. We create works on topics that touch us essentially, and the healthy spleen, in which the healthy Yi resides, helps us to articulate them clearly.

When the EARTH phase is harmonious in us, our thoughts are anchored and constructive. When it is unbalanced, thoughts revolve around something; they cannot free themselves from their object and cannot find their way to peace. They do not bear any meaningful fruit, and this condition begins to develop into passion or excessive anxiety and this is very weakening for the spleen. Excessive thinking, which we also call *pensiveness*, knots Qi. Qi then cannot circulate smoothly through the meridians; it knots and stagnates somewhere in the body, which can manifest itself, for example, as bloating, coughing and, ultimately, stagnation of thinking.

Ordinary thinking is not harmful to the physiological activities of the body, but excessive reflection is. Even excessive study, in which the mind works excessively, greatly depletes the spleen. It is therefore necessary to combine study with physical exercises in which energy can be evenly distributed throughout the body and flow in it regularly. Supplement the spleen Qi, for example, with a suitable diet, herbal mixtures or moxibustion. In particular, moxibustion of the *Zusanli* point, an excellent point for supporting the spleen and stomach and all their functional aspects, is very suitable.

STOMACH AND ITS MASTER POINT *ZUSANLI*

So far, it has been mainly about the spleen. However, the stomach (in Chinese, *Wei*) is just as important. In ancient medical texts, it is considered *a minister, an official responsible for a public store of grain* and *a provider of the five flavors*. It is also called *the Sea of food, Qi and blood*. It manages the intake of solid and liquid foods and their initial processing. It is responsible for pre-digestion, which is the basis of the transformation of food into Qi. It controls the permeability of food pathways through the digestive organs. It is in charge of the descent of food, which means that it is responsible for ensuring that food does not stagnate in it and descend into the intestines. If this does happen, stomach dilation and pain may occur, but also a syndrome of upward Qi flow, manifested by, for example, excessive gurgling, hiccuping or even gastric acid leaking into the esophagus and oral cavity. The stomach is also called the *master of the intestines* because it significantly determines their good function. The stomach Qi is the essence of man. In medical practice, it is essential to constantly take care of its protection.

The importance of stomach input into our system is also evidenced by the fact that one of the most used acupuncture points of the body is located in its meridian. It is *Leg Three Li* or *Leg Three Miles* (in Chinese, *Zusanli*, ST36). Due to its enormous power and great abilities, it is the alpha and omega of every practitioner of acupuncture, Shiatsu or moxibustion, but it is also beginning to become known to ordinary people. It is located below the knees and is indicated on the image of the Stomach channel below.

Why is it so special? It is located on the Stomach meridian, the channel of the organ that is the basis of our lives. It therefore has a strong effect on the state of Qi, but also on the stomach and spleen. By stimulating it, we can influence everything related to digestion and the transformation of substances from food into vitality. It is therefore used, for example, in poor digestion associated with anorexia, with undigested food residues in the stool, with bloating, diarrhea, constipation, feelings of dilation or distension in the abdomen after eating, accumulation of food in the stomach, vomiting or intestinal problems. As nutrients from food nourish the blood and *Zusanli* benefits the nourishment of the blood, it is used for problems such as anemia, weak or interrupted menses, dryness of the skin and internal mucous membranes. *Zusanli* helps the spleen hold the organs in place as well as keep the blood in the veins. It is therefore also used for excessive bruising. It strengthens the body in states of weakness and lack of Qi, which we feel as fatigue. It also helps these organs to function well. In some texts, we can also find it under the second name *Xiaqihai*, translated as *the Lower Sea of Qi*. As indicated by a name in which the word *sea* appears, it is a great source of Qi.

With its reach in support of Qi, *Zusanli* also supports our Defensive Qi (in Chinese, *Weiqi*). Weiqi is a kind of energetic armor that, according to Chinese medicine, flows in the spaces between the skin and muscles and strengthens the surface of the body against the entering of climatic influences into the body—especially cold and wind—which will be discussed in the next chapter. Stimulation of *Zusanli* ensures that the body strengthens enough to withstand adverse weather conditions, but also viruses. It is therefore related to immunity and ranks among the most important immunostimulatory points.

While one could continue to list its strengths and abilities, I will mention one more important example. *Zusanli* strongly supports thinking and intellect. It can support mental activity; on the other hand, it also suppresses excessive unconstructive thinking. It will help us, for example, to relax the stomach if something or someone lies heavily there—for example, a grumpy boss, a neighbor, or anything else that comes to our mind. The point helps us to get to the center, to anchor in the Earth, not to fly too much in the clouds and to deal with essential ideas. It also helps us to handle difficult situations and quickly adapt to life changes, whether they are changes in work, residence, relationship or when traveling.

Zusanli has a huge impact on prevention. Moxa is mainly used for preventive strengthening of Qi and for defense against diseases.

The relationship between the spleen and the stomach is the strongest of all the organs. Their functions sometimes overlap, and the Spleen channel is often used for gastrointestinal disharmonies. Even in the old writings, their inner unity is often mentioned in the common term, while other organs are discussed separately. Together, they form the root of Postnatal Qi obtained daily from food.

A MOVER ON A JOURNEY

The life of a mover, especially a freelance mover, is accompanied by a suitcase always at the ready. The mover does not even take some of the things out of the suitcase—it is not worth it. Traveling is as much a part of our life as a warm-up before training. Many of us cannot imagine our profession without traveling. However, this chapter is for everybody, because every one of us travels from time to time, and so we all fall out of our normal rhythm. Travel, besides all the benefits, causes the disruption of rhythm—it disrupts regularity, resting in the center, rooting, eating—simply everything that the EARTH phase and the spleen need. It affects some of us more and some of us less. What does it depend on?

When we are young, we do not feel some special intervention to our organism during and after traveling. Usually, a young body adapts to changes very quickly and does not feel any notable tiredness or health issues. We mostly feel pleasant excitement from discovering something new. But this latency of consequences is tricky. Based on my communication with many dancers and actors of movement theater from all around the world, I know that, with age, every one of us starts to look at traveling differently. While we are young, we crave possibilities to travel; when we are older, we find that traveling drains us more and more. We start to calculate the time we spend traveling, and begin to think more about the relaxing or recovery days and how to organize

them. The journey for us is not only merely relocation; for us, traveling starts to be work itself.

What is happening during travel?

First, let us look at it from the Western scientific perspective. When we go very fast in a car, bus or train, let alone an airplane, our nervous system knows that it is being exposed to danger. Thanks to its ability to suppress feelings, the brain overcomes it, of course—it is a way of adapting the organism to new conditions and it was given to us so we could survive. We are trained for it from childhood; we teach it to small babies when we are buckling them into their car seat. But the body knows its mind, because the *vestibular system* tells the body how fast it moves. The body is naturally afraid—afraid in the deep, subtle structures—and so, obviously, a reaction of our system must happen. The majority of the time we are tired because our body needs to compensate for the stress with a total shutdown. So that is why resting after travel is reasonable.

During flights through time zones, something even more serious happens to our system. What is known as *jet lag* is a state of total scatter of our body's daily rhythm. Our *circadian rhythm* is disrupted, which is one of the biorhythms. It lasts approximately 20–24 hours, depending on the individual and the conditions. This rhythm is responsible for managing physical functions such as alternating between sleep and vigilance, regular changes of body temperature, secretion of hormones and blood pressure. This rhythm is directly dependent on the amount of daily light. If we deprive ourselves of an amount of this light with a "jump" through a time zone—or, on the other hand, we prolong it—it will influence the secretion of the sleep hormone melatonin, which is responsible for the feeling of sleepiness and allows us to fall asleep. If it is disturbed, we have problems. Our natural circadian rhythm, which we were functioning with for the past few months or years, suddenly breaks. And with this, all the physical processes that are dependent on it become confused and damaged. The more time zones we cross, the worse the manifestations of jet lag are. We can experience buzzing in the head and muscle or joint pain; we can be grumpy and hypersensitive to light and sounds, lose our appetite, or generally not feel like ourselves. Problems with sleep are guaranteed—during the day, we feel strong tiredness and fatigue; in the middle of the night, we wake up. We cannot fall asleep again, and yet we are so tired that we are unable to stay awake either. Women can experience disruption of the menstrual cycle, which can be prolonged by a week or two.

The manifestations of jet lag are generally less with flights to the west because we actually prolong the day. The adaptation happens faster, but it is also strong. The symptoms are worse and longer with flights to the east. Depending on the individual, the state of the organism and the number of time zones crossed, jet lag can last one to three days, but in some cases even a week. If I point out that some of us fly through time zones four or five times a year, we can see that it is a big challenge for the organism.

How do Taoists look at it through Chinese medicine?

The ideas expressed in this book are thousands of years old. Airplanes did not exist, yet alone the possibility to relocate to another hemisphere of our planet at such a high speed. But traveling always existed; even in ancient China, people were traveling long distances for business, even outside of China.

Chinese medicine cannot measure hormone levels, and it did not discover the vestibular system or circadian rhythms, but it looks at this topic with its own perspective and its own terminology. If we understand it, we discover that it is not far from the Western point of view. First, by traveling we disrupt the EARTH phase in a human. As we know, the EARTH phase is dependent on regularity, on rhythm; with traveling, this rhythmic chain breaks. The intensity of the break is proportionally dependent on the length of traveling and conditions in which we are traveling, and where we are traveling to. The organs of the EARTH phase, the spleen and stomach, must function excessively, so that regularity is re-established. The second domain that is influenced by traveling is the WATER phase and the kidneys—our prenatal source. The kidneys, as our deepest source of Qi, are responsible for our deepest and most subtle processes, hence for our biorhythms. If our biorhythm is interrupted, the kidneys must function markedly more to take us back to our normal biological function. When it comes to the fear of speed, we also involve the kidneys. Fear from the perspective of Chinese medicine is related to the kidneys—it weakens them. The kidneys themselves are the basis of our vitality and our health, and if we over-drain their Qi, we are dipping into our reserves. Speed itself is Yang. During harmonization of this state, the kidneys are sending Yin to the system. It is Yin that, in other circumstances, would be used differently—for example, for the regeneration of the organism or blood nourishment. It is therefore over-consumed. So it is logical that after traveling, we feel tired. Even though we are sitting on our bottoms, the system of our body is functioning at full speed. That is why I repeat that it is necessary to give yourself deep relaxation after traveling! Therefore, I repeat again—after traveling, you need to take a long rest!

Finally, the heart is involved in this process too. As we know, the heart is the residency of the Shen, our soul. Although during traveling our body relocates very fast somewhere else, the soul needs a little bit more time to "catch up" with the body. Maybe it sounds too esoteric, but the well-known feeling of "not being in our own skin" is exactly what I am talking about. It can be accompanied by various strange dreams. After traveling to your destination, it is necessary to give yourself time to relax; that means not involving yourself straight away and doing too much. That way, we give the soul time to catch up with the body and unite with it.

The consequence of all of this is that a person with a strong center, with good Qi of the stomach and spleen, and also with good kidney Qi, handles traveling better. Thus, it is logical that an older person, who is generally losing Qi, will feel more discomfort from traveling.

Other factors connected to traveling
Home
The feeling of home is incredibly important for us; it is also very important for the EARTH phase. Home is our external center which we can lean on. There can be times when performers do not have a home; their home is temporarily their suitcase. It requires a big dose of adaptability. Or they are changing homes several times in a short period. Or some of them have several homes at the same time, which also requires the ability to adapt because during this time the EARTH phase organs are on the alert.

The older we get, the less we experiment with the absence of home and the more deeply and strongly we feel our roots. Our increasing age creates the need for us to spend more time at home, and if we need to travel somewhere, we make sure that it is reasonably organized and as short as possible.

Nutrition
The second factor that is strongly influenced by traveling is the change of cuisine and so the influence on eating habits and eating needs. In a new place, we do not have our own kitchen, and often we do not have a kitchen at all, and so we cannot eat and refill our Qi according to our needs. It can be a part of the game of how to manage to adapt in those conditions, but it is undeniable that it excessively influences our state and Qi. So, we solve our eating needs with restaurants. Sometimes it can be freeing, but it is not always advisable. Since it is not always possible to buy what we need in the shops, we often deal with or hunger by buying junk food. It is a heavy load for the organism.

Traveling is not the right time for work
Many of us perceive traveling as time for work, time that should be used productively. When we are very busy, it is often the only time to respond to emails or plan our work and personal life. Many of us, as soon as we get into the means of transport, open our laptop, look at the screen and work. I would point out that surfing or scrolling through Facebook statuses is also a mental job that makes the body tired. We can suppress the symptoms of fatigue very quickly when we are young; with growing age, however, we start to perceive the journey itself as work and that is why we do not add any other work to it. Fortunately, the body is sometimes more wise than the mind. Even if we plan to work on trains or buses, we fall asleep after a few kilometers. In some cases, we are not capable of focusing on work, and so we only listen to music or observe the scenery. The fact that the body is forcing us to sleep during travel indicates that traveling actually is not the right time to work. By relaxing, the body is balancing the fact that it has more than enough work with this situation.

Coffee

Covering tiredness with coffee, or possibly with other stimulating substances, is very dangerous. What does our body tell us when we are tired? It gives us a message that our system is overworked and that if we do not want to wear it out very quickly to the point that it can no long serve us, we should respect the inner voice and relax. During tiredness, the kidneys are "screaming" the most; they are the source of our Prenatal Qi and they do not want to use it all up. They want to save it for the next years of our life. The body wants to protect us from more exhaustion with this feeling of tiredness. After coffee, we feel excitement, but only for a short time. In the end, we reach into our reserves and therefore we exploit our kidneys. If we do this regularly, we are paving a way to many illnesses that otherwise would not have to manifest.

In conclusion

- Travel in a way that allows time for rest and relaxation. No work during traveling!
- After reaching our destination, where we are to teach or perform, ask the organizers for free days. Do not see them as a luxury, because arriving somewhere in the evening and starting to work the next morning is a great burden for the body.
- Never fly by plane on the day of the performance or teaching.
- Try to think about the possibilities of catering in advance; ask the organizers beforehand and request that they secure basic conditions for us.
- Keep hydrated while traveling.

A few tips on how to better handle jet lag

- A few days before the flight, start gradually changing for the time zone that you are traveling to.
- If possible, take a night flight with arrival at your destination in the early morning.
- Avoid drinking alcohol during the flight.
- Drink plenty of water.
- Try to sleep during the flight.
- Do not work during the flight.
- Soon after arrival, take a walk in the fresh air and daylight.
- Do not go to sleep after arrival, but try to stay awake until the evening of the place of arrival.
- After flying over time zones, secure a minimum of two days of rest before you start working.

After arriving home from the business trip permit yourself:

- a lot of sleep
- passive relaxation
- walks in fresh air
- at least two days of relaxation before you start working again (even longer, depending on the length of the journey)
- good-quality and regular food.

From the perspective of Chinese medicine, how can we help ourselves?

With any traveling, but especially with longer and intense traveling, it is important to look after your center—the organs of the spleen and stomach. One of the recommended ways is with moxibustion of the above-mentioned point of *Zusanli* on the Stomach meridian. You can read about moxibustion in Chapter 8. It is advisable to start with moxibustion a week or two before the flight and continue it after arrival. The choice of nutrition to support these organs is also a good solution for supplementing Qi. Chinese medicine also offers several herbal mixtures to support these organs. Strengthening the center is essential. If the center is strong, we will not draw into the reserves of our kidneys. However, a supplementing treatment can also help the kidneys through the point *Yingu*, the tenth point on the Kidney channel. It is located at the knee pit, between two ligaments on the internal sides of the knees. These are the points of our biorhythm; you can press or use moxibustion on them. I teach these basic skills in my seminars.

OTHER CONNECTIONS WITH THE FUNCTIONAL CIRCUIT OF THE SPLEEN

We have not yet exhausted the effect of the functional circle of the spleen. In the medical texts of Chinese medicine, we find the following information.

The spleen opens into the mouth

The mouth and everything connected with it—lips, tongue, gums holding the teeth and the palate (the roof of the mouth)—are related to the Qi of the spleen. At the same time, we taste and eat through our mouths. If the Qi of the spleen is insufficient in this respect, it will affect our ability to distinguish tastes or we will not have an appetite. Teeth in the mouth, so-called *bone protrusions*, are linked with the kidneys, but the gums, the fleshy component of the teeth, are connected to the spleen. In the case of gum problems, attention should be paid to the functional circuit of the spleen.

Spleen manifests in the lips

The gloss, color and shape of the lips reflect the condition of the spleen. If the spleen Qi is sufficient, the lips are nourished, and thus normally fleshy, shiny and of a normal color. Paleness of the lips, weakness and dullness indicate the weakness of the spleen Qi. Excessive red indicates heat in the heart.

Spleen controls saliva

This is logical, because saliva is the first body fluid to come into contact with the food we have chosen to consume. Saliva is very important for starting digestion. It is alkaline, so if we do not want to suffer from gastric hyperacidity, we must mix food in the oral cavity well with saliva and its alkaline component. The best way to do this is to chew, which produces a lot of saliva. Solid food must be sufficiently chewed and moistened with saliva so that it becomes liquid; before swallowing this liquid, it should be mixed with saliva, as if we were chewing it for a while longer.

Connection with the opposite end of the digestive tract

The weakness of the functional circuit of the spleen is also reflected in the final "station" of the process of the transformation of food into nutrients—in the quality of our stool. If the Qi of the spleen is sufficient, the stool is compact, thick and firm in consistency. On the other hand, when the spleen Qi is weak, the stool is soft and pale, and it is possible to see undigested food in it, or the stool sticks to the toilet bowl. When this organ is weak, a person also suffers from flatulence.

Yellow is the color of the EARTH phase

The color of late summer is the color of ripe grain or fertile soil. It is a yellow, golden yellow, ocher to orange color like a Hokkaido pumpkin, which is typical of the late summer. We feed the EARTH phase organs with food of this color. However, an excess of this color is harmful. If a person has a slightly yellowish tinge to their face, this suggests that the Qi of the EARTH phase of this person is not in balance.

The taste of the EARTH phase is a sweet taste

The spleen loves the sweet taste, but it is a naturally sweet taste that some vegetables and cereals contain. The excessive sweet taste harms the spleen, which weakens the whole digestive system. You can read more about the sweet taste and risks of sugar in the section on diet.

Suppressed emotions attack the EARTH phase

Modern Western medicine also confirms that chronic gastritis, such as gastric ulcers, has psychosomatic causes. Those affected by this are people who do not process emotions sufficiently, and often suffer due to both important and insignificant issues; they lack a solid center. Due to their inability to confront, they avoid conflict or suppress their feelings. A constructive exchange of views leading to a conclusion is appropriate; it purifies feelings and emotions. Delayed emotions, among other things, cause stomach ulcers. If the stomach Qi is weaker, emotions will attack it and prevent it from working under normal conditions. This disturbs the balance between the amount, composition and secretion of digestive juices, but also changes the ratio, amount and quality of protective mucus in the stomach and duodenum. This disparity causes gastric acidification, which is the perfect condition for ulcers. However, ulcers can also be caused by innate genetic predispositions that subconsciously affect eating habits such as overeating, irregular food intake, selection of unsuitable foods, etc.

RELATIONSHIP OF THE EARTH PHASE TO OTHER PHASES

According to the Sheng controlling cycle, which we discussed in Chapter 7 on the Five Phases, it is clear that the "mother" of the spleen is the heart. At the same time, there is a close, even anatomical relationship between the stomach (EARTH) and the small intestine (FIRE). When the preparation of food (EARTH) is enriched with the quality of FIRE, so the food is prepared with love, we feel it in the taste and energy of the food; it is tastier and has more value for us. The EARTH phase must also be controlled. In nature, it is the roots of trees and plants that hold the soil together; in the area of digestion, it is the flow of Qi and its ability to pass through the liver (WOOD) so that Qi does not accumulate in the stomach and food moves where it should. The harmonious Qi of the EARTH phase is able to nourish the METAL phase well and at the same time limit excess in the WATER phase.

CONCLUSION TO THE EARTH PHASE

The organs of the EARTH phase need to be cultivated throughout the year, because the EARTH is the center and support for everything. If we are bothered by indigestion, let us try to get it in order as soon as possible, because digestion is the basis for the quality and quantity of Qi. Let us also pay attention to regularity, whether in the diet or in other things. It does not have to be too strict, but a certain order will help us in the right grounding, from which we can draw even in more demanding periods. Cold mornings and evenings announce the arrival of autumn. Think therefore of warmer clothes, albeit thrown into a bag just in case, even if it seems that they will not be needed. Autumn outdoors reminds us that during the late summer it is advisable to start cleansing the large intestine to prepare it for autumn. The clean intestine will also help the lungs to carry out their activity. For example, regular use of charcoal is suitable. Avoid mucus-producing foods such as milk and dairy products. They would cause mucus congestion of the lungs and large intestine, which could encourage various infections during cold and humid autumns. Start to relax more and focus on yourself. Strengthen the EARTH in you with regular treatments in the 18 days between the seasons.

Table 11.1 Main correspondences of EARTH phase

Year season: late summer	Yin and Yang stage: center
Day time: afternoon	Direction: center
Evolution of Qi: descent of Qi	Growth cycle in nature: transformation, maturity, fruit
Life cycle: life maturity	Working cycle: utilization
Yin organ: spleen	Organ clock for spleen: 9 to 11 a.m.
Yang organ: stomach	Organ clock for stomach: 7 to 9 a.m.
Psychospiritual aspect: Yi	Virtue: truthfulness, confidence
Emotion: pensiveness	Climate: dampness
Color: yellow, orange	Taste: sweet
Smell: fragrant, sweet	Number: 5
Tissue: soft tissue, flesh, muscles	Body fluid: saliva
Other body tissues: long muscles, mouth, lips	Other body fluid and excretion: lymph, intestinal lymph, thin saliva, digestive juices and enzymes
Joints: hip joints	Entry point of disease: spine
Sense organ: mouth	Sense: taste
Indicator: lips	Detrimental action: too much thinking
Sound: singing	Mental attitude: honesty, stability, self-identity

MERIDIANS

STOMACH CHANNEL (ST)/YANG

The Stomach channel is a paired Yang pathway, leading from top to bottom. In the image on the right, it is shown on one side. It begins on the face, under the eyes, as a continuation of the flow of Qi from the Large Intestine channel. It descends down the jaw, from where one branch protrudes up into the hair. The second branch descends from the front of the neck and torso, where it passes through the nipples and the inner branch connects with the stomach and spleen itself. It continues through the groin to the front of the thighs. It passes through the anterior sides of the knees, the calves, where its flow is dynamized by a short return up and back down. Below the knees is the already mentioned point of *Zusanli* (*Leg Three Li*). The channel advances to the ankles and leads through the instep to the second toes, where it ends. On the insteps, its inner branch follows the Spleen channel. Another inner branch pours into the middle toes. Its main branch has 45 acupuncture points.

> The channel affects all types of stomach problems, including duodenal ulcers, digestive problems, upset stomach and vomiting, weight problems, aphthae, appetite disorders and overeating. It is used in the treatment of mental anorexia to support the psyche, as well as to stabilize digestion. It also affects the breasts—for example, with breast inflammation and breastfeeding problems. In connection with grounding and centering, it also affects the irregularity of the cycles. Because it supports digestion, it significantly affects the immune system.

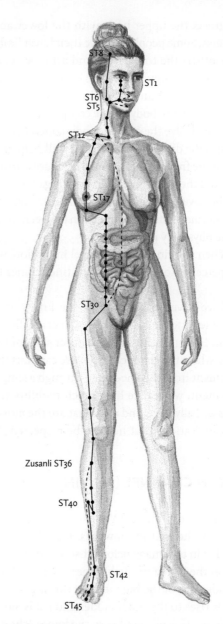

Stomach channel

STOMACH CHANNEL IN MOVEMENT

The channel offers us many possibilities for movement, as it is one of the longest channels and includes the whole body from the head to the toes. By passing through the front, it invites us to stretch it, to the various bends that help Qi in the channel to open more and thus flow more smoothly throughout its course.

It is interesting to work with the area of the groin in movement and physically perceive how this part of the body has the ability and strength to connect the upper body with the lower and vice versa. Some people perceive their lower limbs more, others the torso, head and arms. Moving from the groin upwards to the head or down to the feet will help unify the Yin and Yang in the body and feel the body as one complex unit.

If we involve the eyes and their concrete look in a specific direction in space, it will help give them more fresh Qi and develop the clarity of our steps and the direction we are walking.

The navel and nipples can also be involved in the movement and the connection between them can be physically perceived.

When working with the navel in motion, we also perceive how Qi in the intestines comes to life.

If we have problems with the knees, it is advisable to focus on the knees, specifically on the kneecaps (patellas) and the outer sides of the knees, where the channel passes. We can start the movement from the knees, and through a simple movement, we realize how much mobility the knees actually have, and also what are the movement limitations that need to be respected. In this way, we can also observe how much stability the knees receive from the surrounding tendons and muscles. This work usually helps to release tension in the thigh and calf muscles and thus create a smooth flow of Qi in the channel. The knees often hurt because they do not receive Qi as it is blocked somewhere at the level of the groin or thighs.

The channel leads through the insteps. It is an area that should be moved sensitively. The feet and insteps commonly suffer from tightness in shoes, which prevents the smooth flow of Qi in the stomach channel.

Of course, conscious work with the Stomach channel in movement improvisation also has a significant effect on digestion. In addition, it helps with grounding, which can be practiced in motion by the flow of Qi itself in the channel from up to down. Working with the channel will help us to feel its Yang quality in an excellent way. After prolonged improvisation, Qi is strongly activated in the channel. Let us enjoy this flow of Qi in motion, but also in the stillness that occurs after movement.

SPLEEN CHANNEL (SP)/YIN

The Spleen channel is a Yin pair pathway, leading from the bottom upwards. It is shown on one side in the image below. It starts at the nail bed on the inside of the big toes. It leads along the side edge of the big toes and the arch of the feet. It rises to the inner ankles and leads along the inner sides of the tibia to the knees. Then it continues up the inner sides of the thighs into the groin. In the area of the lower abdomen and navel, the inner branch connects with the Conception Vessel, one of the extraordinary channels. It sinks into the spleen, pancreas and stomach itself. This inner branch passes through the diaphragm to the heart and extends to the throat and to the tongue. In this way, these organs energetically connect with the mouth and the ability to taste. The surface main branch continues along the ribs towards the shoulders, turns sharply downwards and ends at the side of the ribs in the sixth intercostal space. Its main branch has 21 acupuncture points. On the trunk, Qi pours from this channel into the heart channel. The channel is specific as it connects all Yin channels of the foot (spleen, kidneys, liver) at the point of *Three Meeting of Yin* (in Chinese, *Sanyinjiao*, SP6).

The channel affects digestive problems, including increased or decreased secretion of digestive enzymes, diabetes and hypoglycemia, overeating or loss of appetite, weight problems. It is also in charge of muscle tone. It affects the uterus—it influences irregular, painful or strong menstruation, or its absence, anemia and bleeding conditions.

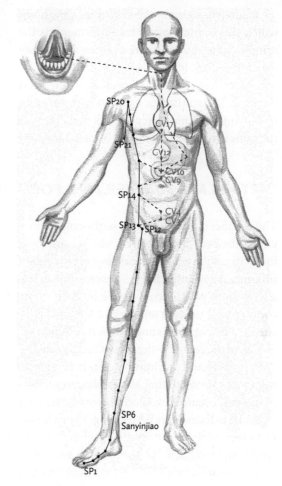

Spleen channel

SPLEEN CHANNEL IN MOVEMENT

The Spleen channel is also relatively long. It has a Yin character—it protrudes from the bottom up and it is located on the inside of the lower limbs and torso. It offers us work with the inner sides of the feet, the inner sides of the ankles, calves, knees and thighs. In movement, we can experiment with what happens to Qi when we begin to lead the movement from the inner sides of the lower limbs or just their individual sections, and how we perceive Qi when the movement in these areas ends.

Since the channel has a connection to the navel, we will use the movement of the navel for our movement, or, vice versa, we will direct the movement to the navel area. The channel also enables us to work with the external pectoral muscles. If we focus on the movement guided by them, it will beautifully expand our chest. This will naturally give us the opportunity to take a deep breath and consciously use the breath even when moving. It will make us physically aware of how the production of the food Qi is linked to the air Qi.

Undoubtedly, an interesting area of the body, which this channel offers for movement, is the armpit. Here, Qi is "poured" from the Spleen channel to the Heart channel. Let us move the body and arms so that this area of our body comes to life, so that we can give it more space by moving it. In movement, let us perceive how the arms in the body are deeply "rooted" and how

their movement passes through the transfer of Qi from one channel to another.

After longer improvisation, Qi is strongly activated in the channel. It offers a physical feeling of its different quality. Let us enjoy this flow of Qi in motion, but also in the stillness that occurs after movement.

DIET IN LATE SUMMER AND FOR THE EARTH PHASE ORGANS

The weather is already colder, so the cold—Yin—enters the body more easily. Thus, we are more likely to catch various diseases—colds, coughs, inflammation, infections. Therefore, it is not advisable to get the cold inside by consuming cooling food in large amounts, such as yogurt, cheese, raw vegetables and fruits. It is important to "warm the center"—the spleen and stomach—with neutral and warming foods. It is good to minimize raw salads, but also cooling vegetables (tomatoes, cucumbers, zucchini/courgette, etc.), and start to focus more on cooking. Warm breakfasts (porridge or soups) are excellent for the spleen and stomach. We should also avoid synthetic nutritional supplements and avoid overuse of vitamins in tablets, because they also cool down. Regularity is needed in the diet.

According to Chinese medicine, the late summer and the autumn that follows are not suitable periods for long fasts. We need to lightly "get plump" to prepare for winter. Round vegetables are suitable—kohlrabi, pumpkin, onion, celeriac. We can sweeten our lives a bit more, because it is starting to be gloomy outside, but mainly because the sweet taste is connected to the EARTH phase. However, I do not mean chocolate and other sweets containing white sugar, which deplete the spleen.

The yellow color
Yellow is the color of the EARTH, so yellow and its shades (orange, brown, ocher) will lead us in the

diet towards suitable foods for the EARTH phase organs. Among the round or orange vegetables we include carrots, onions and pumpkins. They also taste naturally sweet. The sweetest vegetable of this period is Hokkaido pumpkin. It is suitable for soups, porridge, sauces, broths or even pastries. It is suitable for people with poor thermoregulation, for diabetics, for people suffering from a lack of vitality—it contains a lot of natural sugar, and its Qi lasts for a long time.

Recommended foods for the EARTH phase organs and the support of the center
Grains
Grains are generally suitable for supporting the center. Millet is the best choice for the spleen. It is suitable for morning porridge and congee, but also as a side dish to the main course, for puddings, for thickening soups and the like. Barley effectively reduces the volume of moisture in the body; it also lowers blood cholesterol. It removes digestive blockages, thus creating space for the intake of vital substances. It has slightly laxative effects. A recipe for Tibetan porridge, tsampa, made from barley can be found below. Oats or wholegrain rice are also suitable, especially round sweet rice. Long-grain rice grows more in the south, so it is more cooling. Short-grain rice is smaller and, as it grows more in the north, it is more warming. Refined (double bleached) rice creates heat in the body;

sticky Thai rice and long-grain rice support heating. Sticky rice causes the production of mucus which is not desirable. A combination of rice with legumes (soy, red beans, peas, lentils, adzuki beans) is very suitable and we cook them together with rice. A very valuable combination for our center is rice with legumes and corn. Pearl barley (hatomugi) boosts the spleen Qi; we can buy it in health food stores. Sorghum is one of the best cereals because it is also anti-inflammatory and gluten-free, although it is no longer commonly grown for human consumption. Buckwheat is also excellent. Its sweet taste expels moisture from the body, detoxifies and cleanses. Compared to other cereals, it is cooling. Cereal carbohydrates are most valuable when the meals consist of whole grains, flakes or grits; however, you can also eat them in the form of pasta or wholemeal sourdough bread.

Legumes
Legumes remove moisture well, especially adzuki and mung beans. Chickpeas, lentils, peas, soy and soy products—tempeh and natto—are also suitable for the EARTH organs. Tofu is colder in nature, so consuming it too often is cooling. Sprouted mung beans also cool the body and are not suitable for digestive blockages from the cold.

Vegetables
As for vegetables, Hokkaido pumpkin is excellent, but also other types of pumpkins, carrots or turnips—they contain a lot of carbohydrates and are warming. Cabbage is an excellent tonic of Qi. Potatoes support Qi of the center; mashed potatoes are suitable. To support Qi, we can add garlic, onion, leek, ginger and black pepper, but the character of the dish should remain sweet.

Mushrooms
It is also suitable to add shiitake mushrooms or oyster mushrooms to vegetable dishes. They can be stewed in butter. The best therapeutic properties have wood-destroying fungi, such as the common chicken of the woods or the mushroom known as jelly ear or wood ear.

Fruit
Raw fruit is not suitable for those who have poor digestion, because it is cooling and thus slows the digestion. Stewed and cooked compotes are a more suitable version, especially if heating spices are added (e.g. cinnamon, cardamom, star anise, cloves). Stewed apples, plums and dates are suitable as a "sweetener" for porridge. Of the Chinese fruit, red dates (Chinese jujube) are very nutritious for the EARTH organs. Their taste is sweet and neutral, and they affect the spleen and stomach, replenishing Qi, nourishing blood and curing weakness from the emptiness of Qi and blood connected with fatigue. They are also excellent in the treatment of shortness of breath, anorexia, irritability and general restlessness of internal organs.

Meat
For those who eat meat, chicken, duck, pigeon, beef, turkey, lamb, goat (ideally all organic) are suitable for strengthening the center. They are energetically warm, even hot, and provide a lot of strength. It is advisable to stew them in butter. Meat generally supports the center, if it is not eaten in excess, baked or fried. These forms of preparation bring heat and moisture to the body. We therefore prefer stewing or cooking. Fish, especially mackerel, plaice and tuna, are also suitable. However, tuna already contains a lot of fat.

Nuts and seeds
Nuts and seeds are also excellent; they have a sweet taste and therefore support the spleen. However, we have to pay attention to quality, because they can go bad quickly and become rancid, and they often contain molds. The expiration date should always be checked. Almonds, walnuts, hazelnuts and cashews are excellent. However, we prefer to avoid them if we are overweight, suffer from

lipomas and cysts—we especially avoid peanuts. Pistachios contain a lot of iron, so they support blood production. Pine nuts are suitable for asthma and Brazil nuts if we lack essential fatty acids. Hemp seeds and black sesame are excellent for joint nutrition. They support blood production through the nutrition of the Jing essence.

All these foods are naturally neutral and warm in nature, which nourishes the spleen, stomach and pancreas, harmonizes digestion and gradually tonifies Qi. They are also suitable for the formation of body fluids. Body fluids include all the juices we have in the body—blood, lymph, various digestive juices, various nourishing and moisturizing fluids of the mucous membranes, but also synovial fluids in the joints, fluids nourishing tendons, cerebrospinal fluid, and light fluids nourishing and moisturizing the skin. We need them so that we are not dry, not only at the level of the skin, but also in deeper structures—in tendons, bones, joints and fascia. Steaming is the most suitable way of food preparation to support the formation of body fluids. We can steam vegetables as well as fruit. Even bread can be made by steaming instead of baking it. The crust will not be as crunchy as after baking, but the steamed bread itself is delicious. And instead of cooking or stewing vegetables, try steaming them.

Sweet taste

To protect the EARTH organs, we should avoid the following foods that are more or less moisture-forming and cooling:

- Flour and flour products—because they quickly create heat. The heat thickens the moisture into mucus, which causes food stagnation and a feeling of fullness. Flour products are particularly unsuitable for allergy sufferers. We should avoid raw fruits, raw vegetables, yogurts, mucus- and moisture-producing foods such as cow's milk, cow's milk cheese, cold and chilled drinks, fruit juice, cola and other sweetened drinks. Modern raw food is not suitable for people with impaired digestion.
- Furthermore, we should minimize cooling foods, which include tomatoes, cucumbers, tropical fruits, white sugar and artificial sweeteners. Frozen foods are logically cooling, damaging the digestive fire (i.e. Qi that organs need in order to be able to process the food). In addition, they contain much less Qi than fresh food. Regarding drinks, green and black tea, coffee and mineral water cool the organism down. Cold and chilled drinks and drinking during meals are not advisable.
- Freshwater algae, such as chlorella, and also seaweed are also cooling. Various sprouts are also cooling but they are full of enzymes and vitamins, so they should form part of our diet. Therefore, it is advisable to add warming spices to a dish where we use the sprouts—dried or fresh ginger, chili, curry, cinnamon, star anise, cloves, cardamom. Almost all smoothies are cooling as they are made from raw fruits.

According to Chinese medicine, the sweet taste belongs to the EARTH phase. It is neutral in nature, energetically supports the spleen and thus creates Qi. However, it is not the extremely sweet taste of refined white sugar, found, for example, in chocolate, common sweets, fruit juices or in the sugar we put in coffee. It is the naturally sweet taste of vegetables, fruits and grains.

The sweet taste supports the production of body fluids—everything that moisturizes us. It relaxes the psyche, evokes a feeling of harmony. It helps with stress by returning the Qi to normal when stress intensifies the Qi. No matter how beneficial it is, however, it must be in balance. Nowadays, finding this balance is a pretty difficult task. The sweet taste in the form of refined sugar does more harm than good. A sudden craving for sweets is a signal for a lack of Qi in the body.

Sugar

Sugars—carbohydrates—are irreplaceable substances for the human body and belong to a balanced diet. They are an important component that supplies Qi to the body; together with proteins, they help build and renew cells, muscles and tissues. Anyone who works hard naturally feels like eating something sweet. The body asks for what it needs. However, we should know what is good for us and what harms us.

Carbohydrates are divided into complex carbohydrates, *polysaccharides* (mainly starches), and simple carbohydrates, *monosaccharides*. Monosaccharides are the *glucose* contained in grapes, pineapple or honey and *fructose* in fruits; there are also *disaccharides* which are mainly lactose (milk sugars), maltose (sugar contained in malt) and saccharose (commonly known as beet or cane sugar).

For health, we need a diverse range of carbohydrates, especially polysaccharides (compound sugars), which are an irreplaceable supplier of energy to our body. The most important polysaccharides include whole grains (wheat, natural rice, spelt, oats, sorghum, barley, rye, maize polenta), legumes (peas, lentils, chickpeas, beans, soybeans and soy products: tofu, seitan, natto, etc.) and vegetables. Compared to simple sugars, they have a completely different effect on the human body. Sorghum, mentioned above, is a good choice for movers. It has a balanced character, and the sugar is released gradually for up to six hours (longer than other grains). Millet removes excess water and reduces swelling, so it is very important for pregnant women.

Simple sugars supply energy to the body immediately. After a piece of chocolate or drinking sweetened fruit juice, we feel replenished with energy. However, simple sugars cause a rapid rise in blood sugar. This strains the pancreas, which produces insulin that is flushed out into the blood, where it must regulate the amount of sugar. Therefore, with regular use of simple sugars, blood sugar problems may occur. Polysaccharides (compound sugars) supply us with energy by gradually supplying sugar to the blood, and thus ensure the maintenance of a stable blood sugar level. Consuming simple sugars is a way to go from one extreme to the other. If we feel extreme fatigue or an extreme craving for sweets, we quickly consume something that will refresh us quickly. But it will cause an extreme state at the level of blood composition. Consumption of compound sugars is closer to the golden mean. This helps maintain a longer feeling of satiety, but also a balanced psyche and calmer behavior. And it is, of course, a prevention against obesity.

Almost all commonly used sweeteners are simple sugars. The exceptions are cereal malts (barley, rice or corn malt), because they also contain a certain amount of compound sugars. Cereal syrups contain less complex sugar than cereal malts.

White sugar is considered to be one of the "white poisons." During production (refinement), it is deprived of most minerals, vitamins and fiber. If we consume white sugar and refined foods, we are short of calcium, magnesium, phosphorus, iron and B vitamins—all important minerals for our profession. This is one of the reasons why sugar is associated with osteoporosis. This happens due to intake of white sugar, which does not contain those minerals; consequently our body takes them from our reserves, from the bones—that is, from itself. However, white sugar, which we usually use to sweeten our tea or coffee, is also found in white and some dark chocolates, biscuits, desserts and juices. Until recently, people consumed it only in very limited quantities. Nowadays, however, it is an alarming approximately 40 kilograms per person per year, leading to an increase in obesity, digestive problems and fatigue syndrome. By the action of microorganisms in the oral cavity, sugar is converted into organic acids, which etch the surface of the teeth. Another toxic effect is the fact that sugar is an acid-forming food, thus causing the body to over-acidify. In such conditions, the intestinal microflora are also easily disturbed, which can lead to yeast infections—their elimination is impossible when refined sugar is consumed. White sugar also negatively affects the immune system; the acidic environment is a suitable substrate for various infections. It weakens the spleen Qi, which then cannot maintain immunity by its influence on the formation of Postnatal Qi. It also causes restlessness and inability to concentrate, which is very common with children—it is often the hidden reason behind poor results at school. White sugar is also found where we do not see it. Hidden sugars are in durable pastries, semi-finished products, ketchups and even meat products. They are added to these products because they are good preservatives. Therefore, it is important to read the labels of purchased products. And beware—although cane sugar is more considerate towards the body than beet sugar, its excessive consumption leads to the same health problems.

So what to do with it?

A certain amount of sugar (i.e. carbohydrates) is necessary for the function of each individual's organs, especially the brain. Lack of carbohydrates in the diet can lead to hypoglycemia, which is manifested by feelings of fatigue and inefficiency, and can also lead to digestive problems. So what to do when sugar is everywhere, and we should avoid it, but we need carbohydrates?

I recommend going sugar-free carefully, gradually and wisely. It is not advisable to stop eating sugar overnight. It would be a shock for the body. Reduce sugar slightly and gradually. Start building the golden mean—the harmonious gradual release of sugar from food into the blood. This is done by regular consumption of cereals, legumes and sweet vegetables. Consumption of two tablespoons of roasted and crushed black sesame a day will reduce sugar craving to 20 percent after a month. From my own experience, by including a regular and larger amount of these foods, I realized after a few months that I had completely lost my interest in the sweet aisle in the supermarket. This does not mean that I never go for anything unhealthily sweet, but I can resist and have control over it, and, most importantly, I know how I can balance this sweet shock in the body. And, if from time to time I feel that my appetite for sweets has increased, it is a signal that I should again enrich my menu with foods that give me the necessary sugar in a different way.

Instead of white sugar, let us start sweetening differently. Ideal are cereal malts (not cereal syrups) such as barley, rice, spelt, wheat or corn malt. They also contain a certain amount of compound sugars. Other sweeteners, such as fruit malts—for example, date, agave, plum, blueberry or maple syrup—are simple sugars. They are certainly a better choice than white sugar, but they cannot be compared to cereal malts when it comes to delivering complex sugars to the body. Honey is also a simple sugar, so it is not suitable as a standard sweetener. Moreover, as we know, honey is a medicine, so it should remain a medicine. It has a wide range of uses as a medicine, but if our body is used to it as a sweetener, it will no longer act on us as a medicine. Honey should be consumed by older people, because it contains a lot of ether, the air element of bees; it lightens, moves and promotes activity. It is therefore not suitable for children with impaired concentration and hyperactivity.

Breakfast celebration

Our grandmothers were already telling us about the importance of breakfast. Even from the Chinese medicine point of view, breakfast is a very important component of our eating habits and overall lifestyle. First, we should have breakfast by 9 a.m., because 9–11 a.m., according to the organ clock, is the time of maximum activity of the spleen. At that time, the spleen needs to have food in the body digested by the stomach so that it can extract essences from it, which we will then use, in the form of Qi and nourished blood, for our activities throughout the day. Second, what kind of breakfast we should have?

The importance of warm food for good digestion was discussed in Chapter 4. From the Chinese medicine point of view, fruit juices that cool the digestive tract are not suitable for breakfast. People with poor digestion should definitely consider a warm breakfast. In traditional Chinese hotels, you will not find bread, pastries, toast and a chunk of butter, margarine, jam or sausages, salami and cheese on the table. And although in well-known tourist locations these things appear on the breakfast table for Western tourists, there are always mainly cooked breakfasts available. You can choose from soups, warm pasta with vegetables or an egg, warm eggs prepared in various ways, steamed buns stuffed with vegetables or meat and especially porridge. Even today, the Chinese maintain old Taoist dietary habits—start the morning with a warm endearment of the stomach.

Nowadays, muesli or yogurts are considered a healthy form of breakfast. Yogurt cools the digestive tract. Muesli is harder to digest. It can be purchased in different versions, with different flavors, but it is usually based on cereal flakes. It is usually prepared by mixing with hot water. In terms of digestibility, this is not suitable for the stomach; therefore, the flakes should also be cooked. In addition, muesli is full of sugar. When you read what muesli consists of, you will find that sugar is often the second, sometimes even the first item in the list of ingredients. This will not please our spleen.

I have a very good experience with morning porridge. We prepare it also for students on our dance camps, which are very physically demanding. We always go through training without much hunger until lunch. I also consider soups to be excellent for breakfast. Fresh miso soup with mushrooms and vegetables is excellent (you can find the recipe in Chapter 8 on the WATER phase), but because of the proteins, it should also contain legumes. However, other soups are suitable; it is best if they are thickened with grain, so that we also take in the necessary carbohydrates. Freshly cooked soup is ideal, but this is not always possible due to time constraints. You can prepare the soup in the evening, have it for dinner and just warm it up in the morning. If the soup is not fulfilling enough for us, we can have a nice sourdough bread with it, or thicken it with grain during cooking.

Sweet porridge can be cooked in water or cereal milk and served with fruit, ideally stewed, not raw. You can cut apples and stew them in a little water with a pinch of salt and stevia (or malt), cinnamon, star anise and cloves. Then there is no need to sweeten the porridge. The porridge can also be flavored with jam (without sugar), chutney, compote and the above-mentioned malts. For the required dose of fat, it is advisable to sprinkle it with seeds or nuts. For better digestibility, it is better to soak the nuts overnight and cook them with the porridge. The best way of preserving fruit is drying it—it does not require sugar. However, sugar is generally added to compotes.

With regard to sweet porridge, it should also be mentioned that cereals in combination with fresh fruit over-acidify the organism. The only cereal that is alkaline in combination with fruit is millet. And the only fruit that does not over-acidify in combination with grain is pear. Which means that sweet porridge must be alternated with salty porridge and soups. Sometimes, of course, we can also have a classic Western breakfast for a change.

It is not difficult to prepare salty porridge. Cereals or flakes can be cooked in water with a little salt, in broth, or flavored with soy sauce or miso paste at the end. We serve it with vegetables of our choice, either slightly stewed, blanched or fermented, sprinkled with seeds and chopped haulm or sprouts. Certainly the porridge still needs to be "fattened," because we need a certain amount of fat, especially in winter. One of the options is to add seeds and nuts or a little fat into the porridge—coconut oil, butter, ghee and the like—or a few drops of good-quality cold-pressed oil: olive, poppyseed, pumpkin, avocado, etc.

Rice porridge congee

Congee is the most important recipe of Chinese cuisine. It is the most common Chinese breakfast dish at home, but we can find it served for breakfast in hotels and even on planes. During my travels in China, I was in several hotels, even in those for Western tourists, and congee was on offer in each of them.

The prevalence of this dish is surprising as it does not have an interesting taste. So why do the Chinese have nothing but praise for it?

Congee (in Chinese, *Xifan*—i.e. water rice), also known under by the Cantonese name *Jook*, is the food that gives the body the most Qi and juice. The body needs very little Qi to digest it, and it induces a perfect balance of Yin and Yang. It is suitable for sick people, for convalescence after illness, but also for those who have a problem consuming other foods. It is therefore also suitable during fasting, because it helps to lighten and cleanse the body and at the same time supplies it with Qi. In the form of a puree, it is suitable even for infants who do not tolerate breast milk or if breast milk is not available for them.

The basis of congee is rice and water. The Chinese nowadays use exclusively white rice for its preparation, but congee also works with natural rice, red rice or other cereals, such as millet. When rice is cooked without ingredients, it is really tasteless. We can therefore add something else to it, such as dried fruits, nuts, vegetables, legumes, and cook them with rice at the same time. Depending on what we choose for the combination, we can create congee for any health problems—lack of Qi, bloating, weakness of the spleen, stomach, kidneys, etc. Congee is consumed warm; it is the ideal first meal of the day. Significantly, it strengthens us and harmonizes our center.

The simplest recipe for congee is to add 8–10 parts water to one part of rice (or another cereal), let it simmer, turn down the flame and cook it slowly under the lid for at least four hours. We cook congee in a large pot, as the foam, which is formed in a relatively large amount during boiling, could boil over. We can pre-cook it for two or three days in advance, but it is ideal to have it fresh. For congee, long boiling is important, during which all alchemical processes between rice, water and fire have the opportunity to take place. The average Westerner will not like this porridge at first, but as soon as they discover its effects, they will love it. You will find some tips for its preparation in the recipes in this chapter.

Tibetan tsampa

Tsampa is used in Tibet not only as a morning porridge but also as a basic side dish. It can be served as a porridge, or in the form of balls or patties. Tibetans also carry it in a loose form in a bag and add it to their tea. This creates a kind of thick greased soup, which is very strengthening in the harsh mountainous Tibetan climate. Tsampa is not actually cooked. The barley is dry roasted until slightly brown and fragrant, and ground in a grain mill. Then this flour is salted, mixed with butter from yak's milk and kneaded. Instead of yak butter, cow butter or ghee can also be used. Tsampa should be kneaded either with your hands or with a spoon in a bowl. It can be flavored with broth or diluted with tea. Tsampa is great for hunger. Barley flour is very nutritious; aromatic butter greases it and roasted grain will give us the necessary Yang. A few balls can stop hunger.

SOME TIPS AND RECIPES FOR BREAKFAST

Millet porridge with Hokkaido pumpkin

Ingredients: ½ cup millet, 2 slices of pumpkin cut into pieces, pinch of salt, 2–3 cups of water.

Method: Rinse the millet. Place all ingredients except the pumpkin in a heavy-bottomed saucepan and bring to a boil. Cook over low heat for 15 minutes. Add the pumpkin and cook for another 15–20 minutes. Stir a little before serving. Serve topped with sesame salt gomashio (see the recipe in Chapter 8) and sliced leek rings or slices of seaweed. The porridge tastes delicious with a little fat such as coconut oil, butter or ghee. You can also drizzle it with a little oil.

Benefits: It replenishes Qi, adds a sweet taste, and thus heals the spleen, pancreas and stomach. Millet helps get rid of excess water.

Oatmeal or rice flakes porridge

The quickest way is to soak the flakes overnight in rice or oat milk (water will also do). In the morning, bring them to a boil, season with a pinch of salt and simmer on a low heat for about 10 minutes. If cooking on low heat, there is no need to stir them. If you have not soaked the flakes overnight, they will need to be cooked for about 25 minutes. If you cook them in milk, the taste will be pleasantly sweet even without additional sweetening. It can be cooked with carrots, bananas, Hokkaido pumpkin, etc. Finally, sprinkle with seeds, nuts, dried fruit and drizzle with a little fat.

Benefits: Warm morning porridge replenishes Qi and warms the digestive tract.

Savory variant of porridge, called "savery"

Porridge cereals are also delicious in salty form. The word "savery" has its root in the English word *save*—to save, to preserve. Hence, in the form of breakfast, such porridge gives us a lot of strength.

To prepare it, you can use any grain, add a little salt, vegetable broth or miso paste (add miso after cooking). You can sprinkle it with various seeds (pumpkin seeds are excellent for a salty taste), nuts, nori flakes or sesame salt gomashio (see the recipe in Chapter 8). Also, you can add any vegetables you have at home, either blanched or steamed, such as carrots, Hokkaido pumpkin, leeks, broccoli. It is also delicious when this porridge is served with some pickles. Finally add a little fat—in addition to those mentioned above, fresh homemade duck lard goes well with it too.

Benefits: Savory porridge replenishes the spleen and kidney Qi.

The fastest morning porridge

Ingredients: 1 part of wholemeal grits (spelt, wheat, rice, corn or buckwheat), 4 to 5 parts of water or cereal milk, pinch of sea salt.

Method: Bring the water or cereal milk to the boil and season with a pinch of salt. Slowly add the grits and start stirring immediately, preferably with a whisk or fork. Cook over a low heat, stirring constantly, for 3–5 minutes. If you have time, you can let the porridge "sleep" in a pot covered with a lid for about 20 minutes. It will thicken and swell.

Benefits: It replenishes Qi and warms the digestive tract.

Barley groats and hatomugi pearl barley porridge

Ingredients: ¾ cup of barley groats, ¼ cup of pearl barley, 3 cups water, about 5 cm of kombu seaweed, 4 shiitake mushrooms, finely chopped scallions/spring onions.

Method: Wash the barley groats and pearl barley. Soak them together in water in a pressure cooker overnight. In the morning, add the kombu seaweed and the shiitake mushrooms. Pressurize the pot and cook the ingredients for 45 minutes. Once cooked, chop the mushrooms, finely slice the kombu seaweed and mix with the grains and spring onions. If you do not have a pressure cooker, just cook longer.

Benefits: The porridge replenishes Qi, adds a sweet taste, and thus heals the spleen, pancreas and stomach. It cleanses, dissolves mucus deposits in the body, moisturizes the skin.

Sweet rice congee with walnuts
Ingredients: Sweet rice, walnuts, pinch of salt, warming spices, water.

Method: Cook the rice with the walnuts in ten times as much water. Add cinnamon, cloves and ginger to taste.

Benefits: It warms the center, disperses cold and strengthens the spleen, the pancreas and the stomach Qi.

Carrot congee made from wheat or rice
Ingredients: Wheat or rice, grated carrots, pinch of salt, water.

Method: Cook one part rice or wheat mixed with the carrots in ten parts water.

Benefits: It replenishes the center, stimulates Qi, relieves abdominal distention, transforms stagnation.

Congee with adzuki beans
Ingredients: Rice, adzuki beans, pinch of salt, water.

Method: Cook equal amounts of rice and adzuki beans with ten times the amount of water.

Benefits: It wicks away moisture and relieves urination.

Tsampa
Ingredients: 1 cup of hulled barley, water, butter or ghee, salt or vegetable broth.

Method: Dry-roast the barley until lightly browned and fragrant. Grind it in a grain mill. If you do not have a grinder, have someone grind it for you or use the barley grits. Mix with water in a ratio of 1 part of flour to 3–4 parts of water, season with salt and boil. Serve with butter, ghee or sprinkle with sesame salt gomashio (see Chapter 8). Garnish with seeds, nuts, chopped chives and spring onions. It is delicious with blanched carrots and leeks.

Benefits: Tsampa is very nourishing, replenishes the spleen, the pancreas and the kidney Qi. Roasting adds Yang, which is needed especially in winter or when cold.

A FEW MORE TIPS AND RECIPES

Tea from kuzu
Ingredients: 1 tsp kuzu, a cup of water, salt or soy sauce.

Method: Dissolve the kuzu in a small amount of cold water. Gradually, add more water and keep stirring to dissolve the kuzu evenly. Meanwhile, bring a cup of water to the boil in a saucepan, add the dissolved kuzu and stir well. Cook for 5–7 minutes until the liquid starts to have a gel-like translucent consistency. You can add a little salt or soy sauce.

Benefits: It soothes the stomach, helps with all

kinds of headaches, colds and flu, lowers fevers at temperatures up to 38°C. Kuzu detoxifies. It is used to relieve menopausal symptoms. It relieves headaches after consuming too much alcohol, and also helps with addiction to alcohol.

Kuzu drink for digestive problems

Ingredients: 1 tsp kuzu, cup of water, 1 umeboshi plum.

Method: Dissolve the kuzu in a small amount of cold water. Gradually, add more water and keep stirring to dissolve the kuzu entirely. Meanwhile, bring a cup of water to a boil and simmer the umeboshi plum in it for 5 minutes. Stir in the dissolved kuzu and stir well until the cloudy drink becomes clear. Drink warm and eat the umeboshi plum.

Benefits: It soothes the stomach and intestines. Kuzu detoxifies and the umeboshi plum dissolves various hardenings (e.g. fibroids, cysts, polyps).

Hokkaido soup—basic recipe

Ingredients: 1 medium-sized Hokkaido pumpkin, 2 large onions, water, sesame oil, salt.

Method: Clean the onion, chop it finely and fry in oil. Wash the pumpkin, cut it open, remove the seeds and cut the flesh into pieces. There is no need to peel the pumpkin. Add water to the onions, add the pumpkin, bring to the boil, season with salt and cook for 15–20 minutes. Let it cool and blend. Reheat again slightly and serve with soy cream, drizzle with soy sauce, garnish with something green (e.g. parsley, coriander, chives) and peeled dried pumpkin seeds.

Benefits: It replenishes the spleen and the pancreas Qi. Coriander and parsley get rid of heavy metals; their sprigs also support blood formation.

Hokkaido soup—variations

The soup tastes delicious in this simple form, but it can be varied in different ways. For example:

- Add a boiled potato, sweet potato or some root vegetables to the pumpkin.
- Add dried ginger, masala, curry, nutmeg, cinnamon, etc., to roasted onions, depending on what you like or have at home.
- With the cooked pumpkin, blend some leftover legumes, which will also enrich the soup with protein and thicken it at the same time.
- Wheat, couscous, bulgur or other cereals can also be used to thicken the soup.
- You can also cook it with seaweed.
- It can be flavored with miso, tahini sesame paste, coconut milk.
- When the soup is thick, it can also be used as a sauce.

Roasted Hokkaido pumpkin with onions and potatoes

Ingredients: 1 Hokkaido pumpkin, 2 large onions, 4 potatoes, olive oil, spices, soy sauce.

Method: Wash the pumpkin, cut it open, remove the seeds and cut the flesh into equal-sized pieces. Peel the onions and potatoes, chop and arrange on a greased baking sheet or in a glass dish. Drizzle with olive oil and soy sauce. Bake in a preheated oven for approximately 25 minutes. Serve with sour cream, yogurt and pickles. It is simple, quick and very tasty. It is a typical dish of late summer and early autumn.

Variations:

- Omit the potatoes, add garlic. Do not peel the garlic, just separate the cloves and roast them in their skins with the pumpkin.

- Toss the vegetables in a mixture of oil, herbs and spices before spreading on a baking sheet.

Warm drink made from pumpkin seeds

It is a pity to throw away the seeds from the pumpkin we used for the soup. They contain many nutrients, especially selenium. Boil the seeds and the tender flesh in plenty of water, add a pinch of salt. Boil for at least 30 minutes. Drain and drink while still warm.

CHAPTER 12

The METAL phase

Moving inwards and acknowledging values

About: breathing and gaining Heavenly Qi / value and evaluation / sorting and cleaning / lungs and large intestine / voice / skin / protective armor and immunity / flu and cough / smoking / ability to let go / touch and bodily boundaries / sadness / the Corporeal Soul Po / diet for autumn and for the METAL phase organs

---

Concentrate your mind and Qi and use the balance of autumn Qi. Don't focus your efforts on the outside and brighten the lungs.

THE YELLOW EMPEROR'S CLASSIS OF MEDICINE

AUTUMN IS ABOUT THE JOURNEY INWARDS

We are slowly approaching the end of the year. However, it is necessary to prepare for it—to complete and evaluate our supplies, draw our energy inwards and, slowly but surely, close the door behind the year. The Qi of autumn and the Qi of the METAL phase help us, as they naturally condense, directed from the outside inward. Just as a tree draws its Qi from the surface to its depth, and therefore it loses its leaves, so does our planet move its Qi to its depth and brings autumn. The exuberance of the FIRE of summer gradually succumbed during the EARTH phase to calmness. All things that have matured are used during the METAL phase; some are even destroyed. Everything is subject to transformation, even decomposition in the positive

sense of the word. Everything around dries up, becomes brittle, breaks, falls, because Qi is less on the surface. Everything contracts intensively inside. This is happening around us, but also within us, in the metabolism of the physical body, but also at the mental level. The period from the autumn equinox (approximately September 21), when Yin definitely seizes its power, to the winter solstice (approximately December 21), when Yin is at its highest, is a time directed inwards, into our insides, into our dwellings, into the circle of our families. It is time to reap the benefits of everything that has matured in previous months—from subsistence through relationships, implemented projects, to health. No wonder we get used to being less sociable in autumn; we prefer to spend time at home with ourselves. Sometimes we get caught up in nostalgia and maybe even depression, because moving inward creates tension. These are the accompanying phenomena of this period and the preconditions for cleansing. There is no need to be afraid or to feel weird when we are a little sadder than usual, when we are more focused on ourselves or if we even feel the need to cry. The METAL phase is a time to discover what is truly valuable and worthy in our lives. We will not find this on the surface, and the METAL phase, by directing us inwards, helps us to immerse into ourselves, so that we can find the quality of our essence. It is therefore related to our ability to choose a quality that is of value to us.

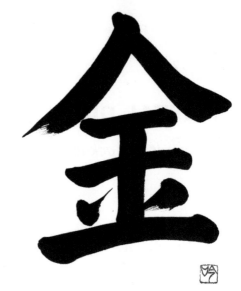

Chinese character for METAL

METAL LIKE A MACHETE

One of the similarities of METAL phase Qi is a sharp knife that can trim, cleanse, reduce and thus revive, rejuvenate and clear. When we allow the METAL phase to work in us, the ability to get rid of the unnecessary and dysfunctional is evoked in us. The METAL phase is a time and space for internal summarization, inventory, sorting, evaluation and subsequent cleaning. We mostly live in internal conflict because we are afraid to let things out of our lives. We tend to cling to material things, people and animals, but also to dysfunctional habits or relationships. We often cling to the projects of which we are a part, and it is difficult for us to admit that they no longer bring us what they once did. And yet, if something no longer works—and that can be a partnership, a working relationship, a relationship to food, hobbies, etc.—it is just one of the normal manifestations of its development. Everything has its beginning, ascension, peak, descent and extinction. This rule cannot be avoided. This extinction can bring about either complete cessation or recovery. At the same time, if we allow ourselves to activate METAL Qi in us, we can also get rid of the knowledge, beliefs and principles that no longer serve us, because we have already transformed their meaning into something new. We need to empty ourselves first in order to be filled with something new. We need to exhale first so we can inhale.

This purifying potential of autumn has long been known from the ancient philosophical book *The Book of Changes* (in Chinese, *Yi Jing*). Hexagram No. 64—*Weiji*—says that no other season has such preconditions for sorting and purification as autumn. It encourages us to decide what to keep and what to throw away. We get rid of what is unnecessary so that there is room and peace for what is to remain. And what we keep will come to an end in the winter. In the spring, it will become part of a new cycle. The order, which was created in the autumn, will appear before the eyes of all in the spring. Changes in the cycle occur in autumn; in this case, spring is only the result of continuity. In the spring, everything processed and prepared in advance reaches the surface. Even in the autumn of our lives, we cut unnecessary things away. Our experience so far allows us to perceive the value of ourselves, and so to choose only the best for ourselves. We no longer accept every job offer that comes, but we consider each of them. We value ourselves, our energy, our body and our time, and based on the evaluation of that particular thing, we decide whether to deal with it or not. In the autumn of our lives, we have the opportunity to pay more attention to ourselves. After all, the children have already flown the nest, our partner is an independent being who can take care of himself or herself, so we find the greatest value in ourselves.

FILLING AND EMPTYING

This mechanism can be beautifully observed in both organs of the METAL phase—the lungs and the large intestine. The lungs can be optimally filled with new inhaled air only when they have been emptied before, thus when they exhale. When the large intestine is affected, it cannot be emptied, and excessive retention causes constipation. Diarrhea, on the other hand, lets out what is valuable. We can feel the relationship between the two organs, for example, in a situation where we lose a loved one and are not yet able to accept that loss. In that case, we still cling to the person, which over time manifests itself in difficult breathing. The breath then takes the form of moaning or sighing. Instead of releasing our breath freely and smoothly, we hold it back. This is, of course, happening on a subconscious level.

Thus, the METAL phase typically manifests in these two organs. Both receive, but they also get rid of what is unnecessary. They clean, they sort, and they let go, so that they can receive the new and the fresh. The Yin lungs and their Yang companion, the large intestine, form a cooperating pair. Together with other connections and parts of the body, they form the functional circle of the lungs.

> **Functional circuit of the lungs:** lungs, large intestine, skin, breathing, body hair, nose, nasal mucus, sense of smell, mucus, dryness, the Corporeal Soul Po, integrity, honesty, courage, emotion of sadness.

THE LUNGS ARE THE MASTER OF QI

The Yellow Emperor's Classic of Medicine characterizes the lungs (in Chinese, *Fei*) as follows: "The lungs are the master of Qi. They serve the ruler (the heart) as the chief chancellor, the highest dignitary."

Where does this sovereign post come from? From a Western point of view, the lungs are responsible for air intake. For Taoists, however, air is not just ordinary air. Air is primarily *Heavenly Qi*, the substance of the cosmos, which, thanks to the lungs, can enter our body and act there. The received Qi of the air and the Qi of food together form what's called Original Qi (in Chinese, *Yuanqi*), the primary substance of our Postnatal Qi. Thus, air Qi is a very valuable component, and the lungs are the organ in charge of disposing of this component sensitively—receiving it, distributing it throughout the body and excreting dead substances from it in the form of exhalation. At the same time, the lungs are the uppermost organ, closest to Heaven. They surround the heart, and thus actually protect the emperor. They also protect other organs like a canopy. The lungs are a bridge to the outside world for the emperor (the heart).

BREATHING

According to Taoist philosophy, breathing is one of the most important life functions. It is an exchange between us and the world around us. With each in-breath, we inhale the Tao, and with each exhalation, we communicate with it from our inside. The lungs are responsible for breathing in Heavenly Qi and distributing it throughout the body through oxygenated blood in the bloodstream. The rhythm given by exhalation and inhalation has a significant regulatory effect on Qi movements in the body in directions up, down, out and in. When the lung Qi is all right, every other organ smiles with joy. Regular and barrier-free breathing is a basic condition for the formation of Qi and the harmonization and regulation of the entire Qi mechanism. If breathing is impaired, it also affects the production of Postnatal Qi, which makes Prenatal Qi more depleted. This can be manifested by respiratory disorders, coughing, shortness of breath, wheezing, gasping for breath or by lack of Qi. The importance of breathing is obvious on a physical level, and every mover is dependent on its quality. We need breath for movement as well as vocal expression. However, the lungs are responsible for the ability to receive even at the mental level. Breathing is associated with receiving without judging and releasing without feeling sad.

Breath has always been associated with longevity. Taoists believe that one has only a limited number of breaths, and when they are used up, life ends. The length of life also depends on the speed at which air enters and circulates through us. They claim that those who breathe fast, live short. Breath has always been an important factor in Qi exercises. We can use breath in Qigong as a strategy for conscious and effective Qi guidance, and this is another reason why I involve Qigong in my work with the body.

Respiration is a complex function involving several organs and several body systems in addition to the lungs. These are the diaphragm, the respiratory and expiratory muscles, the blood that binds and transports oxygen and carbon dioxide, the blood circulation and the central nervous system. However, the Taoists found that the lungs, when breathing, energetically cooperate also with the kidneys. It is written in the *Yellow Emperor's Classic of Medicine* that *the kidneys are the root of the inhalation, the lungs are the root of the exhalation*. We know that the kidneys are a storehouse of Prenatal Qi. This source treasure is energetically connected to the lungs because the prenatal source needs to be connected to the postnatal source, and so the kidneys draw Heavenly Qi towards themselves. The lungs are their mediator and subsequently what excretes used air. Therefore, Chinese medicine has, for example, two ways of treating asthma. If the asthmatic has a problem with inhalation, the treatment is to support kidney Qi. If the asthmatic has a problem with exhalation, the treatment is more focused on the lungs, although the treatment, of course, takes into account the relationship between the two organs. In connection with respiration, it is also worth mentioning that there is a need for deep abdominal breathing—that is, breathing into the Lower Dantian, into the area that is connected to the kidney Qi. Our body naturally needs to breathe into the lower abdomen. Compared to this, chest breathing is shallow; it does not provide a connection between Heavenly Qi and the kidney Qi, nor does it provide us with sufficient oxygenation. Breathing into the Lower

Dantian also helps to strengthen mental grounding, and thus mental stability. In the event of any disturbances, breathing into the Lower Dantian is a suitable way to calm down.

The "bonus" that breathing brings us is an internal massage of the abdominal organs. At the same time, breathing movements create chest elasticity, which helps the heart to function well. Proper breathing also relaxes the thoracic spine, and thus it does not irritate the nerves that branch out between the vertebrae from the spinal cord, so it is a prevention against back pain. Through breathing, the body can get the most out of each of its activities.

One of the factors that inhibits a good-quality breath is stress. Stress and anxiety tighten the chest. The breath of a stressed person is fast and superficial, similar to the breath of a dog. What volume of Heavenly Qi can such constricted lungs inhale? With normal, calm breathing, an adult exchanges about 500 ml of air with one inhalation and exhalation, so from a Taoist point of view that is 500 ml of the Heavenly Qi. During stress, the volume decreases rapidly.

Breathing also performs cleansing work for the body—it removes carbon dioxide, but also many impurities. In addition to distributing Qi throughout the body, the lungs also direct Qi outwards. The result is exhalation through the nose and elimination of impurities through the skin and skin hairs. This pushes the used Qi out of the body. Thanks to the respiratory movements, the used air is eliminated from the body, and if this does not happen sufficiently by itself, we can help such cleansing. Induced coughing—the conscious rapid expulsion of air—is a form of purification of the breath. Laughter is also a great remedy. The large intestine assists the lungs with the cleansing function. It eliminates waste and at the same time the harmonic large intestine Qi helps the lungs work better.

SMOKING

The lungs control the Qi of the whole body and spread Heavenly Qi, which they inhale, throughout the body. Polluted air affects their proper functioning and weakens them. In this context, a few words about smoking are appropriate. I do not say anything new when I point out that smoking is harmful. It is without debate a way of polluting the internal environment and weakening the lung Qi. It damages the lungs by destroying them mechanically and by bringing fumes into them that are carcinogenic. Inhaled smoke causes *heat* in the lungs, which creates a dryness there. The lungs do not like dryness; for their harmonious functioning, they need a certain humidification.

However, smoking also affects other structures, too. In Chapter 11 on the EARTH phase, we mentioned that smoking also damages the vitality and function of muscles because it prevents oxygenation of the blood. However, smoking harms the whole system, all organs and their mutual cooperation. When I see young dance or acting students filling their lungs with cigarette smoke in between classes, it tears my heart out.

SUPERVISION OF TWO GATES—NOSE AND THROAT

The lungs are the uppermost organ of all the Yin organs, and the only internal organ directly connected to the external environment via nose and throat. Therefore, they are easily and quickly attacked by external pathogens and are sensitive to the influence of climatic factors. The nose is the gateway for Heavenly Qi to penetrate the lungs. However, it is also a gateway for external pathogens that can invade the lungs directly through the trachea. Therefore, the lung Qi must guard this gate. The passage of air through the nose, including smell, depends on the activity of the lung Qi.

If the lung Qi is all right, the nose is permeable; we can, in addition to smooth breathing, also smell and recognize scents and odors. If it is not all right, harmful substances can enter the body through the nose, or the nose can become clogged with mucus, breathing difficulties appear, and there is deterioration or loss of smell. Some moisturizing of the nasal mucosa is necessary. If lung function is normal, the nose is moistened but nothing leaks. If the lungs are affected by cold and wind, clear mucus leaks out. If they are affected by wind and heat, the mucus is cloudy. If they are dry, the nose is dry with or without little secretion.

Lung Qi is also responsible for the ability to "smell" that something is going on. This is not a real scent or odor that we smell; it is more about scenting something we should be careful about. We express the ability to feel that something is interesting for us or that something is going to happen with the phrase "to have a nose for something."

The second gate to the penetration of Heavenly Qi into the lungs is the mouth and throat. The lungs must therefore also supervise the "passability" and humidification of the throat and the clarity and intensity of the voice. All possible throat obstructions, ranging from scratching in the throat through cough to voice problems, are evidence of insufficient or blocked lung Qi. Harmonic lung Qi makes the voice resonant and clear. The larynx is the gateway to respiration and the vocal organs. The Lung channel passes through the larynx, so the passage of air through the larynx and the formation of sounds are related to the lungs. However, the Taoists also claim that *the voice comes from the lungs, but the root is in the kidneys*. The Kidney channel encircles the tongue. If the essence of the kidneys is sufficient, it rises to the vocal cords and allows sound to be produced. If it is insufficient, the intensity of the voice is obviously reduced or even lost. When the lung Qi and also the kidney Qi are emptied, the voice changes to quiet and powerless and may even be lost.

LARGE INTESTINE

The main partner of the lungs is the large intestine (in Chinese, *Dachang*). The relationship between the lungs and the large intestine is clearly evident in a situation known to smokers. When they cannot empty their intestines in the morning, a few puffs of a cigarette are guaranteed to help. Although this nicotine solution is not the best, the intense inhalation of smoke and the immediate need of the body to eliminate this dose of toxin causes a strong activation of Qi in the lungs, which in turn affects the Qi of the large intestine. Large intestine Qi is released, and the bowels are emptied. Other connections between the lungs and the colon are evident in therapeutic practice. From my practice, I can confirm that the problems with coughing and congestion of the throat and bronchi cannot be completely solved unless the large intestine is cleared. The lungs and colon are also related in connection with thinking, with the state of our brain. The lungs provide the brain with oxygenated fresh blood, which conditions and supports brain function. The state of fullness of the large intestine also affects the state of the brain and thinking. After eating (i.e. after filling the intestines), it is more difficult for us to think. A clean and passable bowel is the basis for a clean, clear and fast-thinking mind.

The large intestine measures about 1.5 meters; it is about four fingers wide and narrows in the folds. It begins in the right lumbar pit with the appendix, it surrounds the loops of the small intestine, passes to the left side of the abdomen, and through its descending part connects by an esophageal loop to the rectum. The task of the large intestine is to eliminate everything unnecessary from the body. *The Yellow Emperor's Classic of Medicine* characterizes the large intestine as the *main official in charge of passing and conducting, much as a sewer manager would, determining what has changed and what will exit.* This means that it manages the transport of waste and its disposal. Even though it is at the end of the whole digestive process, it should definitely not be at the end of our interest. The quality of our ability to excrete and get rid of deposits and toxins indicates the quality of our health. The large intestine receives the decomposed mushy remains of undigested food. Although the food components in the upper parts of the digestive tract have been sorted several times, the large intestine sorts them again and separates the last necessary substances. These are left for the body and the rest is thickened to form a stool, which is then eliminated.

"PASSABILITY" AND HEALTHY INTESTINAL MICROFLORA

The "passability"—the ability to allow things to pass through—of the intestines and their good condition are extremely important for our health. About 400–500 known species of bacteria live in the intestines, forming the normal intestinal microflora. This not only participates in the final phase of digestive processes and protects the intestine from the inside, but thanks to fiber, it produces many important vitamins, amino acids, enzymes, hormones and other nutrients. A weak acid environment and sufficient fiber are required for the normal functioning of colonic microflora. The bacteria are kept in the villi of the intestines. The intestinal villi are small finger-like projections that move the digestive mass towards the rectum, but during this journey they extract everything that is still needed into the body. When the villi of the intestines are in poor condition, the bacterial intestinal flora is disturbed, which can cause problems such as bloating, flatulency, skin problems or even reduced concentration and impaired thinking.

The intestinal villi are destroyed by everything aggressive we take in. Artificial sweeteners or other flavorings, various preservatives in food and the like. White flour and flour products clog the villi, making it impossible for them to move and operate. However, the disturbed bacterial balance can be restored with food—for example, Japanese umeboshi plums, miso paste or fermented dishes, preferably fermented vegetables, and the consumption of root vegetables.

In addition, the large intestine controls body fluids. This means that after receiving the liquid and solid waste, it still absorbs the residual fluids from it and sends them back to the body. Thus, by its reabsorption of water into the body, it is involved in the metabolism of body fluids and affects their condition in the body. It controls overall dryness because it likes moisture and does not tolerate drought. It also helps to get rid of water in cases of swelling, in which it cooperates with the kidneys.

The result of strong activity of the large intestine is also beautiful skin as well as a clear nose and the associated sense of smell. According to Chinese medicine, the nose is the signifier that there is something wrong with the lungs and the large intestine. The large intestine controls scents and odors. It is directly energetically connected to the nose via the meridian. In the immediate vicinity of the nasal wings are the last points of the meridian of this organ, the point *Welcoming the Scents* (in Chinese, *Yingxiang*, Ll20).

ABILITY TO LET GO

If the large intestine Qi is weak, or if its excess is caused by food or emotions, it stagnates, and the intestine cannot excrete the stool. Constipation occurs. This is also manifested on a psychological level. People who cannot let go of something in their lives have disharmonious large intestine Qi. In my therapeutic practice, I often find that people suffering from constipation have a habit of clinging to something or someone excessively. Whether it happens consciously or unconsciously, they do not know how to let go on the mental level, and this is also manifested on the physical level.

SKIN

We usually do not even realize that the skin moves with us during training, rehearsals, on stage or in competitions. We usually forget about it, because we do not need to warm it up for the movement action itself. After the performance, we shower our sweaty skin and that's it. However, let us remember that our skin is what the viewer looks at. On the stage, we are connected with our colleagues, scenography and the floor through the skin. Skin is more important to us than may seem.

The skin is the largest body organ. If we spread out the skin of an adult, it would be almost two square meters. It makes up 7 percent of the total body weight—about 4–5 kg. Its thickness ranges from 0.5 to 4 mm, approximately. It is thinner in places that are not exposed to pressure and friction as much, like the inside of the forearms. It is stronger and thicker on more stressed surfaces, such as the feet. Skin is a kind of complete outfit that is waterproof, airtight, compact and yet flexible, with an amazing ability to self-renew. This admirable structure brings our body several important benefits. It is our protection, and it participates in respiration, in the excretion of harmful substances from the body, in the absorption of beneficial ingredients from remedial ointments and in the regulation of body temperature. Last but not least, it allows us to feel the world around us through touch. Let us discuss its functions in more detail.

Breathing through the skin

The body breathes through the skin and thus helps the lungs in their breathing activity. It has been shown that if during emergency first-aid treatment, instead of artificial respiration, the skin of the patient is exposed, the body starts breathing sufficiently by itself and then only chest compressions are needed. *The lung Qi evaporates like dew*, the Taoists say. This means that the lung Qi gathers beneath the surface of the skin as a form of protection. On the other hand, Qi enters the body from the outside through the skin. The skin thus breathes, and the main places of this exchange are the pores. The fact that the skin is indeed a respiratory organ, and that it is involved in breathing, I have verified with my own skin—both figuratively and literally. In one performance, I played the character of a very fat woman. My costume was lined with several layers of foam. Dancing for an hour in this constricted way, when my skin was not in contact with the air but with the material, really prevented me from breathing. No matter how hard I tried to breathe through my nose and mouth, I did not have enough oxygen to dance. We had to intentionally adapt my actions choreographically on the stage by me leaving the stage, where, behind the scenes, I could undress, at least for a while, and allow my skin to breathe. Only then could I return to the stage and continue. It is therefore appropriate to consider whether it is really necessary to perform physical activities in leotards, mostly made of artificial fibers, which squeeze the skin and prevent it from breathing. We usually associate ballet or yoga with this clothing. The skin is very sensitive, and even if it does not look like it, contact with chemical textiles, but also chemical make-up, injures it. And since the skin is connected to the lungs, they themselves and their Qi are injured too. In contrast, in natural materials, the skin feels sufficiently safe and is also able to fulfill its breathing function.

Cleaning

The large intestine is mainly responsible for cleaning and removing waste. The lungs are energetically connected to the large intestine; they help in cleansing by exhaling, thus eliminating unnecessary substances. Constant cleansing of what is created by metabolic processes and also cleansing of toxins that we inadvertently absorb from food and air are really very important. These are continuous and demanding processes, and so our body has another organ available to it—the skin. The skin significantly helps to excrete toxic substances from the body. The path of excretion is the lymphatic glands and pores, and the way of excretion is through lymphatic vessels, which are abundant in the skin. So just imagine what a block we create in this mechanism by using antiperspirants. We want to prevent the excretion of smelly sweat, but this pushes the impurities deeper into the body. So sweating is good, although how we sweat gives a picture of the state of our lungs and digestive tract. Instead of preventing our skin from sweating, we should put our digestion and lung function in order. Only then will our sweat not smell unpleasant.

The Taoists call the pores *the Gates of Qi*. Their role is to manage the protection of the body against external pollutants, to excrete sweat, to moisturize the skin and to breathe. When they open, they can eliminate harmful substances from the inside out, and it must be admitted

that through the skin, all sorts of things can come out of us. Many people do not like it because we want to smell nice and have beautiful clean skin. However, the connections need to be seen. Our surface is always a picture of what is going on inside, so cleansing and supporting the lungs and large intestine, which are in charge of the skin, is important. When the lungs and large intestine are working properly, we have no skin problems. If they stop performing their function, the skin wants to help them and starts some way of elimination. It can take the form of rashes, itchy skin with a constant need to scratch, eczema, etc. The elimination rate is proportional to the degree of Qi disruption of these organs and the clogging of the organism by waste. In the case of severe clogging, disharmony can also be created at the level of other organs, such as the liver or gallbladder. Skin problems need to be thoroughly diagnosed, and afterwards focus must be put on those organs that have deviated the most from balance. Ointments often do not work because the cause of the problem is somewhere deeper, and what is manifested on the surface is only a consequence and communication with us.

One of the easiest ways to clean the skin is to scrub the whole body with a brush that should neither be too soft nor too hard. The gentler version is to dry the skin after each shower with a hard terry towel.

Skin as armor

In addition to opening and eliminating impurities, the pores must be able to close perfectly so that they do not allow any external pathogens into the body—such as cold, wind, moisture and viruses, and sometimes the energy impact of another person. The skin thus forms a defensive layer of the body, acting as armor against external harmful influences; it is a barrier that prevents the penetration of microorganisms and absorbs ultraviolet rays and the like. It gets the strength to do this from the lungs. Lung Qi controls the skin and the space between the skin and the muscles. This is the dispersing function of the lungs, which directs the Qi under the skin. In the space between the skin and the muscles, there is a layer called *Couli* in which Qi circulates and strengthens the armor from the inside. We call it *Defensive Qi* (in Chinese, *Weiqi*).

The main task of Weiqi is to protect the surface layer of the body against the attack of pathogenic agents from the outside. It helps us to withstand these influences, but also turns on a mechanism to expel them if they have already entered. It is Weiqi that works hard when, for example, we catch a cold. If Weiqi is strong enough, it causes a fever, opens the pores and sweats the cold out of the body. It is therefore also connected to the immune system.

Because the lungs, skin and autumn are related, it is natural that we are more sensitive to various colds, flu and infections in the autumn. The contracting METAL phase Qi naturally draws them inwards. Unlike summer days, when viruses and bacteria penetrate us through the mouth and nose, in the cold weather of autumn and winter, their zone of penetration is also the skin. If Weiqi is strong, we can resist or quickly eliminate those pathogens, but if Weiqi is weakened, we have problems. The "defensive company" of the body surface is weak and we become less resistant to adverse weather conditions. Protecting ourselves from the winter with suitable clothing is one thing, but in order to ensure the "bulletproof-ness" of our armor, we also need to work from the inside. From the inside, our armor is strengthened by quality digestion, which can sufficiently transform food into Qi. We can help digestion by warming instead of cooling it down. In autumn and winter, we should exclude cooling foods such as dairy products, but also raw vegetables, raw fruit and especially tropical fruit and fruit juices. Although we are used to claiming that tropical fruit contains a lot of vitamins

needed to keep us from getting sick, its cooling effect is much more damaging than the missing vitamins. We can replace them with enough stewed vegetables, stewed fruit, vegetable haulms and the like, but especially by building internal warmth with a warming diet. The basis is a warm breakfast in the form of porridge, or we can eat vegetable or meat broths. It is better to simmer the fruit for our porridge with a little warming cinnamon. At the same time, it is good to add cinnamon to as many dishes as possible, but do not overdo it. Boiled ginger also has a significant effect on our internal heating during this period.

> If you get caught in cold and windy weather, take a warm shower at home, being sure not omit the back of the neck. Make elderflower or linden tea with a bit of spirits (e.g. peach brandy, plum brandy, applejack) to help with sweating. Snuggle under blankets and rest, and drive out these Yin pathogens lying down and sweating. It is simple but very effective. Alternatively, you can rub yourself for a few minutes under the seventh cervical vertebra, where is a point by which the elimination of the pathogen can be supported. This is a *Guasha* method, for which special scrapers are used, but an ordinary teaspoon can also be used.
>
> Do not stop the fever sooner than is necessary. After the penetration of cold or wind into the body, its automatic reaction is to raise the temperature to open the pores, through which these pathogens can be excreted from the body by sweating. It is a natural search for Yin and Yang balance. It is advisable to support this appropriate fever and not to stop it with medication.

If something is already creeping in on us or if we are already sick, we should try to awaken Qi in our depths and send it to the surface to "fight the enemy." This will ensure sweating. When the body sweats, it pushes the Qi clogged with pollutants to the surface of the skin and from there it is excreted from the body. Sweating greatly helps the healing process. If we block it because we do not have time and have to go to work, we create the conditions for subsequent long-lasting colds, coughs or even bronchitis. A good starter for sweating can be hot linden, elderflower or ginger tea. There are also mixtures of Chinese herbs that push Qi to the surface for this purpose. Whatever it is, do not include lemon in this treatment. Lemon has a sour taste and has a tendency to direct inwards. Thus, during the course of the disease, it draws the harmful pollutants from the surface inside the body, instead of being able to eliminate them outside. So, according to Taoists, the oft-used lemon in tea during flu or colds is only harming us. If we are sick, we need to give up both physical and mental work, and calm our emotions so that the body can work on healing without disturbing influences.

Regeneration

The skin can also be injured in our profession. It could be said that abrasions and burns caused by rubbing against the floor are part of our normal routine, especially in contemporary dance, where dancers move barefoot, or when doing floor work where the whole body is moving on the floor. The skin can be easily injured by being bruised on an object on the stage. I could write a whole book about blisters and bloodied toes from ballet shoes. However, nature has equipped us with a regeneration mechanism. It is the mechanism of Qi itself.

Have you ever wondered how it is possible that a cut or burn can heal over time? How is it possible that, without hesitation, a self-healing process begins immediately, in which, unless it has extreme dimensions, we do not have to intervene other than cleaning the wound with water? It is Qi that works on regeneration. The Qi itself is not visible, but its manifestation is visible.

These include, for example, the formation of a protective inflammatory process, the formation of pus to excrete impurities, cicatrization, the formation of scabs and its peeling, and finally complete healing. Of course, if a deeper wound occurs, it should be stitched. But even then, Qi conscientiously works on regeneration. And it should be noted that the rate of regeneration is proportional to how fit we are and the condition of the lungs.

The regeneration process can also be helped. In addition to caring for the wound on the skin itself, Chinese medicine provides several methods to support its healing by strengthening the lung Qi. It can be through diet, the use of herbal remedies or Qigong. The easiest way to help the lungs and the skin is to quit smoking or not to start at all. Appropriate cleansing of the large intestine also helps the lungs. I recommend preventive cleaning using charcoal, at least once a year, from the end of summer until November. If the problem already exists, it can be used at any time.

There is even an acupuncture point on the Lung channel that significantly speeds up skin regeneration. It is the point *Broken Sequence* (in Chinese, *Lieque*, LU7), located near the wrist and you can find it marked on the image of the Lung channel below. We can also stimulate it ourselves, because we can easily reach it. It is the first to be used for various burns, even burns from an iron, because it accelerates the healing of the skin. I have verified that it also helps with the regeneration of the skin in abrasions caused by rubbing against something during movement.

Communication and touch

The skin is a direct physical structure through which the body comes into contact with the outside world and receives important information about it. It is a valuable sense organ. Through the skin, we perceive cold, heat, dryness, humidity, etc., but also various extrasensory vibrations. One of our most important senses related to the skin is touch. Touch is managed by the large intestine Qi. The state of this organ defines the state of our touch. When the intestines are more or less empty, the touch is more sensitive. After eating, or, more precisely, after overeating, sensitivity through touch is weaker. During my early studies of Qi perception, we did exercises to determine the tactile sensitivity of the fingertips.

We laid a few fine hairs on the base and covered them with a sheet of office paper. With eyes closed, we had to count with our fingertips how many hairs were under the paper, what was their length and whether they were the same thickness. The success rate showed the state of the large intestine Qi.

THE PO—THE CORPOREAL SOUL

From a psychological point of view, the lungs are very important for any mover, but, of course, they are important for everyone, because they contain an aspect of the soul that is close to the physical body. The lungs reside in a spiritual essence called the Po. It is the only aspect of the soul with such a close relationship to the body, which is why it is also called *the Corporeal Soul*. The role of the Po is to encourage the soul to reside in the body and feel at home there. It does not allow it to travel excessively in the etheric world, and thus it ensures that it is in this material body on Earth and uses everything that the body offers for its mission.

The Po connects us with our physical aspect through the automatic habits of our body. It is in charge of survival instincts, primary physiological processes such as breathing, limb movement, digestion control, suction reflex, crying, crawling, etc. Thanks to the Po, the baby can orient itself on the mother's body after birth and find the breast milk. The Po connects the soul with the body mainly through the feeling of the body and helps us to orient ourselves in physical feelings. It brings us the ability to feel pain, bodily well-being, tickling, itching and other delicate sensations of touch. It brings us back to the skin. Through the skin and through pleasant feelings of touch, it builds in the body a feeling of security and boundaries.

The Po is like a computer storage disk, a depository in which, from the moment of our birth, all bodily information and all the kinetic experiences that the body goes through in life are saved. It ensures the use of the body's memory to perceive and use everything the body has learned since birth. In addition to instinctive habits, it also preserves habits acquired during life, such as skiing, swimming, dancing—just about anything the body learns. The Po encodes these automations, stores them on a disk and controls them at the same time. It is the physical memory of a particular individual's body that stores the physical experience gained during life. All this information is stored in the lungs through the Po, and the lung Qi shifts the experience into use, according to our needs. If we want to learn a skill, such as swimming or dancing a certain choreography, we must first perceive and understand what the body will have to learn to do, even though we do not yet know how to achieve it. This is followed by practicing and constant repetition by the body until we learn it and it is etched in our physical memory of the Po. So, if we learned to swim as children and then we do not swim for a certain period of time, we just need to enter the water and the Po will initiate the habit of the body and we will swim automatically. Or if we have not danced a choreography for a long time, all we have to do is play the music to it and the body will start remembering the movement habit with the help of the Po itself. Sometimes we wonder how it is possible to remember that choreography for so long. This information emerges to the surface of our needs because it has been encoded into the body by the Po.

The Po codes kinetic experience based on constant repetition and therefore it no longer disappears. This can naturally be transferred to the level of kinetic routine and subsequent reluctance to innovate and change. This is the negative side of the Po. This means that certain entrenched, incorrect childhood habits, such as improper posture, improper walking or improper skiing technique are therefore very difficult to transform into proper habits. The same is true for any movement technique that the mover automated incorrectly in the past. Correction is difficult. It is not impossible, but it takes longer and more intense reprogramming of the body's memory, and if the Po is weak, it is even harder. The new programming takes place on a mental, emotional and spiritual level, of which the Po is a part. It is no coincidence that many of the meditation techniques that offer us immersion are associated with the lungs and breathing. The Po is thus activated to change its structures. Usually, such work for change also requires a change in personal attitude. For this reason too, it is important for movers to pay sufficient attention to the health of their lungs.

The skin is the largest and most distinctive structure of the body, through which we present ourselves to the outside. The Po essence is also connected to the skin through the lungs. The Po helps us perceive our physical boundaries through the skin. It determines whether we like the touch or not. The METAL phase, as already mentioned, is about value, so the Po helps us to evaluate and then decide who we let come close to us and who we do not, who can touch us and who cannot. However, this decision must sometimes be suppressed in our profession. We very often touch each other without having time and space to deal with the decision of whether we like it or not. On the other hand, we must handle mutual contact professionally so that any kind of closeness does not develop in a personal manner. In plain terms, if we play a role, we have to submit to it. However, our subconsciousness—and, of course, the Po—knows about everything, and if we do not show our possible dissatisfaction or sympathy, our inside does. This can manifest as weakening of the lung Qi, shortness of breath when moving and sometimes even skin problems. If we do not want someone to touch us and our wish is not respected, the body will create a barrier on its own. Our touch routine can also manifest itself in the fact that sometimes we approach the other person's body somehow automatically or mechanically. The performer should be aware of these contexts and be able to work with them sensitively and flexibly. I know dancers who do not like touch. Because of this, for example, they do not even get massages, even though they need them. When I first encountered it, I was very surprised. How is it possible that a person who works with the body and touches someone and is touched on a daily basis does not like touch? I understand it today. This is possible precisely because we approach the act of touching professionally and mechanically. We have become used to this kind of model.

In conclusion to this discussion of the Po, I will mention two more things. Through the connection to the physical body, the Po is naturally connected with our animal part, with physical instincts and sexuality. On the mental level, the healthy presence of the Po is manifested in us by feelings of wholeness, integrity, everything being in the right place; we have feelings of correctness, honesty, responsibility for ourselves. When there is a lack of quality of the Po, we immure ourselves; we feel anxiety, sadness, guilt and shame. We may even be unable to state our boundaries, and thus allow others to interfere too much with us mentally or physically.

How to deal with the large intestine and skin problems

First of all, it is necessary to put our large intestines in order. Gentle cleansing of the intestine consists of the use of activated charcoal, regular use of psyllium fiber from the Indian plantain (of course, with breaks), occasional cleansing of the intestines with green clay. Consumption of ordinary fiber is necessary. When cleansing the skin, animal products should be completely avoided, but also buckwheat and extremely Yin foods such as sugar and fruit. Moreover, we should eliminate white flour for at least two months from our diet. Whoever wants to clean the skin should eat cooked food, but never reheated food. Food that is not fresh always contains the germs of various bacteria, which are activated by heating. Until the intestinal microflora are in order, they cannot deal with them.

The large intestine also likes regular cleansing with enemas, which is suitable if the large intestine does not have any pathology. A liquid suitable for enemas is, for example, warm bancha tea or your own urine. Enema does not suit every large intestine, so do not push yourself into it.

These tips for harmonizing the large intestine should be a regular part of our lifestyle. They help the intestine itself, and the result visible on the skin is "only" a bonus. If you want to treat your skin from the outside, rubbing with a slice of white daikon radish works for itchy skin problems. After taking a bath, soak a towel in ginger water and rub your skin with it thoroughly.

SADNESS

The METAL phase includes the emotion of sadness and its various shades—grief, anxiety, hopelessness, disappointment. Some amount of sadness is natural and a part of the diversity of our emotional experience. However, when it lasts too long or it is extreme, we find that it is a reflection of a certain degree of clinging to something or someone. The METAL phase is characterized by the direction of Qi inwards. Autumn is a challenging time in this sense, because the increasing darkness and cold bring us the prerequisites to enter into our inner selves. The result is various sensations, sadness, depression. The deeper we are, the more the pressure increases—PRESS, dePRESSion. Sadness is not destructive; it serves to calm, reflect and internalize. It helps us evaluate, see, realize. However, it should be followed by acceptance and subsequent release, because if grief lasts for a long time and to a great extent, it consumes Qi constantly. For example, the death of a person close to us—the fact that this person no longer exists in the material form via which we were in contact with him or her is a normal manifestation of development. Everything has its beginning, ascension, peak, descent and extinction. This rule cannot be avoided. Not even the deaths of our loved ones. Healthy grief and its expressions are, of course, a necessary part of a farewell. Sadness is also related to the term "value." A state of sorrow occurs when we lose something that we consider valuable to us, and that can be a material thing, a person close to us, an experience or a feeling. Sadness also comes in relation to the value of ourselves—when we feel separated from the world, when we stop seeing our role clearly, when our value is diminished. Paradoxically, even people in a good position, whether at work or in the family, are able to feel the sadness that stems from a lack of their own value. Excessive sadness is thus a manifestation of clinging.

OTHER CONNECTIONS WITH THE FUNCTIONAL CIRCUIT OF THE LUNGS

We have not yet exhausted the effect of the functional circuit of the lungs. In the medical texts of Chinese medicine, we can find following information.

Dryness belongs to the METAL phase

The lungs, large intestine and skin do not benefit from dryness. Dryness in the lungs limits the intake of Heavenly Qi. In the large intestine, it is mostly seen in the form of constipation. Dry skin can be caused by weakness of the lung Qi, but also by weakness of the blood. Dryness is a natural quality of outdoor weather Qi. If it is in excess, it can harm us. However, it is natural and necessary. It is a demonstration of the METAL phase, when the Qi cycle ends the active part of its journey. The drying leaf is no longer able to absorb water in the autumn, just like old human skin can no longer be refreshed by water. The leaf and the skin are still beautiful, but in a different way.

The white color tones of the METAL phase

The white color harmonizes the organs of the METAL phase. White is associated with air. It is a color of transparency, pure energy. Even the autumn fogs cover everything in silvery white. To support the Qi of METAL phase, we wear white clothes and eat white or pale food.

The physiological fluid of the lungs is mucus

If the function of the lungs is normal, natural mucus in the right amount moisturizes the nose without the mucus leaking out. The production of mucus is always associated with the emptiness of the spleen Qi, and it begins in digestion. The lungs only store mucus.

Coughing is a defensive function of the lungs and the whole organism. It cleans the air passages of mucus and dead cells. It can be irritating, dry and unproductive, which does not remove mucus from the air passages. Or it can be moist, productive, containing irritants and bacteria, and thus it helps to cough it out. It is always associated with weakening of the lung Qi. It is common in colds, flu, bronchitis and pneumonia, but also in sinusitis. Irritants can also cause a non-infectious cough, which happens with asthma, hay fever or smoke inhalation and the like. Dry coughs should be suppressed, whereas productive coughs should be supported. We can help with herbs to dilute mucus, such as wild thyme, coltsfoot, horehound or angelica. Dried lotus root is excellent. The similarity between the cross-section of the lotus root and the cross-section of the lungs is not accidental. Adequate fluid intake is always required to treat coughs.

In autumn, not only the cold but also the heat can show up. If, during the summer, we overheated the whole organism—for example, by excessive grilling and intake of overwarming food—and did not supplement Yin with a sufficient intake of fluids, heat will be generated in the autumn. The heat increases the function of the mucous membranes, which swell, get red, fill with mucus and cause coughs. The autumn will show how we treated ourselves in the summer.

Coughs can also be a psychosomatic issue, of course. What does a person sneeze at or what should one sneeze at? What cannot one say due to a cough and sore throat?

RELATIONSHIP OF THE METAL PHASE TO OTHER PHASES

According to the Sheng supporting cycle, which we discussed in Chapter 7 on the Five Phases, it is clear that the "mother" of the lungs is the spleen. The METAL phase has its hidden source of life in the EARTH phase. The quality of the spleen Qi subsequently determines the quality of the lung Qi. This relationship is evident in relation to mucus. As we already know, if the spleen does not have enough Qi, it cannot process difficult-to-digest components in the diet and instead turns them into mucus. So if we want to get the lungs in order, we have to work with the spleen as well. The harmonic Qi of the METAL phase can sufficiently nourish the WATER phase and at the same time limit the excess in the WOOD phase.

CONCLUSION TO THE METAL PHASE

The increasing Yin in the form of cold and darkness will keep us more in the warmth of our home. Let us not be afraid of this period, nor of the nostalgia and sorrows that sometimes catch us. They are part of internal cleaning. Autumn is a good time to summarize the past year in our heads, to pause and have the opportunity to see what we have done, achieved or forgotten. It is also a good time for processing this information. We can devote the time we are no longer spending in society to reorganizing our apartment, clothes, household items and deciding what we still need and what we do not, and we can get rid of the unnecessary. It is recommended to go to sleep earlier than in previous seasons, to indulge in relaxation and a real rest. During walks in nature, let us perceive how everything calms down and returns to itself, how nature is beautifully colored by the colors of peace. Protect your head with a hat—at the very least, protect your ears and neck from the wind. Eat longer-cooked meals and fermented vegetables. Limit raw vegetables, frozen foods, cold drinks and tropical fruits. Do not forget about your skin; give it various kinds of cleaning.

Table 12.1 Main correspondences of METAL phase

Year season: autumn	Yin and Yang stage: Lesser Yin/Yin in Yang
Day time: twilight	Direction: west
Evolution of Qi: Qi directed inward from the outside	Growth cycle in nature: harvest
Life cycle: appreciation of life, ageing	Working cycle: assessing, evaluating
Yin organ: lungs	Organ clock for lungs: 3 to 5 a.m.
Yang organ: large intestine	Organ clock for large intestine: 5 to 7 a.m.
Psychospiritual aspect: Po	Virtue: integrality, fairness
Emotion: sadness	Climate: dryness
Color: white, silver	Taste: pungent
Smell: rotten	Number: 9
Tissue: skin	Body fluid: mucus
Other body tissues: mucous membranes, vellus (skin and skin hair)	Other body fluid and excretion: protective nose excretion
Joints: arm joints	Entry point of disease: back, shoulders
Sense organ: nose	Sense: smelling
Indicator: skin hair	Detrimental action: too much laying
Sound: weeping, crying	Mental attitude: courage

MERIDIANS

LUNG CHANNEL (LU)/YIN

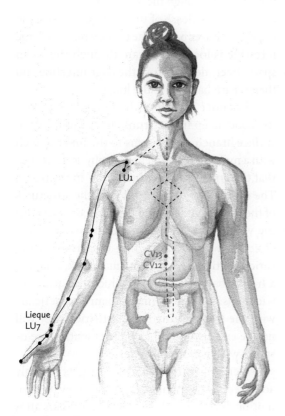

Lung channel

The Lung channel is a Yin pair pathway, leading from the chest along the inside of both arms to the thumbs of the hands. In the image below, it is shown on one side only. It starts in the lungs area. From there, the inner branch connects the lungs with the large intestine; on the way back, it also connects with the stomach, penetrates the diaphragm and goes to the lungs themselves. From there to the neck, it turns and goes towards the shoulders. Under the collarbones, it rises to the surface at the first point of its surface branch. From there, it penetrates the shoulders, passing along the biceps on the inner sides of the hands to the elbows. It passes through the forearms towards the thumbs of the hands. In the wrist area, it connects to the Large Intestine channel with an internal flow line. It ends on the inner side of the thumbs at the nails. This main branch has 11 acupuncture points. The picture shows the above-mentioned point *Broken Sequence* (in Chinese, *Lieque*, LU7).

The channel affects all respiratory disorders and the lungs themselves, including asthma, cough, susceptibility to upper and lower respiratory tract diseases, irritation and sore throat, nasal congestion, hay fever, all skin manifestations including burns, eczema, spots or dry skin, olfactory problems and all physical problems along the channel. At the mental level, it is related to identification with one's own boundaries and self-value, the ability to accept touch, the ability to create and follow rules, with a sense of order, courage and honesty, and the ability to deal with grief.

LUNG CHANNEL IN MOVEMENT

The pathway of the Lung channel is relatively simple. The surface branch leads from the upper part of the torso only to the upper limbs, so here the range of motion has its limitations. However, it invites us to work internally and to work on details. It gives us the opportunity to work with our thumbs and whole arms. The flow of Qi can be blocked here by excessive use of the thumbs during frequent work on a computer or mobile phone. An interesting area for realizing the flow of Qi is the section on the bone radius (forearm bone on the thumb side), especially at its lower end, where Qi branches off the pathway to the above-mentioned point *Broken Sequence* (*Lieque*), LU7. Working with this area in motion helps to release stiffness of the wrists and thumbs. The channel also offers work with the inner sides of the elbows, especially with an awareness of their Yin quality, and with the pectoral muscles and the outer ends of the collarbones. Conscious work with Qi, which floats around the collarbones, naturally opens up the space between the collarbones and the upper tips of the lungs, which helps the lungs increase their space and thus fill them with more new air.

Since the inner branch of the Lung channel leads through the throat, during the movement we can try to imagine the throat as a vital tube through which Qi air passes into our interior and through which we can exhale Qi from our interior. At the same time, we can use it to communicate with the world by words.

The lungs themselves can also be involved in movement, and we can observe how the movement affects the breathing and diaphragm. Fast and sharp movement works well as it forces the body to exhale quickly and suddenly. In this context, movement can be associated with laughter, which significantly activates and revitalizes the diaphragm. By activating the passage of Qi in the channel through the diaphragm, it is possible to realize the release of the passage between the upper and lower part of the torso, where the large intestine is located. Qi can, through this open space, freely descend into the large intestine and then return back up to the lungs.

The inner branch of the Lung channel has its "root" deep in the trunk. If we connect the surface branch on the arms to the inner branch with a movement, it will help us physically realize that the arms also have their "root" in the trunk. The connection of the arms with the structures of the torso helps them to be more compact with the whole body, which proves to be especially effective when overloading the arms during various actions, such as manual work, carrying a heavy load or a sport in which the arms are widely used. If we connect them energetically with the torso during these activities, they will not be exhausted, and the movement, dance or sports will be more effective.

After longer improvisation, Qi gets strongly activated in the channel. Enjoy this flow of Qi in motion, but also in the stillness that occurs after the movement, and physically feel its Yin quality.

LARGE INTESTINE CHANNEL (LI)/YANG

The Large Intestine channel is a Yang pair meridian. It is shown only on one side in the image below. It starts on the inner sides of the index fingers and proceeds to the outer Yang side of the arms, along the elbows and biceps through the deltoid muscles to the shoulders. It penetrates into the shoulder joints. From there, it progresses through the nape of the neck and to the face. Meanwhile, the inner branch connects with the other Yang meridians below the seventh cervical vertebra. From there, it returns to the main pathway to the pit above the collarbone. From there, it drops its branch down into the lungs and through the diaphragm into the large intestines. This inner branch descends below the knees, to the Stomach channel. The main branch separates from the collarbone upwards to the throat and to the face. It crosses under the nose, so its right branch goes to the left side of the face and the left branch to the right side of the face. It ends in the small hollows next to the nasal wings. The main branch has 20 acupuncture points. The picture shows the mentioned point *Welcome Fragrance* (in Chinese, *Yingxiang*, LI20).

The channel affects all problems associated with large intestine function, including constipation, diarrhea, and irritable bowel syndrome. It also affects skin problems and increased mucus secretion. It supports the activity of the lungs, so it is also used for breathing problems, hay fever and stuffy nose. It also affects the treatment of sore throats and asthma. It has an effect on toothache, gingivitis, pain and redness of the eyes, nosebleeds, upper limb paralysis, nape pain and general pain along the channel. At the mental level, it influences the ability to let go, and thus the ability to get rid of the unnecessary, identification with one's own limits and value.

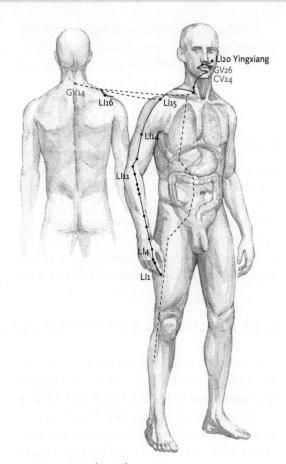

Large Intestine channel

LARGE INTESTINE CHANNEL IN MOVEMENT

The Large Intestine channel offers us the opportunity to connect the upper limbs with the neck and face. Since it ends next to the nostrils, we can involve the nose in the movement—either to guide the movement with the nose or, conversely, to end the movement in the area of the nose. Focusing on the nose will help deepen nasal breathing and consciously connect the nose to the lungs.

As the channel begins on the index fingers, using the index fingers to lead the body into motion will help activate Qi in this channel. This will give the upper limbs a different dimension.

If we lead the movement from the index fingers in a spiral (from the index finger, we rotate the arm inwards), we will physically feel the Qi in the channel naturally passing through the elbow, shoulder, neck and jaw to the opposite nostril. At the same time, this spiral movement "forces" us to turn our heads to the opposite side, thus activating the flow of Qi of this channel in the neck area.

Guiding the movement from the outer sides of the elbows or the top of the shoulders also puts the neck and upper torso into motion, which naturally engages the lungs and deepens breathing.

It is also worth noting the area of the philtrum (groove under the nose), where the pathways intersect. Working with this area of the face will enliven the whole face and its expression, and any tension in the lips and jaws will be released.

The principle of crossing can also be used in movement improvisation, where we guide the movement with the arms from the index fingers so that the right arm moves to the left side of the body and vice versa. This movement creates pleasant moving spirals in the body, in which the chest and the lungs themselves are also involved. They are naturally compressed by movement, so they are subsequently stimulated to inhale more and thus Qi circulates more in them. If we increase this movement to the maximum extent, the energy spiral will pass to the large intestine, hence connecting this organ itself with the flow of its channel on the hands. This way, we actually work with the inner branch of the channel running through the trunk.

The inner branch, which connects the surface channel on the arms with the lower limbs, will help us to ground well in movement improvisation.

After longer improvisation, Qi is strongly activated in the channel. Enjoy this flow of Qi in motion, but also in stillness and enjoy its Yang quality.

DIET IN AUTUMN AND FOR THE METAL PHASE ORGANS

With the increasing cold, we need to warm up more from the inside with our diet in order to strengthen our defensive Weiqi and be able to withstand the cold weather. Therefore, the preparation of dishes is prolonged and boiling is longer, which gives them more Yang Qi. We can also supply Yang by cooking in a pressure cooker. We use more warming and heating foods and spices such as ginger, curry, chili, black pepper, dried herbs, cardamom, cinnamon and cloves.

Root and round vegetables
Autumn is a time when nature moves inward "to its roots." Therefore, we find many important substances in root vegetables. Since the color of the METAL phase is white, we can also consume white vegetables—parsnip, kohlrabi, celery, cauliflower. However, we also continue to eat round, orange and yellow foods from the late summer, such as Hokkaido pumpkins, carrots and potatoes.

Legumes
We also choose legumes of lighter to white color—white beans, light lentils and the like.

The taste of the METAL phase is a spicy, sharp taste
The typical spicy taste of our region is radish. In addition to the traditional red radish, white radish is suitable for organs of the METAL phase. Round white radishes are sweeter; oblong ones (such as daikon) are spicier. Do not avoid radish leaves either, they are pleasantly spicy and contain a lot of nutrients. Radish root tips also do not belong in compost: they contain a huge amount of vitamin B, including B12. Horseradish, which warms the digestion and lungs, also has a typical sharp taste.

Cereals
From cereals, white rice is suitable, but also dark natural rice. However, in order for rice not to have an overly tightening effect on us, we can also vary our diet with other cereals. In the autumn, we should start cooking grain in a pressure cooker. On colder days, we can roast it dry or in a little oil before cooking, which will give it more Yang. During this period, congee or tsampa porridge are excellent. Barley, from which tsampa is made, helps moisturize the body, mucous membranes and skin.

Meat

Poultry is suitable, but other types of meat are mucus forming. The lungs do not like dryness, so for their necessary moisturizing components we also consume in moderate amounts slightly moisturizing foods, such as pears, apples, almonds, sesame seeds, mushrooms, sour milk products (natural and in moderation) or soy milk products. Miso, green leafy vegetables, root vegetables, fermented vegetables will also do. We can include a classic sauerkraut, but also other types of pickles. Ginger tea with honey is excellent for warming and softening the lungs.

Foods supporting the lung Qi

Rice (in excessive quantity can draw Qi in), oatmeal (in excessive quantity can produce mucus), carrots, green leafy vegetables, broccoli, cabbage, mustard leaves, sweet potatoes, garlic, leeks, onions, walnuts, grapes, sesame seeds, fresh ginger.

Avoid mucus-forming foods

In general, we avoid mucus-forming foods—mainly cow's milk and products from it (cheese, yogurts, sour cream, etc.). Also, we avoid sweets, especially if we suffer from chronic rhinitis, lung congestion, coughs or slight coughing and allergies. An excess of oats and oat products also produce mucus, as does soy milk, particularly its dried version.

We need to warm up in the autumn. Breakfast should be warm and cooked. We limit raw fruit, but instead gently stew the fruit as an additive to our morning porridge, because everything raw cools our body. Tropical fruit naturally cools the human body in a tropical environment; in cold climates in the autumn, it is no longer suitable. However, some have the necessary effects on the lungs, such as mandarin and grapefruit, but we should eat them sparingly.

The intestinal microflora should be constantly taken care of, but this is doubly true during the autumn. Regular consumption of miso paste, fermented vegetables and a diet rich in chlorophyll—found, for example, in green leafy vegetables—helps to keep the intestinal microflora in order. Japanese umeboshi plum vinegar, a by-product of the fermentation of umeboshi plums, is an excellent medicine for the large intestine. In the morning, it is recommended to drink a glass of warm water with 1 teaspoon of umeboshi plum vinegar on an empty stomach in the autumn. Ayurvedic cleansing of *Shankhaprakshalana* is also suitable for cleansing the intestine, but also the entire digestive tract. Indian kichri—white basmati rice boiled for more than two hours with split mung beans, turmeric and ghee—is recommended as the first dish after this cleansing.

At the same time, as Qi moves inwards in the autumn to rest, so does the Qi of the digestive tract. Dinner time should also be shifted to an earlier time with the darkness coming sooner. We should not have dinner after 7 p.m. in autumn and winter. The digestive tract needs at least 3–4 hours of our wakefulness. When digesting food in sleep, there is a great loss of Qi.

The METAL phase is also about evaluation and purification. Cleaning foods include barley, daikon radish, shiitake mushrooms, fresh lotus root and boiled lotus kernels. If we normally do not include them in the menu, they should at least be part of the autumn dishes.

Foods that eliminate mucus

Seaweed, black radish, umeboshi plums, green leafy vegetables, boiled nettle, pearl barley, grapefruit, mandarin and tangerine, bamboo shoots, lotus root, garlic and other bulbs, fresh ginger, daikon radish, watercress sprouts, turmeric, large-leaf vegetables such as cabbage, mangold and mustard leaves. Corn silk also removes mucus well. We can cook them in water like tea and drink. Daikon radish decomposes mucus. In the pickled form, it is excellent as a side dish to fried or fatty foods.

A FEW TIPS AND RECIPES

Horseradish yummy
Ingredients: Horseradish root, 1 tsp salt, 4 tbsp olive oil.

Method: Finely grate the horseradish and mix with salt and olive oil.

Benefits: It warms up the digestion and lungs.

Lotus decoction
Ingredients: 1 slice of lotus root, cup of water.

Method: First infusion—boil for 5 minutes and drink. Second infusion—boil for 10–15 minutes and drink. Third infusion—pour double the amount of water and boil to the original amount. This will extract the most inaccessible minerals. The root can then be eaten or put in soup.

Benefits: This decoction clears and soothes the lungs.

Cleansing decoction
Ingredients: 1 tbsp grated carrot, 1 tbsp grated daikon, water.

Method: Cover the grated carrot and daikon with boiling water and boil for 30 seconds. Drink and eat. Drink daily.

Benefits: It detoxifies.

Lotus decoction with daikon
Ingredients: 2 slices of dried lotus root soaked for 10 minutes in advance, 1 tsp fresh juice of grated ginger, 1 tbsp grated daikon, 1–1½ tbsp soy sauce, 2 cups of boiling water.

Method: Boil the lotus root for 5 minutes in the water in which it was soaked. Turn off the heat, add the other ingredients, let it stand for 10 minutes. Drink while it is still warm.

Benefits: It replenishes the lung Qi, relieves congested lungs and bronchial tubes, has a special effect on pneumonia, removes hoarseness and unpleasant smell from the mouth.

Brewed fresh ginger tea for sweating
Ingredients: Fresh ginger, water.

Method: Cut 7 slices of ginger and boil them for 5–10 minutes.

Benefits: Cooking activates the immune-stimulating substances in it. Do not drink it with lemon or honey.

Lime or lemon juice for diluting mucus
Ingredients: Lemon or lime, honey.

Method: Pour warm water over lemon or lime juice with honey. Drink while warm.

Benefits: It warms, dissolves mucus and helps to remove it from the body. It is suitable only when one is not acutely ill, as the sour taste would push the pathogen even further inside. It can be used in the after-care phase.

Pickles of daikon radish
Ingredients: Daikon radish, sea salt.

Method: Wash and slice the daikon radish. Place the slices one by one in a preserving bottle, salting them layer by layer. Weigh down for 24 hours and leave to ferment. Once fermented, it can be eaten immediately; what is not eaten can be put in the fridge to prevent further fermentation.

Benefits: Pickles strengthen the lungs and large intestine, help to thin mucus and process fat.

Rice porridge with poppy seeds

Ingredients: 1 cup of sweet natural rice, 4 cups of rice milk or water, 1 cup of ground poppy seeds, 1 cup of raisins or other dried fruit, pinch of cinnamon and salt, rice, maple or oat syrup, ginger.

Method: Cook the rinsed rice with the raisins in the milk or water; once it boils, turn down the heat and cook covered for at least an hour. If you cook on a gas stove, put a simmer plate under the pot so that the rice does not burn. If you prefer a finer consistency, you can blend the rice. Sprinkle with poppy seeds or season with syrup. Add cinnamon for a warming effect. A piece of ginger can be added to the porridge to warm the stomach and dispel any chill. It also makes the food easier to digest.

Benefits: The porridge strengthens the lungs, large intestine, spleen, pancreas and stomach. It generates Qi and expels cold.

Cleansing chicken soup

Ingredients: Fresh organic whole chicken, star anise, turmeric, fresh ginger, garlic, lotus kernels, leek, lemon, salt, rice pasta.

Method: Boil the chicken in water for 2–3 hours with the star anise, turmeric, fresh sliced ginger root, garlic and lotus kernels. About 10 minutes before the end of the cooking, add the leeks, sliced into rounds about 1.5 cm thick. Season with salt if necessary and bring to a boil. Sprinkle with a little lemon juice. Serve with rice pasta.

Benefits: The soup warms, dissolves mucus and draws it out of the body.

Baked apples

Ingredients: Apples (ideally organic), cinnamon.

Method: Wash the apples, remove the core, cut them into slices, sprinkle with cinnamon and bake at 160°C for about 15 minutes.

Benefits: Baked apples are warming and great for our mental well-being in autumn.

CHAPTER 13

The realm of the Five Phases of Transformation

Many of us are fortunate enough to have the opportunity to witness such notable differences and qualities of Qi throughout the year for the different phases in relation to the seasons. Many people ask me how it is in tropical countries where they do not have winter, autumn or even spring. In these countries, nature and people do not experience such striking changes of the seasons, but the transformations are still present. Seasons are characterized by the awakening of Qi, its rise, culmination and then descent and time for regeneration. The transformation is present, but in a different way. Otherwise, nature could not regenerate and bring sustenance to humans in the long term.

Therefore, after this journey through the seasons, I would like to emphasize that the message offered by the Five Phases theory is not limited to understanding the Qi of the seasons. It is certainly evident there, yet the basic principle occurs in everything around us and within us independent of the seasons. The tremendous cycle of these transformations is our very life itself. We enjoyed the WATER phase in the prenatal period and we will return to it again after death. Our childhood is a clear and typical manifestation of the WOOD phase Qi, when, thanks to the Ethereal Soul Hun, we learn a lot, we discover, we build our own path and independence, and if something stands in our way, we fight for it and show our dissatisfaction or even anger. In the FIRE phase, we are extremely active—traveling, working, building

careers, starting families, raising children; the Qi is peaking and the Shen Spirit is fully realizing its plan. What has gone more slowly and been hidden beneath is now manifesting faster and more on the surface. The EARTH phase is the time when we are harvesting the fruits of our efforts thus far. The children are already leaving the nest; we can go back to ourselves, to our own needs. The METAL phase is the autumn of our life. It is about appreciating what has gone before. We are no longer as active, we are more with ourselves, we see the value of our life and reflect. We preserve Qi rather than spend it due to our ageing. The WATER phase is the culmination of life's wisdom and enjoying this treasure. It is also a resting and then a passing away, a death—a return to the Tao. In the WATER phase, we began our prenatal life; with the WATER phase we close the circle to begin the new cycle.

The dynamic of the Five Phases is evident in everything we begin to observe from this angle. Browsing through this book, we have learned that in each phase, different organs of our body are more active or, conversely, more vulnerable. This also reflects in the different life cycles and settings of our psyche. If we are starting a project, the liver and the Ethereal Soul Hun are working the most. Once the project is underway, the liver can rest and the heart and the Shen Spirit come into play. The heart, filled with realization, can glow with joy. The spleen and the Yi aspect must ground it all to prevent the heart from becoming too exhausted. Afterwards, they pass the initiation to the lungs and the Corporeal Soul Po, which will evaluate it all.

All of us in our personal or professional lives go from one phase to another. Each phase has its own special time for development. However, if we stay stuck in one phase for too long, it can slow down our growth. Conversely, if we fly through a phase too quickly, it will not give us as much "fruit" and experience as it could, which will also slow down the progress. We will find out that even if we have accelerated something because of our impatience, we have to go back to make up for what we have missed. However, sometimes such a return is not possible, so the opportunity to learn or experience something essential is lost.

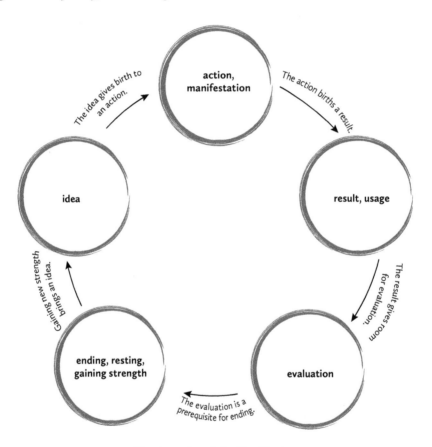

The dynamics of the Five Phases

I would like to come back to the phases and the seasons. Year after year, I have been working intensively with my students to observe the qualities of the phases during the seasons. We meet in nature on a regular basis at every single season of the year, absorbing the particular Qi of the countryside, observing what is happening in nature and how its needs are changing. At the same time, we also allow ourselves to perceive our own needs related to the changes of the seasons, we strengthen the Qi of a particular season in our own body through Qigong exercises and we get to know the Qi of the different organs belonging to the seasons. And we learn that these needs are denied by the society we live in and are part of. It forces us to function at the same rhythm throughout the year and to be equally efficient regardless of the Qi state we are in. Together, we are looking for ways to return to natural cycles. The theory of the Five Phases helps us to recognize them, to physically experience their transformations, to identify with them and to attune to them. To stop blaming ourselves if we start to slow down in the autumn or are less efficient and more inward-looking. To recognize that we need to sleep longer in the winter, and that overall we would rather just lie around and laze about, and that in summer it is as if we are unleashed, always traveling somewhere, exploring the world and often forgetting to take care of ourselves and rest while we do it. The theory of Five Phases helps us to accept that the harder times are an important part of the whole, and without them, the better times would not be as valuable. It teaches us to see the present as it is and to stop fighting life so much.

I personally experience immense fulfillment when I am able to make the most of the season and its Qi. When life circumstances allow me to "get in the boat" and let myself go with the flow. That is when I feel like I am truly living. But life does not always allow us to do that. Some of life's work or even personal situations and circumstances can engulf us so much that we do not have the right setting or time to have any perception of the time and space around us. And so it sometimes happens that spring passes and we do not even have time to notice it. Or the year has somehow slipped through our fingers. But this too is part of life.

In conclusion, within the Five Phases, it is important to realize that the quality of each phase is present in each of us. Some are more significant, some less so. Someone may be more "metallic," others "fiery" or "earthy," or a combination of several of these. What we are like is influenced by our upbringing, and also by our predispositions inherited from our ancestors. It is also influenced by the time we were born. Chinese astrology works with this wisdom, and the knowledge from it is also used by original Taoistic Chinese medicine. It depends on what constellation of stars and planets we were born under, and this influences what we will be inclined to do. These can be tendencies towards physical ailments, but they can also be tendencies towards the way we think, the way we solve problems. This information can help us to understand ourselves better, to respect our inclinations and nature as a kind of predestination. At the same time, however, we always have the opportunity and space in our lives to cultivate our personality. We have the opportunity to regulate, so that those character features and health predispositions which are destructive do not develop to uncontrollable proportions. On the contrary, so that we, and those around us, may benefit from them.